Brain Change Therapy

BRAIN CHANGE THERAPY

Clinical Interventions for
Self-Transformation

CAROL J. KERSHAW
J. WILLIAM WADE

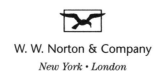

W. W. Norton & Company
New York • London

For information about permission to reproduce selections from this book, write to
Permissions, W. W. Norton & Company, Inc., 500 Fifth Avenue,
New York, NY 10110

For information about special discounts for bulk purchases,
please contact W. W. Norton
Special Sales at specialsales@wwnorton.com or 800-233-4830

Manufacturing by Courier Westford
Production manager: Leeann Graham

Library of Congress Cataloging-in-Publication Data

Kershaw, Carol J.
    Brain change therapy : clinical interventions for self-transformation / Carol J.
Kershaw & J. William Wade. — 1st ed.
        p. ; cm.
    "A Norton professional book."
    Includes bibliographical references and index.
    ISBN 978-0-393-70586-7 (hardcover)
    1. Neuropsychiatry.   I. Wade, J. William.   II. Title.
    [DNLM: 1. Mental Processes—physiology.   2. Mind-Body Therapies—
psychology.   3. Brain—physiology.   4. Consciousness—physiology.
5. Psychotherapy—methods.   WB 880 K41b 2009]
    RC341.K47 2009
    616.8—dc22   2009004506

ISBN: 978-0-393-70586-7

W. W. Norton & Company, Inc., 500 Fifth Avenue, New York, N.Y. 10110
www.wwnorton.com
W. W. Norton & Company Ltd., Castle House, 75/76 Wells Street,
London W1T 3QT

1 2 3 4 5 6 7 8 9 0

To our family

CONTENTS

ACKNOWLEDGMENTS

To create a book always takes a team effort, and there are many people who have contributed to the completion of this project. We would like to thank W.W. Norton's chief editor, Deborah Malmud, for her vision and patience, without which we could not have completed this book. Suzanne Elusorr has been a wonderful editor who played a major role in making this project a reality, and we value her friendship as well. We also want to thank Margaret Ryan for her detailed copyediting, which created a clear and accurate manuscript.

To our students and clients we owe a debt of gratitude. They taught us that people have amazing abilities for change. They helped us take theory and make it both practical and personal.

We owe much to our mentors and colleagues. Among those are Milton Erickson, Carl Whitaker, Steve Lankton, Roxanna Erickson-Klein, Jeff Zeig, Betty Alice Erickson, and our dear friends in Group 17 who helped keep us emotionally honest, connected, and feeling personally supported.

Thanks go to our three children, Chris, Stephen, and Tiffany, who taught us that parenting, like therapy, requires connection, creativity, humor, humility, and the steadfast belief that people can reach their potential.

PREFACE

The human brain–mind is an extraordinary tool. With it, humans have the ability to shape their lives, their environment, and their destiny. As a species, we are still expanding our understanding of that tool's capabilities; what we repeatedly discover is that we have not found its boundaries. Unfortunately, few people know how to use this tool well.

Brain Change Therapy: Clinical Interventions for Self-Transformation offers a psychotherapeutic model based on the scientific understanding that humans emit fields of information in the form of measurable frequencies; that people have unsuspected abilities to heal psyche and soma; and that thriving is a fully possible state. There is an information flow within the body and between bodies that impacts how we feel, communicate, interact, and perceive events. When the client is in an appropriate neurological and emotional state (i.e., a stable arousal state), his or her perspective, attitude, beliefs, and personal narrative shift toward the positive. When we as therapists are in an appropriate state that models for the client either how to elicit personal resources or how to build them through experiences, we could say that we are employing frequency-based techniques to accomplish frequency-based healing.

Internal states govern how well this information system operates. When information flows appropriately in the brain–mind–body, there is a balance of activation between the parasympathetic and sympathetic nervous systems, and emotional states can be managed easily. Anxiety and depression block this system from working optimally, and people begin to suffer symptoms. When chronically experienced, these conditions, commonly tied to memory activation caused by something in the current environment, activate certain neural pathways and shape a person's perception of, and response to, life events. Over time, neural networks become conditioned and turn on with increasing ease in the presence of conscious and unconscious triggers. However, due to neuroplasticity, the ability of the brain to form new associations, individuals have the capacity to inhibit old networks and to condition those that lead toward positive states.

Brain Change Therapy utilizes *state change* to stimulate positive emotional patterns and behavioral alterations. Appropriate corrective information in the context of a secure attachment environment and calm and accepting states from the therapist can allow the client to move into a dynamic stability so that he or she can flexibly adapt to changing environments. *Brain Change Therapy* is a resource-focused psychotherapy that accomplishes the following:

1. Elicits resourceful states (frequencies) for change from the client's past experiences.
2. Builds resourceful states for change from the relationship with the therapist.
3. Improves neural patterning using technologies that model a healthy range of frequencies to which the brain can entrain.
4. Creates resourceful states for change from new experiences in the client's community that lead to new learning.

Through this process the client develops brain–mind–body states that promote stable levels of arousal and the ability to live and thrive in joy.

Brain Change Therapy

CHAPTER 1

Fundamentals of Brain Change Therapy

Early in life we all learn that there are important differences between thoughts, words, and deeds. As very small children, we quickly realize that our thoughts are our own private business; that our words can get us into trouble (and sometimes get us out of it) but that, in and of themselves, they don't *do* anything; and that deeds, such as hitting a little brother, have definite consequences. However, contemporary brain research has found that, at the level of the brain, *thoughts, words, and deeds are all neurochemical acts.* This extraordinary organ, which has no moving parts, registers electrochemical activity with every thought that we ever have, either awake or in sleep; with every word uttered aloud, even in the softest whisper; and with every movement of even the smallest muscle. And contrary to what we learned as children, it may be that the brain's activity creates an electromagnetic field that overlaps, and may be perceived by, other people around us: That is, although the content of our thoughts may be private, empathic attunement may allow others to sense our state (Cozolino, 2002; McFadden, 2002).

Brain Change Therapy (BCT) is a therapeutic approach using brain–mind state change as a focus of treatment. Ultimately, all types of psychotherapy—from psychoanalysis to behavioral intervention—are successful to the extent to which they enhance change in relevant neural circuits (Cozolino, 2002). BCT starts with that working assumption: Effective therapeutic change must inevitably include a repatterning of neural pathways. It utilizes cognitive, affective, behavioral, and interpersonal techniques as they are informed by neuroscience.

Short of direct pharmacological intervention, there are three broad therapeutic modalities through which the clinician can assist the client in changing the brain's neural patterning and shifting attention from negative to positive states. BCT makes directed use of all three. The first is through the conscious refocusing of attention using techniques of mindfulness. The second is by circumventing the conscious mind. To change states and access resources, we access preconscious levels of awareness through the use of hypnotherapy, empathic responses, curiosity, surprise, and humor, which we intentionally employ to inhibit chronic negative states and activate positive ones. The third method, and the one we have found to be the most powerful, is to address the brain specifically. This can be done through the state change therapies of biofeedback, neurofeedback, and deep hypnosis in conjunction with software and equipment that condition brain change, such as Cygnet neurofeedback software and the DAVID PAL device.

We emphasize the value of changing states of consciousness and conditioning the changed state through repetition to access or build internal resources. This process allows clients to experience their own "self-directed neuroplasticity" through the active practice of focusing attention (Rock & Schwartz, 2007b). As an adjunct to those methods, BCT helps clients create new, empowering life experiences that can serve as the basis for new neural patterns. And because the brain generates an electromagnetic field, BCT also requires the clinician to consciously direct his or her brain–mind state within the therapeutic interaction.

Due to the breadth of the BCT approach, it is not only effective in treating clients' problem states but in working with individuals who are interested in shifting and conditioning peak performance states of consciousness.

Neuroplasticity

The brain, a major organ of the body, and the mind, having no material existence, are intimately connected. Some researchers are of the opinion that the mind and consciousness are simply concepts that we use to describe what are essentially artifacts of the brain (e.g., Baars & Gage, 2010). In other words, the mind is "smaller" than the brain. Other contemporary research (e.g., McTaggart, 2002), particularly supported by studying phenomena such as quantum memory and "out-of-body" experiences, strongly suggests that the mind is nonlocal (i.e., not confined to any particular physical location). The concept of nonlocality implies that the mind is "bigger" than the brain. In either case, for most people, most of the time, the mind and brain are not only co-located but inextricably connected.

Daniel Siegel's idea that the "mind is using the brain to create itself" (2007, p. 32) may be remarkably accurate. Studies have now demonstrated that the brain exhibits a lifelong property of *neuroplasticity*: New neurons can be grown, neural networks can be formed, and old networks can be changed (Eriksson, 1998). In fact, contrary to earlier views, the brain continues to grow new cells throughout the lifespan (Restak, 2001). While life experience constantly shapes the brain, the brain can also be intentionally changed through attention training (Schwartz & Begley, 2002). In fact, Schwartz, Stapp, and Beauregard (2004) note that "an accelerating number of studies in the neuroimaging literature significantly support the thesis that . . . with appropriate training and effort, people can systematically alter neural circuitry associated with a variety of mental and physical states that are frankly pathological" (p. 2). Far beyond the repair of dysfunction, it is also possible to develop the "exceptional" mind, wherein deep states of concentration lead to profound experiences of stillness, calm, and equanimity. In short: The brain can be changed through the mind; reciprocally, the mind can be changed through the brain.

Negativity Bias

Gordon et al. (Gordon, Barnet, Cooper, Tran, & Williams, 2008) and Williams et al. (2008) described the brain's organizing principle as moving toward reward and away from danger or threat. The brain is constantly scanning the environment and, on the basis of incoming data, making decisions about what to move toward or away from. However, the "negativity bias theory" (Baumeister, Bratslavsky, Finkenauer, & Vohs, 2001) states that the brain–mind has a negative bias; that is, it is easier for it to give attention to negative feelings (the "FUD" factor—fear, uncertainty, doubt) than positive ones. Clearly this attunement to potential threat would have survival value and therefore, evolution has presumably favored it. But the result is that, left to itself, the mind's innate tendency is to wander to something distressing.

Consistent with the brain's propensity to focus on threats, psycho-physiological arousal occasioned by the perception of threat tends to arise more quickly, be more intense, and last longer than arousal levels associated with potential reward. When calm levels of arousal prevail, we experience empowering states such as joy, pleasure, love, concentration, determination, courage, and clarity. However, the positive feeling states are more fragile; they tend to last for shorter periods and can easily degrade (Baumeister, Bratslavsky, Finkenauer, & Vohs, 2001). In essence, the negativity bias, which selects in favor of survival, *selects against optimal functioning*. However, due to the plasticity of both the brain and the mind, it is possible to moderate the brain's negative bias.

State Change

The term *state change* refers to the capacity to shift the mind from one emotional state to another and to shift the brain from one neural pattern to another—for example, from anxiety/high psychophysiological arousal to calm/low psychophysiological arousal (Panksepp, 1998; Fisher, 2009). Being able to control one's brain–mind state is central to living successfully. When people cannot shift from reactive states to calm ones or activate themselves to accomplish a goal, problematic patterns in living emerge.

As Albert Einstein observed, "We can't solve problems by using the same kind of thinking we used when we created them" (Calaprice & Lipscomb, 2005, p. 292). He was speaking about our problems at a societal level, but the same holds true for individuals. However, with a shift in state, a person can access a different set of emotions and abilities. Often such a shift results in the ability to find solutions where previously none appeared to exist. At other times, the external circumstances simply cannot be changed. Nonetheless, with practice, we can always change internal states. That shift can transform the inner landscape as it is experienced at that moment; it can even transform the inner life.

Focusing on the brain specifically, Siegel defined states as "the total pattern of activations in the brain at a particular moment in time" (1999, p. 208). Brain states permit the organization of mental processes. Grigsby and Stevens (2000) remarked that a state is "an emergent property of the self-organizing activity of the brain, acting as an organizer of experience, and influenced by experience itself in a variety of ways" (p. 164). All mental processes involve neural activation tendencies (NATs), which are located in different memory systems (Grawe, 2007). These NATs are engaged to reduce stress or incongruity in life situations. In turn, the reduction of tension strengthens the neural activation pattern. Grawe (2007) added: "If this process is repeated, the newly formed pattern occurs more and more quickly and easily and is facilitated better with each new activation until finally it becomes part of the individual's repertoire" (p. 222). As these patterns become old and familiar, they also become increasingly difficult to change.

States maintain certain levels of emotional regulation, memories, mental models, and patterns of behavior (Siegel, 1999). The physical indications of a mental state shift include changes in breathing patterns, focus of eyes, posture, skin color, rate of speech, tone of voice, choice of language, and nonverbal behavior. A facial expression or fragment of speech can reflect a person's inner experiential world. For example, someone who feels intimidated by another might have a tight smile while saying "Hello." Each state determines the behaviors in which a person will typically engage.

Numerous factors determine brain states, including "arousal level, point in the sleep–wake cycle, level of activity, mood, sympathetic nervous system activity, current emotional status, body temperature, blood glucose level, current status at that moment in a significant personal relationship, and short-term behavioral goals" (Grigsby & Stevens, 2000, p. 166). Biological cycles are another significant factor. Research has identified three major biological cycles for humans. The *infradian rhythm* is governed by biological factors and exogenous cues such as pheromones and extends over periods of more than 24 hours (e.g., the menstrual cycle); the *circadian cycle*, which recurs every 24 hours (Brown, Graeber, & Curtis, 1982; Rossi, 1986); and the *ultradian cycle*, which recurs every 90–120 minutes (Rossi, 1986). In addition, states are influenced by mood—mood is defined as the "manifestation of relatively persistent neurophysiological activity" (Grigsby & Stevens, 2000, p. 169)—temperament, immediate physical factors such as feeling hungry or tired, and emotional reactions.

Sensory input (e.g., suddenly noticing smoke coming out of your toaster) can also trigger certain states, activating neurochemical responses and tendencies toward specific actions. These actions (e.g., quickly unplugging the toaster) help the individual cope with environmental demands. However, the fight–flight–freeze response that mitigates danger is of little use in the therapeutic setting. In fact, it may be highly counterproductive. "The rational, executive brain, the mind, the part that needs to be functional in order to engage in the process of psychotherapy, has very limited capacity to squelch sensations, control emotional arousal, or change fixed action patterns" (van der Kolk, 2006, p. 5). Instead, low levels of neurological and emotional arousal facilitate openness and an ability to make constructive use of the therapeutic interaction.

"As state changes, so does behavior, and thus state is associated with both adaptive and maladaptive behavior" (Grigsby & Stevens, 2000, p. 362). Neuroscientist Jaak Panksepp (1998) recorded seven different neural circuits that turn on mood states. When a particular neural circuit is active, certain patterns of feeling, thinking, and behavior naturally occur. It is impossible to make changes in the perceived experience unless another circuit is turned on. When a person's emotional circuits have been conditioned to switch on automatically with specific triggers, he or she falls into certain behavioral patterns that are difficult to interrupt.

In a similar vein, Damasio (1999) discovered that each emotion has a specific neural mapping pattern. Sadness, happiness, anger, and fear each has a distinguishable neural pattern that can be activated by the memory of an event that originally evoked the emotion. The parts of the brain that are engaged in the regulation of these feelings, the somatosensory cortices and the upper brainstem nuclei, activate during these experiences. When these emotions switch on and are reinforced over time, their circuit activation seems automatic. Therefore change needs to focus on their inhibition and the activation of alternative states.

Grawe (2007) suggested that the goal of psychotherapy is to bring about neuronal change through incongruence reduction and need satisfaction. He said further, "Neuropsychotherapy strives to shift the brain into a state that enables these basic needs to be fully satisfied" (2007, p. 424), and he concluded that "concepts of traditional therapy schools can no longer be regarded as adequate foundations of psychotherapy" (2007, p. 419).

The Neurochemistry of Well-Being

Davidson and Lutz (2008) researched mental practice and its effects on the brains of monks. Like other research, their study confirmed that the brain can be trained to change its own circuitry. When researchers asked the monks to meditate on unconditional compassion, their brains activated extremely organized and fast-moving gamma waves, which occurred in many different places in the brain. Such complex neural coordination reflects higher mental activity and heightened awareness. Magnetic resonance imaging (MRI) also indicated that, in particular, the left prefrontal cortex was activated by positive thoughts and emotions.

But a monastic lifestyle is not necessary to create enhanced neural patterning; increasingly there is experimental support for the idea that with mental training, anyone can learn to feel happier. General happiness seems to be a constellation of states of well-being. Even if there is trauma in one's background, an individual can cultivate a happiness mindset. When we shift states to the calm center on a regular basis, the happiness quotient increases and our liveliness, clarity, fulfillment, and ability to enjoy life expands; in addition, our health may improve. By practicing state shifting, it may even be possible to access "pure happiness"—a state of happiness that is pure in the sense that it is not necessarily the result of, or dependent upon, any external circumstance. Instead, it exists internally for each person.

Positive psychologist Jonathan Haidt (2012) discovered one brain circuit that activates what he called a state of elation. Elation tends to wipe out all other emotional states for a period of time. It occurs when people witness virtuous acts or a manifestation of humanity's higher moral nature, such as a display of generosity, loyalty, or courage. Haidt first developed the idea of elation from reading Thomas Jefferson's letters, which focused on the practice of virtue. Haidt (in press) said that language can "transport" an audience into a state of elation. Charismatic speakers would easily agree with him. For some people, certain musical compositions may also have the same effect. Haidt found that elation produces oxytocin, the chemical released in the brain during bonding experiences (Silvers & Haidt, 2008). It is not clear exactly how, but the experiences of elation and pure happiness may overlap. One possibility is that pure happiness also involves the release of natural oxytocin.

The Role of Conscious Attention

The 19th-century psychologist and philosopher William James said: "Everyone knows what attention is. It is the taking possession by the mind in clear and vivid form, of one out of what seem several simultaneously possible objects or trains of thought. . . . It implies withdrawal from some things in order to deal effectively with others, and is a condition which has a real opposite in the confused, dazed, scatter-brained state" (1890/1950, p. 403). Forms of attention have since been categorized more specifically as sustained, divided, and selective. *Sustained* attention involves holding the mind on a single focus or stimulus over time. *Divided* attention is the ability to attend to multiple stimuli at one time (or in such rapid and recurrent succession as to be nearly simultaneous). *Selective* attention is the ability to bring a stimulus into the foreground and place others in the background (Raz, 2004).

New discoveries in neuroscience, systems work, biofeedback, consciousness training, and meditation approaches have reinforced the idea that a direct key to change may lie in selecting which type of attention a person uses at any given time and on what that attention is focused. This skill requires learning how to shift brain–mind states in order to activate different neural circuits, different brain-wave frequencies, and, consequently, different abilities (Panksepp, 1998). In short, the ability to shift brain states makes it possible to view the world through a different lens. Schwartz and Begley (2002) state:

> Since attention is generally considered an internally generated state, it seems that neuroscience has tiptoed up to a conclusion that would be right at home in the canon of some of the Eastern philosophies: introspection, willed attention, subjective state—pick your favorite description of an internal mental state—can redraw the contours of the mind, and in so doing can rewire the circuits of the brain, for it is attention that makes neuroplasticity possible. (p. 339)

By shifting the focus of attention, a person can make an immediate change in his or her emotions, mood, perceptions, and behavior. By learning new brain–mind habits, long-entrenched personal patterns can also be changed. Once the shift in internal states has occurred, even on a momentary basis, the therapist can use empowering strategies to help

the client access commonly overlooked internal resources or build missing developmental experiences.

State Stability

Shifting attention toward some aspect of a situation that can be considered in some sense positive (rather than strictly negative) is important
in repatterning habits both at the neurological and the personality levels.
Fredrickson (2001) suggested that developing an internal "reset button"
to move from negative to positive states could be done by noticing the
part of a situation that was benign or "better than bad." The ability to
change states and "look on the bright side" tends to enlarge a person's
perspective and improve coping ability.

For positive state *stability*, however, attention training may be necessary. Whatever a person focuses on—a fear or an insight, a dear friend or
a personal nemesis—tends to maintain the brain–mind state associated
with the experience (Rock & Schwartz, 2007a). Learning to hold a focused attention will contribute to stabilizing brain circuits and improving
the brain–mind's ability to maintain a state associated with a particular
positive experience. Intentional and practiced state change shifts emotion and "drives appraisal and reflection" (Baumeister, DeWall, Vohs, &
Alquist, in press), such that state stability is more likely and more easily
activated by the associated brain circuits. Through attention (state)
training, one can become able to regulate thoughts, emotions, and behaviors and achieve goals even in the midst of distraction or situations
causing high levels of arousal.

Mihaly Csikszentmihalyi, known for his work in positive psychology,
observed: "What we pay attention to, and how we pay attention, determines the content and quality of life" (1990, p. 43). Similarly, the Span-
ish philosopher and humanist José Ortega y Gasset wrote: "Tell me to
what you pay attention and I will tell you who you are" (1962, p. 94). As
a person focuses awareness and gives attention to the inner and outer
matters of life, he or she creates the moment-to-moment experience of
living. When a client can witness a powerful feeling, turn down the intensity, learn to change states, and condition more positive circuits, new
levels of self-awareness and mental flexibility emerge.

Circumventing the Conscious Mind

Long-entrenched neural pathways, however, are difficult to dispel. Additionally, many clients find that they have difficulty implementing direct therapeutic suggestion and are often subtly resistant to changing their habituated thought patterns. Because of this, a conscious approach to changing problematic patterns can backfire, causing the pattern to become further entrenched, particularly if a client feels that his or her personal choice is being taken away. Therefore, BCT also includes numerous techniques that address the brain while circumventing the conscious mind.

A particularly effective means of "flying under the radar" of the conscious mind is the use of integrative hypnosis. Milton Erickson viewed trance as a common, naturally occurring, and everyday experience. As an example, a person might be driving on the freeway while listening to the radio and thinking about an upcoming luncheon meeting. Arriving at her destination, she might have no memory of driving from her point of departure to her destination. This was similar to, if not precisely the same as, a formally induced amnesia. One of Erickson's many contributions to therapy and hypnosis was his recognition that therapy can utilize these everyday trances with or without a formal induction. Instead of suggesting directly that a person would experience something, Erickson often embedded or interspersed suggestions within a prolonged monologue. He altered the tone of his voice in such a manner that the client's unconscious mind would hear the suggestion, while his or her conscious mind did not pick up on the fact that anything had been suggested (Erickson-Klein, February 15, 2003, personal communication).

Listening attentively to the client and then offering a completely unexpected, positive response is another method of "making an end run" around the conscious attitude of the client. This tack achieves three purposes. The surprise element immediately shifts the client's state; simultaneously, the fact that the response was unexpected calls into question the client's sense of the unquestioned "rightness" of his or her perspective; and the "novel" response models the possibility of seeing the situation in a completely different way. As examples of an unexpected response, curiosity on the part of the therapist can counter a client's fear and anxiety; gentle humor can defuse frustration; and pleasant surprise can offset negativity.

Addressing the Brain Directly

In the 1970s Barbara Brown (1974) demonstrated that subjects could turn on subjective states to make a biofeedback machine light up. Going further, the Greens discovered that people can become aware of very subtle internal sensations that normally go unnoticed until they are hooked up to a biofeedback device. What can then be sensed and controlled is a state of consciousness that contains sensory cues (Green & Green, 1977). During their research, Elmer Green noted that although it is possible to be aware of corresponding physiological conditions such as muscle tension, cold extremities, or a pounding heart, it is impossible to detect one's own brain-wave patterns. However, by incorporating different types of brain feedback and/or brain stimulations, delivered by an increasing variety of specialized devices, training the brain to produce particular wave frequencies becomes readily possible. Deep hypnosis is another means of accessing states of profound inner quiet, which then allows rich material to come to the surface of the mind in the form of hypnogogic imagery. All of these methods can lead to integrative and long-lasting experiences of psychological well-being—which, in the therapeutic context, can significantly increase the effectiveness of state management.

The State of the Therapist in BCT

Science has yet to determine the full extent of the capacities of the human mind. Nonetheless, with recent research in the field of neurobiology, therapists are now able to understand more about the ways in which clinical interventions function at a neurological level and, with new brain-based technologies, can design interventions that are more effective. However, interventions are far from being the sole agents of therapeutic change. In fact, substantial clinical evidence supports the idea that the relationship between the therapist and client is significantly more influential than the interventions, per se (Cormier, Nurius, & Osborn, 2009). Based on this understanding, it becomes clear that the state of the *clinician* must be as intentionally managed as the state of the client. As therapists, when we shift our own internal states and focus attention in the right way, we help the client shift his or her internal state and then keep that desired target state stable. As we are able to witness, accept, and keep the intensity of our feelings managed, the client's functional behavior will follow.

Milton Erickson conceptualized what he termed *response readiness* as the internal state of the therapist in making him- or herself ready to respond to a client and to utilize whatever the client has to offer. He believed that in therapy, response readiness was crucial not only for client change, but also for therapist efficacy; that is, the therapist must be able shift states deftly in order to be effective. Zeig (1992) noted that "problems represent a 'state' of insufficiency in which patients believe they do not have resources to cope or change. . . . The therapist enters into a state of response readiness and thereby becomes a model for the patient to access a similar state" (p. 300). Holding the appropriate state, the therapist models sufficiency back to the client. Response readiness thus becomes a state that creates a bridge between the client's problem and more functional and resourceful inner states.

The BCT Process

The BCT process can be encapsulated in the following steps, which are illustrated in the case that follows:

1. Acknowledge the client's presenting state and the issues driving it.
2. Define the problem as solvable.
3. Identify the target state.
4. Assist the client in changing states and moving toward the target state.
5. Condition and reinforce the new state.
6. Establish the new state as a means of resolving the underlying issues.
7. Assist the client in creating workable solutions as they emerge from changed states and behaviors.
8. Support the client in taking action.
9. Link the action into the client's social context.

Case Example: Using State Change to Reach Therapeutic Goals

Arriving for his therapy session, Roger appeared to be depressed and in a state of negativity. Carol asked Roger where he would like to begin. Roger, looking toward the therapist to start the session, replied, "I don't know. Everything is the same, nothing is better." Hearing the hidden blame couched in sad language directed toward the therapist, Carol responded empathically: "Life feels really difficult when you are stuck and not going in the direction you want. Tell me what 'the same' feels like." [Step 1: acknowledge the client's presenting state]. Roger replied that it felt like a huge, heavy weight.

Roger had lost a good job 4 years earlier and had been unable to find work at the same level of pay. Several dating services had rejected him, and collectively, these blows had been devastating; as a result, he felt helpless and could not summon the motivation to make any significant changes in his life. Questions about his family of origin revealed that in his childhood, Roger had felt rejected by his father and continued to feel judged as inadequate in his ability to take care of himself.

A therapist who had not considered Roger from a neurophysiological perspective might have continued to respond empathically and then explored potential cognitive and behavioral strategies to help him. Using BCT, however, the therapist would include some additional inquiries in an initial assessment—among them would be questions to determine if the client had racing thoughts or lived in such negative states so chronically that it would be difficult for him to switch out of them. In that case, underlying damaged neurophysiology might be a contributing factor. Many clients either do not remember if they had a fall or believe it to have been inconsequential. However, the number of people, clients included, living with some type of undiagnosed head injury is significant (Amen, 1999; Proler, personal communication, May 23, 1998).

Usually, after the initial evaluation, we begin with the simplest neuro-psychotherapeutic intervention to see what response occurs. This intervention entails the use of therapeutic dialogue to determine the range of states to which the client has access. These various states might include anticipation, determination, humor, excitement, happiness, a sense of pleasure, and/or hopefulness.

Roger had difficulty accessing positive feelings, but he was grimly determined to feel better. We asked when he felt the cheeriest, what truly held his interest, and what he found himself passionate about. He had difficulty formulating any answers, but the questions themselves launched him on an internal search (state shift).

Roger felt inadequate, anxious, and depressed and had little access to a sense of humor—the possession of which is an indicator of ego strength and the ability to change states. We hypothesized that if he could experience his own capacity to change states, perhaps through changing temperature in his hands with trance, he might develop enough self-confidence and motivation to explore other potential capacities [Step 2: define the problem as solvable]. The experience of trance phenomena such as developing heaviness or warmth suggests indirectly to a client that the mind's hidden abilities can create the backdrop for solution generation. Roger was intrigued by the idea that he could use his own body as a biofeedback device and learn how to control certain physiological responses.

In designing an intervention, the therapist should identify the emotional circuits that are chronically aroused. Roger was persistently anxious, depressed, and angry; overall, he was caught in a loop of emotional upset that he medicated with alcohol. Because of his chronically depressed and angry mood, we assumed that there was an increased level of activation in his right prefrontal cortex, which generally tends to mediate negative feelings (Davidson, 2000). Furthermore, Roger had responded poorly to selective serotonin reuptake inhibitors (SSRIs). This response fit the research on anxious and depressed people with an activated right prefrontal cortex and low activation on the left, who tend to experience little change in their emotional states with SSRI medications (Heller & Nitsche, 1998). The hypoactive state of the left (since the right prefrontal cortex is activated) prefrontal cortex is associated with a reduced ability in the executive areas of conscious planning and problem solving (Grawe, 2007). We also wondered if he was drinking more than he said.

Carol helped Roger to activate the impoverished brain circuits that were factors in his current inability to nurture himself and to experience curiosity and play [Step 3: define the target state]. This was accomplished first by using empathy and nurturance and then through the experience of trance phenomena. Roger became really curious about not only that experience but about what else he might be able to do. The curiosity circuit turned on, as well as his interest in exploring other abilities without alcohol. Carol also encouraged him to stop drinking. She developed as much rapport as Roger would allow, with the intent to stimulate positive feelings. Because it takes some time for the brain to grow new neural pathways through experience, the activation of positive emotions may take several weeks. Therefore, it is important to keep triggering them over time. Educating the client about the process may also be useful.

This process with Roger was especially difficult in that he consistently blocked Carol's attempt to stimulate positive feelings. When he later reported that he had stopped drinking, he still could not move from the state he was in to a more positive state. Because alcohol can have an inhibiting effect on the neurotransmitter serotonin, Carol surmised that part of his depression may have been due to brain injury sustained from alcohol abuse. In therapy, Carol focused on his ability to raise his hand temperature in hypnosis. This small success allowed him to begin to move into the "access state," that state of mind where there is an openness to new learning. He became curious about what he could accomplish [Step 4: assist the client in changing states and moving toward the target state].

Roger began to be able to shift into more positive states during his therapy sessions but found that he was still unable to sustain those states outside the office. Carol suggested that he try alpha–theta training, using a neurofeedback device to assist him in reaccessing his innate capacity for relaxation and to encourage a more open, optimal learning. This training helped him move into the state just above sleep, which lowered his emotional reactivity. It also improved his access specifically of the alpha frequency, which his alcohol use had diminished. This increased access translated into an increased ability to self-comfort [Step 5: condition and reinforce the new state].

In one of the alpha–theta sessions, Carol suggested the following: "As you relax your mind and drift down to the edge of sleep, try viewing this predicament [his joblessness] on your mental screen. This may come as a symbol or question to be answered. Ask your unconscious mind for an answer to the mystery or for a new path to take."

After 20 minutes, Roger said: "What comes to mind is an image of the most modern computer I have ever seen. I think my mind is telling me I can upgrade my skills and become an expert in a niche." After several sessions of alpha–theta training, Roger began to respond more positively in psychotherapy sessions. Brain training was allowing him to experience a state change that he could practice at home with meditation [Step 6: Establish the new state as a means of resolving the underlying issues].

An important therapeutic goal was to help Roger begin to experience life events that would stimulate positive emotions. Because he had few friends, Carol inquired about the possibility of adopting a pet. She hoped a pet might interrupt the long periods he spent at home ruminating on negative emotions. In addition, learning how to nurture and receive unconditional love from an animal might ultimately be generalized to a human relationship. With an animal, Roger would be able to practice being in a positive state, un-self-consciously, attaching to a responsive creature and feeling the simple pleasure of connection. At Carol's suggestion of acquiring a pet, he immediately smiled and reported that he had been thinking of doing the same. After he purchased a puppy, dialogue about the new puppy took up some of each psychotherapy session and served to stimulate positive feelings [Step 7: assist the client in creating workable solutions as they emerge from changed states and behavior].

The next phase of therapy dealt with Roger's avoidance of his previously stated goals of quitting smoking, starting to exercise regularly, and improving his nutrition. Although he himself had identified these goals, Roger found that he could not stay motivated enough to accomplish them. Therapy was able to help him shift states and be open to experiences that would help him achieve his goals [Step 8: support the client in taking action]. As he began to feel better, he also initiated the process of acquiring several certifications that would qualify him for a higher-paying job.

Without an active focus on continuing to inhibit negative responses and activate positive ones, the BCT therapist would not be surprised to find a client's problems generally recurring. For this reason, homework assignments that activate positive states are important. As an assignment, Carol asked Roger to engage in social conversation at work several times a week. Over time, he began to feel more positive and achieved several interpersonal goals [Step 9: link the action into the client's social context].

Although not appropriate in Roger's case because he lived alone, the BCT therapist may ask family members or other parts of the client's support system to come in. We suggest that these caring members can help the client by paying attention to where they focus their conversations with him. While we are careful not to identify one person in a family system as the source of dysfunctional behavioral patterns, we want to be sensitive to how the client's personal family system operates. For example, the interpersonal dynamics within which the client lives may contribute to a propensity to stimulate negative circuits of fear and panic. Making an intervention in the family dynamics often affects the entire family system for the better.

We also encouraged Roger to practice brain–mind training at home with a brain technology device called the DAVID PAL (see Chapter 6). It was in following this suggestion that he reported that he was able to stop drinking completely. When he wanted to drink, he used the device to handle the urge. In doing so, he learned that his mind could override the physiological sensations of craving.

Chapter 1 has presented an overview of the BCT approach, which uses brain–mind state change as a focus of treatment. It recognizes the necessity of positive state stability, which may require attention training, noting that there are numerous ways in which that can be accomplished. BCT also involves the active monitoring and directing of the therapist's brain–mind state as he or she holds and models states for the client.

In Chapter 2 we lay the foundation for the brain–mind interventions BCT uses by exploring the basics of the brain: its anatomy, neuroanatomy, neurophysiology, and electrochemical processes, and the rhythms of the brain, the body, and nature.

CHAPTER 2
Brain–Mind and Brain–Body Basics

The study of the human brain has a long and august history. In the middle of the fifth century, B.C.E., ancient Greece had three outstanding centers of medical science. The oldest of them was in Crotona, a Greek colony in what is now the Calabria region of southern Italy. Alcmaeon, Crotona's foremost physician, researcher, and lecturer, wrote the first known treatise stating that the brain is the site of sensation and cognition. As a practicing physician, his approach was entirely clinical, developed through the study of brain-injured patients.

Roughly 600 years later, Claudius Galenus (129–199 C.E.), more commonly known as Galen of Pergamum, used piglets to perform the first recorded experiments on the brain (Gross, 1995). As perhaps the premier medical researcher of the Roman period, he devised a number of experiments to demonstrate that the brain controls all of the muscles through innervation by the cranial nerves and the peripheral nervous system (Frampton, 2008).

Ever since then, this organ—with the consistency of a soft-boiled egg, floating in spinal fluid—has continued to challenge medical researchers. From anatomy to physiology and, much more recently, from neurochemical reactions to electromagnetic fields, slowly, the brain has been yielding its secrets.

The brain's neurophysiology is expressed via behavior, affect, and attitude. When the brain is in a state of electrochemical stability, affect is regulated, temperature stays constant, the heart rate functions well, digestion promotes energy management, and a person feels well. When the brain is in a state of instability, a pleasant mood is difficult to maintain, negative thoughts are pervasive, temper is short, and thinking may be foggy. Different emotional or behavioral problems may be directly related to different parts of the brain's electrochemical system which are under- or overfunctioning. Since our task as clinicians is to help people make the changes necessary to experience more fulfilling and productive lives, it is important to grasp the basics of the brain's organization and operation.

Anatomy of the Brain

There are three major structural regions within the brain: the brainstem, the cerebellum, and the forebrain. The forebrain is composed of the thalamus, the hypothalamus, and the cerebrum. The cerebrum includes the cerebral cortex, basal ganglia, and limbic system.

The brainstem contains the medulla (the upper spinal cord), the pons, and the midbrain. Via the cranial nerves, this structure provides innervation to the face and neck. Additionally, all nerve connections for the motor and sensory systems of the body as a whole pass through the brainstem. It coordinates cardiac and respiratory functions and regulates sleep cycles. The brainstem is also critical in maintaining a person's consciousness.

The cerebellum is important to motor control; it doesn't initiate motion, but it assists in motoric coordination, precision, balance, and timing. People with damage to this area make errors in the timing, direction, aim, and intensity of their movements. Recently, cerebellar involvement has been demonstrated in the working memory, that is, the memory involved in implicit and explicit learning and language (Desmond & Fiez, 1998).

The forebrain is the largest part of the brain. Within it, the thalamus relays information between the midbrain and the cerebral cortex, and the hypothalamus controls every endocrine gland in the body. The main function of the hypothalamus, along with the pituitary gland, is to maintain homeostasis by controlling heart rate, vasoconstriction, digestion, and sweating. It also holds temperature, electrolyte balance, fluid volume, blood pressure, and body weight to a precise value called the *set point*. This is a point that can change over time but stays relatively fixed from day to day. Other structures, such as the amygdala, the hippocampus, and the olfactory cortex, send information to the hypothalamus to assist in the regulation of eating and reproduction. In addition, fibers from the optic nerve go to a small nucleus within the hypothalamus that regulates circadian rhythms.

Wrapped around the evolutionarily older parts of the brain, the most prominent part of the forebrain is the cerebrum. Complex behaviors and functions such as social interaction, learning, working memory, and speech and language are mediated through the cerebrum. As noted, it includes the cerebral cortex, basal ganglia and limbic system.

The cerebral cortex integrates information from all of the sense organs, manages emotions, retains memory, and mediates thinking and emotional expression. It is divided into the right and left hemispheres. Communication between hemispheres is managed by the corpus callosum, which connects the two halves and is the largest white matter structure in the brain. For unknown reasons, it is slightly larger in left-handed people (Driesen & Raz, 1995). The right and left hemispheres of the cerebral cortex are each divided into four lobes: frontal, temporal, parietal, and occipital.

The two frontal lobes are involved in higher mental functions. For example, they facilitate the ability to plan for the future; understand future consequences based on present choices; analyze possibilities as to good, better, and best; learn language (Broca's region); and modify behavioral impulses to conform to societal norms. They also maintain the memory system and personality traits such as level of self-confidence, independence of judgment, willingness to take risks, and degree of extroversion.

The temporal lobes assist with memory, language comprehension, retrieval of words, and temper control. They also organize the senses of hearing and smell. These structures are found under the temples and behind the eyes. Problems in the left temporal lobe show up in aggression, dark or violent thoughts, sensitivity to slights, mild paranoia, decreased verbal memory, and emotional instability. The right temporal lobe usually facilitates the assignment of meaning to vocal intonation and the perception of melodies, social cues, and facial expressions. Problems with the right lobe often result in social difficulty, trouble processing music, impaired visual memory, and difficulty decoding vocal intonation. Other problems with either lobe may include amnesia, headaches or abdominal pain without explanation, anxiety and fear, visual or auditory distortions, feelings of déjà vu, religious or moral preoccupations, and even seizures.

The parietal lobes support the recognition of touch, pressure, temperature, taste, and pain. They integrate sensory information and are especially critical for spatial sense and navigation. Problems in the parietal lobes may result in difficulty processing information (verbal, written, or mathematical) or comprehending directions, and problems with spatial recognition.

The occipital area of the brain is responsible for visual processing. The eyes send information to these lobes for image construction. Damage to either side of the occipital area can result in impaired vision in both eyes.

The human cortex is also divided into 52 distinct areas ("Brodmann's areas") based on structural and functional differences. Because the cerebral cortex operates on a contralateral basis, information from the left side of the body is sent to the right brain, and information from the right side is sent to the left brain. The one system that works ipsilaterally (i.e., on the same side of the body) is the proprioceptive system, which operates from the sensory neurons in the inner ear and in the muscles that give us both our sense of motion and our orientation in space (Weedman, 1997). Proprioception is communicated to both the cerebrum and the cerebellum.

The cerebrum also contains the basal ganglia and the limbic system, which lie beneath the cerebral cortex. The basal ganglia are a group of nuclei strongly connected with the cerebral cortex and associated with a variety of functions, including motor control, resting metabolic rate (the body's idling speed) (Amen, 1999), and learning. This structure also controls habit-based behavior. Overactive basal ganglia can lead to anxiety issues; when they are underactive, problems with concentration and motor control may be experienced (Amen, 1999).

The limbic system denotes an area containing several brain structures, including the hippocampus, amygdala, gyrus fornicatus, and their connecting structures, all of which form a kind of border around the brainstem. The limbic system appears to affect motivational and emotional states, long-term memory, and olfaction. It is also implicated in the formation of spatial memory and the ability to create cognitive maps for navigation. Additionally, it maintains various autonomic functions.

Other structures beneath the cortex are involved with other functions. Located on the roof of the midbrain are the inferior colliculus, an auditory structure, and the superior colliculus, which is involved with eye movement and visual attention. The visual system has two subsystems: the visual sensory system, which is used to focus, send, and interpret an image, and the ocular motor system, which keeps images from both eyes aligned. Brain injury to this area can cause symptoms such as double vision, light sensitivity, blurred vision, headaches, visual field impairment, or reading problems.

The cingulate gyrus is located in front of and above the corpus callosum. It becomes active when people engage in cognitive tasks such as problem solving. The cingulate gyrus runs through the middle part of the frontal lobes. It acts to help a person stay focused, shift from one thought to another, and to shift behaviors. When this part of the brain becomes overactive, obsessive thinking and compulsive behavior can occur.

Neuroanatomy: The Building Blocks of the Brain

The brain is composed of two kinds of cells: glial cells and neurons. Glial cells are partner cells for the neurons. They physically support the neurons by forming a mesh and regulating the neuronal environment. They act as scrub brushes to eliminate waste and dead cells produced by neurons. Certain glial cells also prevent abnormal communication between neurons in the spinal cord and central nervous system through an insulating material called *myelin*.

Containing approximately 100 billion neurons, the brain may have more connections than there are stars in the universe (Lubar, 1997). Neurons, or nerve cells, receive and transmit information by electrochemical signaling. Structurally, each neuron is composed of a nucleus surrounded by a branching dendritic formation, which looks somewhat like small tentacles. Each neuron also has an appendage, an *axon*, which stretches toward, but does not quite touch, the dendrites of nearby neurons. From cell to cell, neurons communicate with each other through a process using both electricity and chemical substances known as *neurotransmitters*. Across the synaptic space between neurons, electrochemical "sparks" fly: Chemical ions generate an electrical charge that travels along chains of neurons. On one side of each neural synapse is the *presynaptic neuron*, the axon sending the information, and on the other is the *postsynaptic* neuron, the dendrite that receives the communication. As neurons "fire" across the synaptic gap, constant feedback and adjustment by the brain serves either to release further transmitters or to inhibit them.

Intricate cell-to-cell communication must occur in the brain for learning to take place. As messages move from neuron to neuron via neurotransmitters, changes can happen within single neurons and among neurons at the synapse itself. Changes can also occur in the circuits of interconnected neurons. Learning sensitizes a circuit to react in a certain pattern in order to produce the memory and/or experience again. Over time, the circuit becomes *conditioned*, so that its activation requires a smaller and smaller stimulus to set it off.

Neurons are specialized in function and are grouped in the brain accordingly. Two types of neurons that play critical roles in the maintenance of emotional well-being are mirror neurons and spindle neurons.

Mirror neurons fire not only when we ourselves perform an action, but also when we watch someone else perform the same act. Mirror neurons may actually allow learning through the process of mirroring or imitating another's emotional and behavioral responses to stimuli. Neuroscientist Marco Iacoboni (2008) suggested that when we see others in the grip of a certain emotion, our brains respond similarly in empathic resonance. These neurons may also be partly responsible for the transmission of culture, allowing people to absorb the values and emotional expressions of those around them. Certain social emotions such as shame, embarrassment, disgust, and guilt are associated with activity in the mirror neurons located in the insula (or insular cortex) of the brain. Daniel Siegel suggested that mirror neurons provide a potential neurobiological basis for the psychological mechanisms known as transference and countertransference (2006, p. 1). In addition, Rossi (2006) suggested that mirror neurons may act as a "rapport zone" and that the neural "mirroring system could be an essential mechanism for the sensitive and highly focused empathy between therapist and subject in hypnosis" (p. 264).

Spindle neurons, also known as *von Economo neurons*, have a spindle-shaped nucleus that tapers to a single axon at one end, with only a single dendrite at the other end. They are exceptionally large cells that transmit signals from region to region across the brain. According to neuroscientist John Allman, spindle neurons function as "air traffic controllers" for emotions and seem to be central to the circuitry for social emotions, including a moral sense (Allman, Atiya, Erwin, Nimchinsky, & Hof, 2001). Moreover, they appear to play a central role in the ability of humans to adapt to unstable situations, cognitive dissonance, and difficult problems (Siegel, 2006).

Neurological and psychological disorders may reflect problems either in the development of, or communication between, neurons. For example, the abnormal development of spindle neurons can result in disorders such as psychosis; a dysfunction in mirror neurons may be implicated in some cases of autism (Oberman et al., 2005). When either the necessary raw products or precursors for producing a neurotransmitter are missing, or the body's ability to produce a neurotransmitter is impaired, difficulties in neural communication, including lowered or increased levels of neurotransmitters, affect mood, patterns of thinking, and relational approaches.

Neurophysiology: Assembling the Blocks

From an anatomical perspective, the entire human nervous system has two major divisions: the central nervous system (CNS), comprised of the brain and the spinal cord, and the peripheral nervous system (PNS), including all the nerves in the rest of the body, whose function is to connect the CNS to the organs and limbs.

From a physiological perspective, the nervous system also has two major divisions: the portion of the nervous system that can be controlled voluntarily and the portion that, at least for most people, cannot be. For the PNS, those two systems are called the *somatic nervous system* and the *autonomic nervous system* (ANS), or involuntary system. The somatic nervous system is engaged whenever a person makes a conscious motion, such as walking, speaking, or doing back flips off the high diving board. Of greater interest to the clinician, however, is the ANS, which manages bodily functions that generally occur outside conscious awareness.

Autonomic Nervous System

Like the CNS, the ANS is always "on" to one degree or another, maintaining basic internal bodily processes and working with the somatic (voluntary) nervous system. Functionally, it is further divided into two major subsystems: the sympathetic and parasympathetic nervous systems, which have opposite and complementary purposes.

The sympathetic system controls the fight–flight–freeze response that stimulates dilation of the pupils, increased heart rate, and the suspension of digestion. Although sympathetic neurons are predominantly part of the PNS, the cell bodies of the first neuron (the preganglionic neuron) are located in the CNS, in the thoracic and lumbar sections of the spinal cord. This part of the nervous system uses acetylcholine and norepinephrine as neurotransmitters. People who habitually tend to activate the sympathetic nervous system may find that, over time, it is harder to relax, and sleep and appetite are negatively affected. Sympathetic-dominant individuals often have chronic digestion problems, anxiety, and insomnia.

The parasympathic system controls the "rest-and-digest" response. It works to slow heart rate, constrict the pupils, and stimulate the gut and salivary glands. The first cell bodies of the parasympathetic nervous system are also located in the spinal cord, but in the sacral region and in the medulla.

The third part of the autonomic nervous system is the enteric nervous system, which innervates the viscera (gastrointestinal tract, pancreas, and gall bladder) and releases over 30 neurotransmitters. Underscoring its close connection to the brain proper, the intestine has revealed amyloid plaques and neurofibrillary tangles usually found in the brain and identified in Alzheimer's disease. Some researchers believe that the diagnosis of this disease may eventually be made with a biopsy of the intestine (Gerson, 1999).

The ANS is involved in conditions such as essential hypertension, panic disorders, generalized anxiety disorder, and obesity. Autonomic inflexibility seems evident in the behaviors and states of clients with these conditions (Friedman & Thayer, 1998; Lyonfields, Borkovec, & Thayer, 1995).

Electrochemical Processes

When a neuron is not firing, it has a "resting potential" of roughly −70 millivolts, measured as the difference in electrical potential between the electrical charge of the ions inside the cell and those outside it (Fisch, 1999). Electrical current flows along the membrane of the cell body and the dendrites. When a neuron sends a signal down an axon, a depolarizing current causes an "action potential," or release of electrical activity. At roughly –55 millivolts, the neuron reaches its threshold state and fires. In contrast to depolarization, which involves the activation of neurons and the release of neurotransmitters, hyperpolarization dulls the neurons, and they become less responsive to stimulation by other cells. The process of producing electrical current in the body is a fascinating and complex one; for a more complete understanding, we suggest the *Textbook of Medical Physiology* (Guyton & Hall, 2005).

Rhythms of the Brain

The combined activity of millions of neurons firing in concert produces patterns of electrical activity that can be detected on the surface of the scalp. Because of their cyclic, wave-like nature, the electrical activity is commonly referred to as *brain waves*. The thalamus is believed to be responsible for generating the particular rhythms of brain waves. Sterman (1995) suggested that the generation of cortical potentials measured on the scalp may come from thalamic oscillatory generators occurring in the brainstem.

Delta frequencies, 1–4 Hertz (Hz; cycles per second), are related to hypothalamic functions and appear in deep, dreamless sleep (stages three and four of sleep). Human growth hormone is released during this deep stage of sleep and promotes healing and regeneration. People with attention-deficit disorder often show high delta frequencies when awake (Gurnee, 2003). Delta waves can also occur in individuals with brain injury or various forms of dementia. When people are close to death, they are primarily in a delta brain rhythm, which is a state of suspended feeling and thinking.

Theta rhythms, at 4–7 Hz, are produced in the limbic system. Someone who has been driving on a long open stretch of freeway and discovers that he or she can't recall the last 5 miles may be in a theta state. The theta state has also been called the "twilight state" and is experienced fleetingly upon awakening or while going to sleep. Hypnogogic (going to sleep) or hypnopompic (waking up) imagery is often experienced in theta. Past memory seems to reside in this frequency, as well as access to universal symbols (archetypes), imagery, and information. In this state, traumatic memories that were recorded in the hippocampus can be "decharged" and healed. This brain rhythm is also present in deep meditation and in deep hypnosis. People with dominant theta rhythms are likely to be highly intuitive.

The alpha rhythm, at 8–12 Hz and higher in amplitude, originates in the thalamus. The associated mental state is one of being awake but relatively relaxed. This frequency is considered to be the "idling" rhythm. It is important to note that in this state no hunger is experienced. Because the sensation of hunger activates beta frequency, controlling the appetite with alpha states is one key to weight management. People with overly high alpha states often end up anxious when trying to focus. As people age, alpha waves decrease and, once they disappear, death is imminent (Hardt, 2007). Alpha states are important in brain health and can actually rejuvenate an older brain. Seventy-year-old people who were taught to achieve an alpha state using neurofeedback techniques achieved brain-wave patterns commonly associated with 35-year-olds and evidenced renewed energy and motivation (Hardt, 2007).

The beta rhythm, at 12–40 Hz, has a relatively low amplitude and a high frequency. A person focused on his or her work, in conversation, or shopping would be in beta rhythm. This rhythm is needed for focused concentration and for processing linear information. People with predominant beta rhythm activity are action-oriented: movers and shakers. Beta rhythms are also evidenced during periods of high anxiety, stress, paranoia, irritability, and mind chatter. A shortage of beta frequency activity in the brain has been linked to emotional disorders such as depression, attention-deficit disorder, and insomnia.

Gamma frequencies range from 25 to 100 Hz, but are usually over 40 Hz and indicate intensely focused thought. Research has shown that gamma waves are continuously present during neocortical low-voltage fast activity (LVFA), which occurs during active rapid eye movement (REM) sleep. Buddhist monks who had accumulated 10,000–50,000 hours of meditation practice showed these amplitudes when they were meditating on compassion (Lutz, Greischar, Rawlings, Ricard, & Davidson, 2004).

Lubar (1997) suggested that there are three kinds of resonances in the cortex that produce the different frequencies. *Local resonance loops* occur between narrow macro-columns of neurons and produce gamma frequencies above 30 Hz. *Regional resonance loops* develop between macro-columns that are several centimeters apart and produce alpha and some beta frequencies. *Global resonance loops* develop between areas that are wide apart, such as the frontal-parietal and frontal-occipital regions, and are responsible for delta and theta frequencies.

There is an important relationship between levels of neurotransmitters—specifically acetylcholine, norepinephrine, dopamine, and serotonin—and the resonant loops. Increases in serotonin lead to increases in the slower frequencies in the theta and delta ranges by connecting to the global resonant loops. Increases in acetylcholine, norepinephrine, and dopamine favor the regional and local loops, and higher frequencies are stimulated. Optimal functioning allows the brain to access appropriate frequencies for particular tasks. Higher frequencies are appropriate for tasks that require crisp attention; lower frequencies are appropriate for activities such as creative problem solving and sleep.

Another important electrically-based concept regarding brain function is that of *coherence*, a measure of how well various areas of the brain connect with each another. Lubar (1997) notes that "coherence measures by correlation the amount of phase locking which exists between two EEG signals of specific frequencies and amplitudes over many successive time intervals which are called epochs" (p. 114). According to Robert Thatcher (Evans, 1999), inappropriately low coherence implies that two areas are functionally disconnected. Excessively high coherence means that two areas are somewhat locked in function. For example, when the coherence between Broca's area, which is responsible for speech, and Wernicke's area, which is responsible for the interpretation of language, is too high, it can result in speech disorders.

Robert Thatcher (1997) developed a means of evaluating coherence that may explain certain neurological conditions. Thatcher asserted that analysis of the development of electroencephalogram (EEG) coherence could provide information about the "organization and differentiation of intracortical connections during post-natal development" (as cited in Dawson, 1994, p. 232). He proposed that children experience "growth spurts" of cortical connections within the roughly four-year anatomical cycles from ages 1½ to 4, 5 to 10, and 10 to 14. These growth phases assist in connecting the hemispheres of the brain and developing higher cognitive levels of functioning (Dawson & Fischer, 1994). Based on this information, Thatcher developed a database of coherence patterns for children of different ages that is used today to compare normal brain profiles with people who have sustained brain injury or who exhibit brain dysfunction. This means of brain-profile analysis provides a topographical map suggesting where problem areas may exist. Using this analytical tool, the neurofeedback clinician can be much more selective in working with a client to retrain the brain toward stability. This tool is also being used in psychiatry to assist in the choice of pharmaceutical interventions, supplanting the much less efficient "try it and see" method, based on observing subsequent behavioral change to determine how well a particular medicine may be working (Proler, personal communication, August 18, 2001).

Rhythms of the Body

Just as the neurons of the brain generate an electrical pulse when they fire and, collectively, generate an electrical field, so too do all the other cells in the body generate minute but measurable electrical fields. Because every movement in the body generates oscillating bioelectric signals, or microcurrents, that are conducted throughout the body, all the cells are connected in terms of overlapping electrical fields. These fields also extend out beyond the body and may act as a web of interconnectedness (McCraty, Atkinson, Tomasino, & Tiller, 1998; Schwartz, 2003). Because organ cells tend to fire in concert, organs generate much stronger fields. For example, the heart generates small electrical waves (measured in millivolts) that can be detected by an electrocardiogram (ECG). A different electric current is produced by the skin. The "galvanic skin response," a change in the skin's conductivity caused by an emotional stimulus such as fright, is the basis of "lie detector" tests.

In looking at commonalities that might underlie the maintenance of health and the prevention of disease, Irving Dardik, a cardiologist, proposed that not just the heart, or even the body as whole, but everything in the universe, moves in waves. As a corollary, he hypothesized that illness results when we stifle those waves within our body (Dardik, 1996; Dardik & Lewin, 2005). In other words, maintaining a variability of waves is a key to maintaining health.

It is well known that a healthy heart beats with a degree of variability from one heartbeat to the next. It speeds up with every breath in and slows down with every breath out. Plotted over time, these variations generate a pattern called the heart rhythm or, more formally, *heart rate variability* (HRV). Specifically, HRV is a measure of heartbeat variations in the beat-to-beat rhythm. This variation is driven by an interplay of the sympathetic and parasympathetic systems: the SNS speeds up heart rate, whereas the PNS slows it down. "Although our understanding of the meaning of HRV is far from complete, it seems to be a marker of both dynamic and cumulative load. As a *dynamic* marker of load (i.e., the physiological wear and tear on the body that results from ongoing adaptive efforts to maintain stability [homeostasis] in response to stressors), HRV appears to be sensitive and responsive to acute stress. Under laboratory conditions, demand for high mental functioning—e.g., making complex decisions or public speaking—has been shown to lower HRV. As a marker of *cumulative* wear and tear, HRV has also been shown to decline with the aging process" (MacArthur & MacArthur, 2000, Chapter 9). States of chronic load or stress can result in a generalized lowering of HRV, and a decreased HRV is often an early indicator of illness (Kristal-Boneh, Raifel, Froom, & Ribak, 1995).

By keeping HRV within optimal levels, a person can increase his or her overall health (Dardik, 1996). HRV can be increased by using an exercise strategy of high exertion and recovery. For example, a brief burst of high-speed running alternated with a few minutes of rest several times in a designated exercise period will improve HRV. During the rest phase, study subjects used Benson's relaxation response, whereby a word or simple phrase is repeated while other thoughts are gently ignored (Benson, 2000). Each rest phase was concluded when the heart rate had stabilized for at least 15 seconds (Dardik, 1996).

The Institute of HeartMath has conducted research on "heart rhythm pattern analysis" and found that emotional states influence heart rhythm patterns. Positive emotions such as compassion are associated with coherent patterns in the heart's rhythms. With negative feelings such as anger, heart rhythms degenerate into less ordered patterns, and the body feels stressed (McCraty, Atkinson, Tomasino, & Bradley, 2006). Studies done on the risk of developing heart disease have shown that both those people who vented their anger and those who repressed it tended to significantly increase their risk (Siegman, Townsend, Blumenthal, Sorkin, & Civelak, 1998; Carroll et al., 1998). In terms of heart health, a preferable approach is learning to discuss problematic situations calmly, without moving toward intensity.

Because the body's electrical field extends beyond the skin, other people may also perceive the electromagnetic fields that are generated by someone's coherent or chaotic heart patterns. In effect, a person's emotional states can affect others (McCraty & Tomasino, 2006). Although only a few people perceive these fields consciously, we often register another person's electrical field at a subconscious level. It is what leads us to refer, colloquially, to someone's "good vibes" or "bad vibes." In fact, when two people are connected by proximity or emotional ties, there may be a natural resonance reflected in both brain and heart electrical patterns. James Oschman (2000) suggested that the "heart's biomagnetic field is hundreds of times stronger than that of the brain [and] provides a simple physical explanation for the apparent entrainment of one person's electroencephalogram (EEG) by another person's electrocardiogram (ECG)" (p. 96). In a similar vein, it has long been known that the monthly periods of women who live together frequently become synchronized. Although primarily unconscious, the ability of people to come into a biomagnetic alignment is far-reaching and profound.

HeartMath's use of the term *coherence* describes an increase in parasympathetic activity and alpha rhythms, and entrainment—the process whereby two interacting oscillating systems, which have different periods when they function independently, assume the same period—among heart rhythm patterns (patterns of heart beats and the spacing between beats), breathing, and blood pressure (McCraty, 2002). HeartMath researchers have found that when people intentionally shift their heart rhythm into a more coherent rate, their emotional states improve (McCraty & Tomasino, 2006). Childre and Rozman (2007) said that "coherence is an even more powerful physiological state than relaxation. It is considered an optimal state for healing, learning, emotional transformation, and peak performance" (p. 45). Using a tool such as emWave®, a biofeedback device utilizing a specially-designed software program, users can learn to slow their heart rate and maintain an alpha brain wave, through which a subjective sense of calm can be produced. By generalizing the training, this state of calm can be achieved or maintained in other settings. This method of developing heart rate coherence incorporates learning to breathe appropriately.

Rhythms of Nature

Consistent with Dardik's hypothesis, Fritjof Capra (1997) suggested that rhythmic patterns can be observed in all levels: from the atomic patterns of probability waves to the vibrating structures of molecules to the multidimensional wave patterns found in complex organisms. People are awash in the multilayered rhythms of their own pulsating cells, fluctuating hormones, and cycles of growth and maturity. They are also enveloped in nature's rhythms, cycles, and waves: ultradian rhythms of 90–120 minute cycles, circadian (solar) rhythms of 24 hours, weekly cycles, monthly (lunar) cycles, rhythms produced by the sensory input of sound and light, and so on.

Understanding the clinical implications of many of these rhythms is important. For example, circadian rhythms are related to hormonal changes and weight gain. Research from the National Institute of Mental Health (NIMH) suggested that a treatment for obesity might include normalizing the circadian pattern of light and dark (Rousch, 1995). Exposure to 14-hour periods of darkness can trigger hormone release and foster deeper and more restful sleep. Ultradian rhythms seem to correspond to the periodic release of certain hormones that regulate attention span and hunger. Carol Orlock (1995) described experiments wherein subjects headed for the refrigerator or the coffee pot roughly every 90 minutes in order to forestall, if not prevent, the natural ultradian cycle and switch in hemispheric dominance. This behavior might even be expected for individuals working in areas such as accounting or the practice of law, where a consistent left-hemisphere dominance would be more appropriate to the required tasks. Based on her research, Orlock suggested that the oscillations in hemispheric dominance that occur every 90 minutes affect the ability to reason, think, and exercise spatial skills.

Brain, Mind, and Consciousness

The brain is an extraordinary organ that produces electrical activity at all times; whether a person is awake or asleep, the brain continuously receives and processes information. The origin of consciousness and specifically the *mind* is still a mystery. Some cutting-edge thinkers, including Karl Pribram (1994), believe that the mind is a hologram. Jon Cowan, long-time neurofeedback clinician, hypothesized that the mind is a "multidimensional electroholomorphic field" that exists outside the brain (Cowan, 2006). Siegel (2007) suggested that the mind emerges from the interaction of the brain with relationships. As a simple heuristic convenience, the mind is conventionally said to be comprised of the conscious and unconscious; with finer delineations, it includes the subconscious and preconscious.

The conscious mind holds current information and currently perceived emotions, moods, and attitudes. It can hold about four pieces of information at one time if they are not complex (Cowan, 2001); if complex, the conscious mind can hold only one piece at a time. However, the conscious mind can retrieve and replace stored data with a rapidity approaching near-simultaneity. The conscious mind uses past experiences to direct present emotional states and behaviors; based on those experiences, it evaluates potential futures and makes choices.

The unconscious mind holds memories of the entirety of a person's experiences from the very beginning of life. As such, it forms a substantial repository of resources that can be drawn upon by the conscious mind in any given situation. This part of the mind also processes a great deal of input outside conscious awareness. The unconscious mind has an "internal search" function; when asked for a solution to a problem, it goes on an internal search to come up with the best solution at the time, and it continues searching for the best answer in the future (Rossi, Erickson-Klein, & Rossi, 1970/2008).

Much of a person's mental life, as orchestrated by the unconscious mind, is based on an ability to recognize familiar patterns. The term *adaptive unconscious* was coined by Daniel Wegner (2002) to refer to mental processes that can direct judgment and decision making, but that are inaccessible to introspective awareness. The processing of the adaptive unconscious is differentiated from conscious processing by its superior speed, effortlessness, focus on the present, and inferior flexibility. It can size up people's emotions, character, and intent quickly and accurately. Through the adaptive unconscious, snap intuitive decisions can be made. It may lead a person to have a sudden flash of insight or spontaneous "knowing" that something is about to occur (e.g., the firefighter who suddenly shouts to his team to hurry out of a burning building just before the structure collapses) (Wilson, 2002).

Along with all of the learning an individual has acquired, these unconscious processes become resources that can be tapped for problem solving and living well. Milton Erickson (Erickson & Rossi, 1979) believed that people have many positive untapped resources at the unconscious level that can be accessed by priming the client's associative function through the use of metaphorical or symbolic imagery. A relaxed state of mind allows the unconscious to reorganize ideas, issues, and perspectives, which can generate better decision-making. In a study done at the University of Amsterdam, Dikjsterhuis (2004) found that when people were asked to think hard about a complex decision, they made poor choices. But if they were asked to set the decision aside for the moment and engage in a variety of puzzles before making a decision, they made much better choices with which they were more satisfied. The researchers concluded that unconscious thought leads to improved decision-making. Wegner suggested that "we often experience a thought followed by an action and assume the thought caused the action. However, it may be that both thought and action come from another unconscious process"—that is, from a state that precedes both (p. 47).

Putting Knowledge into Practice

With a general working knowledge of the intersections of the brain, the mind, and the body, the clinician is prepared to approach the therapeutic encounter with a much broader understanding of the underlying neural implications of dysfunction and the healing potential of shifting the brain state. In 1909, Sigmund Freud described psychoanalysis as "the talking cure." Although the connection established between clinician and client through conversation is still one of the most powerful tools for healing, now the clinician also has access to a wide array of additional modalities to support the therapeutic connection. In the next chapter, we discuss the evaluation process for a new client within the context of BCT.

CHAPTER 3

Neuroassessment of New Clients

When we take a car into a mechanic for work, we know what the problem is. Actually, what most of us know is what the *symptom* is: for example, the right front tire keeps losing air. However, we may or may not really know what the problem is. The slow leak may well be due to an easily visible embedded nail or a deep cut to the sidewall. But it might also be caused by damage to the valve stem or by air leaking around the tire bead (where it connects with the tire rim). With all of its "parts" really composing one interconnected system, the human brain–mind–body is far more complex than any mechanical device, and the point is even more valid: A description of the symptoms is not necessarily an adequate diagnosis of the problem. When new clients first begin psychotherapy, they know what led them to seek help, that is, the symptoms, but they may not comprehend the underlying issues involved. Therefore a thorough clinical assessment should always be integrated into the process of establishing client rapport.

Before devising a treatment plan that includes any of the therapeutic techniques of BCT, it is important to assess clients' habitual states—both functional and dysfunctional—because those states relate to the activation of specific emotional circuits. It is equally important to determine the client's flexibility in changing states. The chronic activation of certain neurological states and emotional circuits underlies many problem behaviors as they are expressed in recurrent life patterns. These negative patterns, comprised of attitudes, emotions, and behaviors, are often the default responses when the client is under stress or in conflict. In addition, we want to discover the client's resources for self-soothing and whatever positive life patterns we can then engage, reinforce, and encourage the client to practice.

Optimum Arousal

Because managing daily life challenges us to be in optimally aroused states, we want to assess how well clients can activate this optimal level of arousal. If there is too little emotional arousal, there will be insufficient motivational energy for change. If emotional arousal is too high, people can become overwhelmed and immobilized. The Yerkes–Dodson law, developed by the psychologists Robert M. Yerkes and John Dillingham Dodson in 1908, formally describes the relationship between physiological or psychological arousal and performance. This law states that when physiological arousal is low, performance will be subpar (see Figure 3.1). As a person's arousal levels increase, levels of motivation, energy, and passion also peak. However, arousal beyond the peak point leads to increasingly incapacitating stress and poor performance.

Subsequent research has demonstrated that in overaroused states, brain activity moves from the executive center in the prefrontal area to the primitive part of the midbrain. The result is emotional overreactivity, loss of rational thinking, limited access to memory, and frequently, a complete breakdown of cognitive functioning. This is the "neurobiology of frazzle," or distress from overstimulation (Arnsten, 1998). When the brain becomes overly stressed, "neuro-frazzle" makes it difficult to manage even ordinary tasks; in that state, it is impossible to enjoy them. But when an individual can relate to situations from a calm center, he or she can develop creative solutions and access the motivation to follow through until goals are met. Because the ability to do so is so critical, throughout BCT, we repeatedly evaluate how well the client can modulate states of arousal.

Neural Patterning of Emotional Circuits

In the last 40 years, research has enormously expanded our understanding of brain physiology, neurology, and electrochemistry. New studies are continually refining both what we know and the means we use to ad-

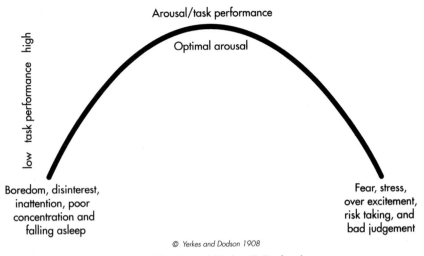

Figure 3.1. Arousal (Yerkes & Dodson).

address brain function through noninvasive modalities. In truth, brain research has only recently emerged from its infancy. However, numerous researchers have now identified various patterns of neural activity directly associated with specific drives, emotions, or behavioral dysfunctions. Numerous studies have repeatedly confirmed a high degree of correlation between neural activity and observable behavior.

Jaak Panksepp (1982, 1998) has identified seven emotional systems that exist in all mammalian brains. In humans, these systems are subcortically situated (Panksepp & Panksepp 2001, p. 146), and each one is associated with particular key areas of the brain (2001, p. 156). Panksepp (2004) also noted that "each emotional system is characterized by its own, at times unique, neuropeptidergic neuromodulators, which may eventually become targets for novel therapeutic strategies" (p. 22). These emotional systems—seeking, rage, fear, lust, care (nurturance), panic, and play—are of use in evaluating neurological dynamics and the states that may be involved in problem attitudes, emotions, and behaviors. Evolution has preserved these systems based on their survival value. However, as Panksepp postulated, each of these systems is also implicated in particular emotional disorders.

1. *SEEKING.* The circuit that mediates seeking behaviors relates to many positive incentives and includes desire, hope, and anticipation.

When this circuit is activated, people experience excitement, curiosity, anticipation, intentionality, purpose, novelty, and, in its darker aspects, craving.

This circuit is responsible for the motivation to seek novel stimuli as the basis for learning. However, it can become problematic when a person seeks novelty at the expense of maintaining a stable relationship or lifestyle. Because this circuit fuels motivation, the process of goal-seeking can deteriorate into an end state in and of itself. For example, clients who have social anxiety may lean toward goal-seeking (e.g., "workaholics") as a replacement for intimacy (Atkinson, 2005).

Overarousal of the seeking system can engender obsessive–compulsive patterns, cravings, and addictive behaviors. In addition, an over-aroused seeking system may result in delusional and paranoid thinking. When this system is overactive, as happens under stressful conditions (perceived or "real"), behavior can become manic as a result of excessive dopamine levels. Drugs such as nicotine, alcohol, amphetamines, and some foods may also overarouse this system. Calming the person—for example, by encouraging slower and deeper breathing—and activating the alpha brainwave frequency are the most immediate means of rebalancing this emotional circuit. With trauma-based symptoms, the empathic therapeutic relationship is crucial to the client's learning of self-soothing behaviors and compassionate self-regard, with a resultant increase in clarity of thinking and improved behavior.

When this system is underactive, as can happen in aging, depression may set in. As a means of reinvigorating this system, the clinician can assist a client in searching through previous life experiences to find some area in which motivation might initially be reactivated. For example, an adult education course may reawaken a long-dormant field of interest. If an individual is anxious or mildly fearful, the stimulation of the seeking circuit through the arousal of curiosity or intention and determination can deactivate the previous state.

2. *RAGE*. The positive intention behind this circuit is usually protection—of the self, of another individual, or of a group with which the individual feels a connection. For example, the rage circuit may appropriately be activated in the face of injustice. In that case, we might suggest that the client attempt to identify what activated this response—for example, a desire to be treated fairly. To manage this state, the client could assess

potential strategies to deal with injustice, as well as the possible consequences of each strategy, and initiate a course of action.

However, if a person cannot successfully manage the feelings associated with this emotional system and dampen the circuit, it becomes
problematic. People often report experiencing an emotional "tunnel vision" and being unable to stop themselves until the rage exhausts itself.
In its less extreme forms, the rage circuit includes irritation, frustration,
indignation, anger, etc. Clinicians need to acknowledge or process a client's intense anger before the person is able to activate a different circuit. The activation of the rage circuit will immediately shut off the
seeking circuit.

3. *FEAR.* The neurological system that responds to danger either by
fleeing or freezing is the fear circuit. Its lesser forms include such states
as anxiety, alarm, foreboding, worry, and dread. The activation of the
fear circuit is an appropriate response when a person is under threat; it
becomes dysfunctional when it is activated under circumstances that
seem benign to most. However, people can feel such intense anxiety in
otherwise benign situations that their only available response is to become immobilized or to leave. The client may need to move away from
the perceived threat to access a calmer state. Prolonged activation of the
fear circuit can lead to hopelessness and despair. Engendering a feeling
of purpose may curtail despair, but it may also, in turn, activate the rage
circuit. Underactivation of fear may lead to excessive risk taking, which
may become equally self-destructive.

4. *LUST.* This system seeks movement toward adult intimacy and
sexual expression. It is set off by visual or verbal cues, hormonal fluctua-
tions, and physical touch. The hormone oxytocin is associated with pair
bonding, and Panksepp (1998) noted that oxytocin levels increase during sexual activity. An inability to appropriately manage this system may
result in irrational jealousy, sexual addictions, or fetishism. In any of
these circumstances, the client will be able to identify what activates
this circuit.

5. *CARE/NURTURING.* Feelings of warmth, concern, empathy, and
tenderness are engendered by the activation of this circuit, which is important in being able to attach appropriately and engage in nurturing
behavior toward others. A lack of early nurturing may result in depen-
dency disorders or inhibit the ability to nurture the self. It may also

cause a delayed or reduced development of empathy and care for others. Overactivation of this circuit may be expressed by the refusal to allow a child to separate properly, a parenting style that "smothers" the child. In the case of a client who finds it problematic to be alone, we would assist him or her in identifying the particular "drivers" of this circuit.

6. *PANIC*. Panic is an emotional circuit that is activated in response to separation. It results in agitation and moves a person to seek social contact, which eventually turns off the circuit. In terms of child development, this is the system that cues the infant when he or she needs to reconnect with the mother. As the infant grows into an increasingly independent toddler, the seeking circuit is activated. As a counterbalance, the panic circuit cuts in when the separation is too great.

Panic may be an appropriate response in the face of imminent threat. An example of managing panic is a pilot's ability to shift into a steady state called "deliberate calm" in an emergency (Gallwey, 2009, p. 45). This shift engages the frontal cortex in a metacognitive process that, with practice, allows individuals to override primitive emotions in a crisis. Extreme panic, as occurs in a panic attack, can feel like a heart attack, with excessive sweating, arm pain, and difficulty breathing.

Rage, fear, and panic are all states of high arousal that occur in response to perceived danger to the self or significant others. Rage generates motion toward the source of danger with the intent to subdue it; fear generates motion away from the source of danger with the intent to escape it; and panic generates motion toward a source of safety.

7. *PLAY*. The feeling of joy is aroused when this circuit is activated. According to Panksepp (1998), ludic impulses are inherent in the nervous system, but a safe environment must be present for this behavior to occur. Activation of this circuit triggers neuropeptides that encourage bonding, creativity, and experimentation. This system produces the "flow" state that Mihalyi Csikszentmihalyi (1990) referred to as a peak state of mind.

Play is appropriate for eliminating stress and providing rest and regeneration. This circuit becomes overactivated if, in the play experience, there is no prearranged agreement with self or other on how to end the game. The play circuit can become problematic if a person responds in an inappropriately playful manner to serious situations, which may communicate dismissal to another, or when it is engaged in to the point of irresponsibility. Fear and hunger can temporarily suppress play.

Valence Tagging

As the brain experiences events, it places positive or negative values on them. This process is called *valence tagging* or "secondary/conditioned reinforcement—the ability of previously neutral events to assume the intrinsic values evoked by emotionally salient events (i.e., unconditional stimuli) through associative learning" (Panksepp & Panksepp, 2001, p. 148). This is the learning process of pairing new, unconditional stimuli that evoke unconditional responses with previously conditioned stimuli and, with reinforcement, producing conditioned responses to the new stimuli. Since Pavlov first discovered this learning process, neuroscience has found that most emotional responses can be conditioned in this way (Panksepp & Panksepp, 2001). In addition, new findings suggest that states cause and regulate certain behaviors associated with them (p. 149).

Table 3.1 summarizes the postulated relationships between the seven basic brain systems, the emotional states to which they give rise, and possible psychological disorders related to these emotional systems. This simplified model of a brain-systems-based typology provides an easily referenced framework for understanding symptomatic states in relation to the various brain systems that have been conditioned to activate through repeated stimulation over time. The plus and minus signs indicate the major types of affective valence tagging that each system can generate.

Panksepp suggested that in addition to these basic mammalian emotional (sub-cortical) systems, humans also have another category of emotions that he called "higher sentiments." These include envy, shame, guilt, empathy, sympathy, humor, and certain kinds of jealousy. Neuroscience confirms that these emotions tend to be mixed with higher-level cognitive processes (Austin, 2006).

Damasio (1999; Damasio et al., 2000) used positron emission tomography (PET) to record brain activity during the recall of certain emotions, such as sadness, anger, fear, and happiness. Although Damasio found that all of these emotions stimulated the somatosensory cortices and the upper brainstem nuclei, each emotion showed a specific neural pattern. For example, sadness activated the ventromedial prefrontal cortex, hypothalamus, and brainstem. More recently, Lai, Daini, Calgagni, Bruno, and Risio (2007) reported on 14 empirical studies that

Table 3.1. Panksepp's Seven Systems and Their Emergent Emotions
          and Related Disorders

Basic Emotional System	Emergent Emotions	Related Emotional Disorder
SEEKING (+ and –)	Interest Curiosity Craving	Obsessive–compulsive behaviors Overachieving Addictions
RAGE (+ and –)	Anger Irritability Contempt Hatred	Aggression Psychopathic tendencies Personality disorders
FEAR (–)	Simple anxiety Worry Psychic trauma	Generalized anxiety disorders Phobias Posttraumatic stress disorder variants Underachieving
PANIC (–)	Separation distress Sadness Guilt/shame Shyness Embarrassment	Panic attacks Pathological grief Depression Agoraphobia Social phobias, autism
PLAY (+)	Joy and glee Happy playfulness State of flow	Mania ADHD
LUST (+ and –)	Erotic feelings Jealousy	Fetishes Sexual addictions
CARE (+)	Nurturance Love Attraction	Dependency disorders Autistic aloofness Attachment disorders

Note. Adapted from Panksepp (2006). ADHD = attention-deficit/hyperactivity disorder.

analyzed psychodynamic psychotherapy outcomes in terms of neural correlates. For example, individuals with borderline personality disorder showed a specific biological pattern, with neurobiological correlates of amygdalar dysfunction, fronto-limbic brain abnormalities, and frontal serotoninergic activity. This pattern has been identified as the neurological signature of impulsivity.

Research to date in cataloging the correlation between brain states and mental states is far from exhaustive, so no list is yet complete. Furthermore, while the activation of certain emotional systems is mutually exclusive of the activation of others, in the experience of "higher sentiments," areas of the cortex may be activated differentially in relation to the activation of the same subcortical emotional system. Therefore, a pure one-to-one, "this equals that" style of conceptualizing these matters would be misleading and severely limiting. What is important here is that the clinician consider the client's situation from the perspective of potential over- or underactivation of primary emotional systems, tentatively identify which circuits might be involved, and keep these in mind when choosing interventions.

Evaluating Clients' Emotional States

In the assessment process, we use an adaptation of Panksepp's model of emotional circuits as a framework for determining which of a client's commonly activated states are related to various emotional systems and ingrained life patterns. The clinician may find it useful to introduce a descriptive or colloquial term for a particularly relevant state or brain pattern (e.g., "deer in the headlights" or "seeing red") to the client. Once a state has been identified and named, the client can be encouraged to inquire introspectively and describe when and under what circumstances that state is experienced.

Emotional and cognitive processes constantly interact. Emotions often are projected onto people and objects and could be considered a form of "valence tagging" that attaches personal meanings to perceptions. Panksepp and Panksepp (2001) suggested that this process may be "a more pervasive and dynamic brain response . . . that operates through some type of global neurodynamic/ neurochemical process in the brain" (p. 151). Interventions that change states by turning on a different circuit can interrupt the negative valence (projection) process.

Problematic emotional states (as opposed to basic emotional systems) are usually characterized by either a generalized low or high arousal manifested as sadness/depression or anxiety/panic. We ask clients to define the problem that caused them to seek help. Frequently the description will indicate the problematic states even if the client is not able to identify them as such. We then ask under what circumstances these states are activated. We inquire about the feelings and behaviors he or she experiences in this symptomatic state. Following this, we examine problems arising from learned behaviors or unresolved trauma, which can include fears, habits, or addictive behavior (Othmer, 2008).

Lastly, we request that the client describe one or more preferred states and begin to collaborate with us on developing state-shifting tools the client can use (Atkinson, 2005). Table 3.2 summarizes these steps and suggests specific clinical questions to ask. In the process of creating a connected rapport with a new client, we use these questions to help direct the "dance" of client and therapist introducing themselves to each other. As such, the questions are thoughtfully woven through the first few sessions.

The evaluation of states is important for the later development of therapeutic hypotheses and the goals that will inform the design of interventions. Based on the client's answers to the aforementioned questions, the BCT therapist may find that, rather than using a problem-solving approach, it would be more productive to help the client rebuild impoverished brain regions by beginning to activate needed circuits and reducing the activation of those connections that lead to problems (Grawe, 2007).

Table 3.2. Clinical Questions for Assessing Emotional States

1. "What states do you experience that cause you distress?" For example: anxiety, depression, pessimism, perfectionism, procrastination, boredom, fear, anger, worry, apathy, or addictions.
2. "Under what kind of circumstances do you experience these states?"
3. "What feelings, perspectives, and activities do you notice when in these states?"
4. "Do you notice any patterns around these negative states?"
5. "When did these problem states begin?"
6. "Describe the preferred state(s) in which you want to spend more time. These target states might include calm, ability to problem-solve without anxiety, or nonreactivity to stressors. When are you in this state? When have you previously been in this state?"
7. "How able are you to focus and hold your attention on an activity?"
8. We also want to know how readily a client can shift states. A playful intervention is a good way to determine how rigidly a person holds a state. For example, when a client is in the middle of a tirade about a partner's behavior, the clinician can interrupt by asking, "Is there anything you want to hear from me or do you just want to pay my fee without any response from me?" If a person continues nonstop, the clinician might say, "Were you out of your mind, intoxicated, or hit on the head when you decided to marry such a scoundrel?" The clinician's tone of voice and facial expression are critical here: The questions must be asked playfully—but in such a way that it is clear to the client that he or she is not being laughed *at* and not being judged. If the question causes the client to stop for a moment, there is a good chance that he or she will shift out of the previous state.

An example might be a client whose parents were emotionally distant or cruel and who has difficulty maintaining stable adult relationships. This person needs to learn how to nurture interpersonal connections and receive love. As part of the therapeutic process, the therapist can ask the client to activate such responses, for example, by volunteering in a Meals on Wheels program. In this way the client will acquire many experiences of doing something which other people will truly appreciate. Learning to give care to, and receive gratitude and affection from, people who are initially strangers and slowly become familiar individuals is a good precursor to attempting to develop an adult relationship. If the client cannot follow through on this activity, his or her reluctance may stem from overwhelming feelings of inadequacy or intense ambivalent attachment issues. In that situation, the BCT therapist needs to find a nurturing activity that is less difficult for the client.

Neural Imprints

We always assume that each person's behavior makes sense within his or her construction of reality. Most behaviors—meaning almost all actions—are *responses*; that is, they usually follow a stimulus, which may be either an external event or an internal state. Generally, a behavior is an attempt to change a state by meeting a human need or reducing a level of physiological/psychological stress. Such behaviors, whether constructive or destructive, are frequently initiated by the activation of a neural imprint.

Neural imprints or life patterns (Young & Kloska, 1999; Wisneski & Anderson, 2005) can be positive or negative. They are usually learned in one's family of origin, where certain emotional responses and perspectives were modeled. Negative neural imprints can form from early trauma or simply hurtful interactions that overwhelmed the person's emotional defense system and left him or her feeling belittled, demeaned, or denied hoped-for opportunities (Bowlby, 1988).

These patterns are attached to different emotional circuits and are neurophysiologically coded with their own "language." Phrases, metaphors, symbols, and sensations trigger specific states and reflect both their persistence and strength as well as the person's flexibility in adjusting to life demands (Grigsby & Stevens, 2000). They can unconsciously direct lifelong behavior and relations with others as well as contribute to negative feelings of anxiety, yearning, sadness, anger, and overarousal. At times, the states initiated by a client's neural imprints do not appropriately match external circumstances; certainly they do not allow for optimal behaviors. However, as long as a psychological problem persists, it will maintain a structure of perceptions, emotions, and beliefs with a concomitant neural imprint. Therapeutic resistance will often have its basis in the chronic and long-term activation of familiar states used for survival.

Table 3.3 presents potential negative life patterns associated with the seven emotional systems. It is useful to identify a client's major negative life patterns and the emotional circuits to which each is connected.

All of these patterns can lead to behaviors that have the potential to become self-fulfilling prophecies. For example, if a person is chronically frightened, he or she may unintentionally take on a victim mentality. Over time, "victim" may become a default state, creating a rigid identity that revolves around being wounded.

Negative neural imprints tend to loop in repetitive patterns and themes. These loops can occur in such areas as the selection of friends, chronic complaints about spouses, financial problems, and issues in the workplace. Clients usually can identify these looped patterns and the triggers that activate them.

It is particularly important for the therapist to identify those self-protective states that are triggered by the activation of fear, panic, or rage and the behaviors and thought processes that accompany those states. However, the activation of the states of seeking, play, lust, and caring should also be identified (Atkinson, 2005). The therapist should note which emotional circuits are chronically turned on—including ones that are positive or potentially positive—and what life patterns are activated in the client's life. In what circumstances does the person experience positive states, and how frequently do they occur?

Filters and Patterns

Besides the psychophysiological elements of autonomic arousal of emotional states, the clinician needs to understand the client's unique structure of filters and patterns for perceiving the world and maintaining symptoms of emotional disorder. As opposed to neural imprints, which

Table 3.3. Negative Life Patterns as Expressions of Activated Emotional Systems

Emotional Systems/ Circuits	Negative Life Patterns
SEEKING	"I need more novelty to feel happy." "As soon as I achieve a goal, I have to go further." "A stable relationship is boring." "I need substances, food, or things to change states."
RAGE	"I never get what I want." "I must retaliate." "Life is a fight—nice guys don't win."
FEAR	"I will be harmed or judged." "I try never to 'make waves,' so I agree to things that I don't really like." "I don't like to try new things." "I don't matter."
PANIC	"I will die." "A close relationship is suffocating."
PLAY	"I must fill life with activity to feel alive." "If it isn't fun, why bother?"
LUST	"I must have sex to feel connected." "I must have sex to feel calm."
CARE/NURTURANCE	"I am unsafe in relationships." "I must cling to my partner." "I am all alone in life." "I can't bear to be alone."

have content, filters and patterns are simply behavioral styles. Deletion, distortion, and generalization are common filters and patterns used by clients. *Deletion* is the tendency to omit certain information; *distortion* occurs when a person projects onto others or misrepresents information to him- or herself; *generalization* is the tendency to assume something is true in most circumstances based on one or two experiences. These filters and patterns are always accompanied by certain states.

Because almost everyone experiences their interpretation of events as an accurate recounting of reality, in the assessment process it is important to accept the client's reality. An evaluation of the person's particular brain states and life patterns can assist the clinician in understanding the basis of the client's experienced reality more fully. It will also be useful for selecting specific interventions to support the client in building needed neural connections.

State Flexibility

Frequently, the brain strings together emotions in sequences that lead to rapid state change. Emotional reactivity begins with arousal, which leads to a problem state accompanied by a habitually informed negative emotion. In the problem state, a person typically loses connection with internal resources, such as the ability to solve problems creatively, and cannot envision a way out. The therapist should assess how well the client can observe this personal process and identify a desired state to access. The clinician may need to educate the client about both observing the process and working with it.

Schore (1994) suggested that we develop "internal representations of human relationships that serve as 'biological regulators' by influencing physiological processes" (p. 293). As children develop properly, they begin to have the ability to manage a whole spectrum of internal emotional and motivational states and the shifting processes between them. The ability to shift back and forth from sympathetic arousal to parasympathetic inhibitory circuits generates psychobiological states. Commonly, this shifting occurs in response to the face of a significant person, either seen or recalled. In anticipated interactions between an individual and a significant person, the imagining of emotional facial expressions prepares a person for the anticipated behaviors. This complicated psychobiological process takes place rapidly.

In the process of shifting, the "emotion-specific state of action readiness is activated and manifested through overt behavior and experienced as moods" (Schore, 1994, pp. 293–294). The person begins to favor certain habitual emotional states and behavioral responses that include moving *toward (safety)*, moving *away from (danger)*, or moving *against* others (Horney, 1950/1991). Note that these echo Panksepp's basic emotional systems of panic, fear, and rage. Wiener and Graham (1989) observed that emotions act to "bridge the past and future" (p. 401). How well a client can switch psychobiological states when needed indicates how self-regulated he or she is.

We can assess a client's state flexibility, level of arousal, and neural imprint by his or her narration of the problem story. If an individual is agitated or depressed, the words selected will reflect the client's state and give an indication of his or her ability to enter into the therapeutic conversation. For example, one woman told us that she absolutely needed to wear a certain brand of clothing to feel confident. When she was not wearing that designer's clothing, she tended to interpret elements of her colleagues' behavior as expressing their negative judgments of her. We surmised that she kept herself out of anxiety states by identifying with the image projected by that designer line. Anxiety had become the default state she experienced when under stress. Once her anxiety was triggered, she had very little flexibility to change her state. Later we discovered the basis for this neural imprint: Her mother had always been quite critical of how she looked and frequently commented on what she needed to change. So, in fact, longstanding attachment issues with her mother were connected to the expensive suits.

Another client with weight issues discovered that once she stopped eating compulsively, she began to distract herself from frightening thoughts or images by watching television or playing computer games. As a teenager, this woman had had very different interests from her family. Her father, a blue-collar worker, loved country music and believed classical music to be snobbish. His way of defending himself from what her love of classical music represented to him was to call her "crazy." As she was unconsciously reaccessing the life pattern around being "crazy," she reported feeling afraid of her own mind. Her disturbing ideation often took the form of fears of becoming ill or of being isolated from her family. Compulsive eating calmed her anxiety temporarily. When we suggested meditation as helpful practice in between sessions, she was afraid her mind would trap her in a darkness she would not be able to handle; nevertheless, she was willing to try it. As she settled her mind, she began to understand how anxiety fueled the eating, and gradually the sensation became a signal for her to relax her mind. By calming the mind, it became possible for her to look directly at the fear, see where it had come from, and interrupt the compulsive eating pattern. She also stopped the compulsive television-watching and computer-gaming; she began to exercise and to use meditation tools, such as calming music and refocusing the mind, to stay in control. We reinforced her ability to manage her fears by turning on her seeking system. We asked her to become curious about how a feeling had been triggered and to observe what happened after that. As she paid closer attention, she discovered the scary feelings began to occur less frequently and with less intensity.

Family System

Knowing the context or system in which a client currently operates is helpful in understanding his or her unique situation. Family-of-origin information is additionally useful in identifying biological predispositions. It may also hint at the client's degree of emotional flexibility and stability, since family dynamics play an integral role in the development of a child's neurological functioning. For example, parents who frequently display angry outbursts or violent behavior will condition children for aggression and hostility or for constant connection-seeking.

In the evaluation process, we are interested in learning how a person's neurophysiology may have been shaped by the original family environment. Additionally, genetic predispositions—which may by shared by other family members—can underlie certain dysfunctional states. A clue to both those possibilities may be found by asking, "Does anyone else in your family have the same problem?"

The family system can continually reinforce a dysfunctional state. For example, if one person in the system tries to lose weight, there may be resistance from other family members—for example, subtle implications that by losing weight, the person is being disloyal. In that case, losing weight must be accompanied by finding other ways to reaffirm commitment to the family. Along this line, because the brain is an interpersonal organ (Siegel, 1999), interactions with family members can help or worsen conditions. The depressive state of other family members may be constantly "reinfecting" a client. If a person lives in an environment of constant criticism, disregard, or emotional abuse, it will be particularly difficult for him or her to effectively shift states in the family environment until that context is also changed.

The clinician will wish to evaluate family dynamics in terms of (1) the level of anxiety in the family, (2) how conflicts are managed, and (3) how feelings are addressed. It is also important to note if there are issues that cannot be discussed directly.

Life patterns at this level might include enmeshed themes—"I cannot share my feelings"; "I must remain loyal to the family at the expense of myself"; "I can only be somewhat successful"—or they might include the overall inability to set and maintain appropriate boundaries. For example, a life pattern might include a daughter's feeling compelled to tell her parents everything that goes on between her and her husband or not being able to spend holidays away from the family of origin.

In some instances, biological factors present from birth impact neural imprint development. As children, these individuals may have difficulty being soothed and may carry this problem throughout life. When working with the parents of a troubled child, it is important for the clinician to avoid a stance of blaming the parents for a child's behavior. Rather, the clinician should focus on identifying appropriate and effective treatment, which may involve parental education. As adults, individuals with attention problems may feel that they are inferior to others. Certainly, people with Asperger syndrome find it difficult to manage social situations. We want to educate clients who have such conditions so that they can better understand how the brain functions and how they can manage their reactions more successfully.

Set Point

In the assessment process, it is important to determine whether an individual presents with symptoms characterized by underarousal, overarousal, or aspects of both, and where the emotional set point resides. A set point is "a predisposition to feel a certain way and a baseline to which we quickly return" (Davidson, 2003, p. 16). Under chronic stress, this set point tends to become less adaptive. Eventually it may take only a very small stimulus to trigger a negative response pattern, such as anxiety, and the cascade of behaviors that are designed to change the person's inner state. Identifying which emotional state a person uses as a default state—that is, in which state an individual lives emotionally—is useful in deciding where and how to intervene.

As a subjective measure of set point, we might ask the client, "In your day-to-day situation, on average, where would you put yourself on a scale of 1–10 in terms of being relaxed versus stressed?

Relaxed_____Stressed
1 2   3   4   5   6   7   8   9   10

We then suggest to clients that *under stress* each person is predisposed to feel either more anxious (overaroused) or more depressed (underaroused), and we ask for them to tell us where they are along that continuum, and what occurs in their case:

Anxiety 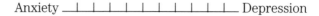 Depression

In overarousal, the patterns of dysfunction include fight, flight, and panic states, including difficulty with focus and the tendency to become immobilized, to "freeze," or to "go numb." In patterns of underarousal, people may become helpless and pessimistic, easily offended, unmotivated, and lethargic. They may easily give up and "throw in the towel."

Even in the relative absence of stress, unstable arousal is sometimes evidenced by a brain that keeps shifting from underarousal to overarousal in an attempt to find balance. For example, "Ring of Fire ADD," as identified by Dr. Daniel Amen (1999; so named because brain scans showed marked hyperactivity throughout the cerebral cortex in a ring-like pattern), cyclothymic disorder, and borderline personality disorder commonly exhibit unstable arousal. The resulting behavior might be characterized as a seemingly sweet and calm person who "spins out of control" with the slightest provocation.

All three of these arousal patterns reflect increased emotional reactivity. Learned patterns of behavior, unresolved trauma, fears, habits, and addictive behaviors need to be evaluated for appropriate interventions. As we get to know more of the client's life story and accustomed stress response, we can deduce which states are chronically activated and later develop interventions to deactivate them and to stimulate positive neural networks. For example, those individuals who have learned to avoid social situations to manage anxiety may have had abusive experiences in the past that have never been resolved. These people may chronically use substances or food to medicate feelings and keep them from conscious awareness.

Diagnostic Refinements

Because a thorough understanding of the symptom complex is important, a complete history should be gathered, including a description of present symptoms, medical and head trauma history, support systems, stress levels, and current medications. This information is important when evaluating potential treatment interventions. Table 3.4 includes

Table 3.4. Diagnostic Questions to Clarify Assessment and Diagnosis

1. Which states can the client turn on easily and which are difficult to turn off?
2. Does the person have a history of physical illnesses or surgeries?
3. Is there any prior drug use? (Consider both prescription and "recreational" drugs.)
4. Is the person taking medications and/or nutritional supplements currently?
5. How well does the client eat? How well does the client sleep?
6. Have any recent medical exams included blood work?
7. What are past and present sources of stress and coping capacities?
8. What gives the client joy and meaning?
9. What emotional/behavioral tasks does the client need to learn in view of the problem he or she describes?
10. Holding in mind that the client's explanation for the symptom is his or her reality, what is limiting about that explanation that may block a solution? Given the client's explanation, how optimistic or pessimistic is the client that the situation can truly be improved?
11. By what major life theme and in what primary state of consciousness does the client live?
12. Does the client have any longstanding family estrangements? If so, what keeps the client from reconciling these broken relationships?
13. Are there secret traumas that have never been discussed?
14. What emotional/physiological resources does the person have? These might include:
    - Confidence
    - Assertiveness
    - Appropriate risk taking
    - Appropriate boundary setting
    - Mastery of tasks
    - Curiosity
    - Compassion
    - Connection and cooperation; ability to attach
    - Appropriate sense of independence
    - Appropriate dependency
    - Flexibility
    - Sense of humor
    - Ability to overcome disappointment and emotional pain
    - Ability to change states of consciousness
    - Ability to self-soothe

questions intended to enlarge upon an initial assessment and diagnosis and inform subsequent therapeutic interventions. As with the previous lines of inquiry, many of these questions need not be directly asked. However, the therapist will want to keep them in mind and lead the conversational exchange in such a way that he or she learns the answers.

Experiences are neurologically "recorded" by the brain in the biosocial state in which they occurred. Through this process, they become locked into various organizations of brain frequencies and neurochemical states (Rossi, 1996). Because of this, information and skills acquired in one state may not be easily accessed from another; that is, they are state-dependent. We assume that although clients have many of the resources noted in Table 3.4, some of those resources will have been acquired and activated only in the context of rare experiences, and, since memory and learning are state-dependent, those inner resources may be associated with, or anchored to, certain physiological/emotional states to which the client cannot readily return without intervention (Rossi, 1993; Overton, 1968, 1982).

Head Trauma

We directly ask a variety of questions regarding possible head trauma that may have contributed to certain symptoms (see Table 3.5). Because clients discount this possibility and many people have had head injuries, we ask this question a number of times during the initial interview and/ or subsequent meetings. Head trauma can occur in many ways: through auto accidents, sports injuries, high fevers, or exposure to toxic chemicals, to name a few. Genetic predisposition may also be a factor.

Even with mild whiplash, the resultant injury can cause difficulty at the level of the midbrain. It has been calculated that in a ten mile per hour rear-end collision, 14,000 pounds of inertial force is exerted on the spinal cord. This impact can cause dysfunction in the sensory–motor connections, and vision can be impaired (Thomas et al., 2003). Mild brain injury is defined as a traumatically induced physiological disrup-

Table 3.5. Questions Investigating Head Trauma

1. Have you ever hit your head as a child? As an adult? How about whiplash? Where was the injury? What was the extent of injury?
2. Did you experience any amnesia? (Amnesia is usually associated with the period of time between a severe brain trauma and the point at which the patient again had clear memories.) How long did it last?
3. Did any problems occur after this event, such as depression, fogginess, or strange physical or mental experiences?

tion of brain function as manifested by at least one of the following: any loss of consciousness, any loss of memory for events immediately before or after the accident, or any alteration in mental state at the time of the accident (feeling dazed, disoriented, or confused) (Thomas et al., 2003).

Quantitative EEG

After an informal evaluation of any possible dysregulation stemming from brain injury, if the problems appear to be related to an injury, we may use a quantitative electroencephalograph (QEEG) or a make a neurological referral (Manstead, 2001). The QEEG provides a digital measurement of electrical patterns at the surface of the scalp. Scalp locations reflect electrical activity in different areas of the brain and provide information on brain function which may be related to symptoms. In that it can disclose neurological problems, the QEEG evaluation may also be a useful diagnostic tool later in the course of treatment for clients who have not responded well to numerous interventions.

The QEEG procedure takes about one hour and is noninvasive. A snug cap containing 19 electrodes, designed to measure electrical activity from selected scalp areas, is placed on the head. Data are collected by having the client keep the eyes open for 5 minutes, closed for 5 minutes, and then spend 5 minutes doing a reading, listening, or math task. Selected areas of the raw data that are free from artifact (eye movements, excessive muscle tension, etc.) are analyzed statistically and compared to normative readings for a person of the same gender and age. The test also gives us information on whether there has been a traumatic brain injury that may contribute to emotional problems.

Prichep and John (1992) have confirmed that the QEEG can reveal profiles of psychiatric disorders. The American Psychological Association has endorsed the QEEG and neurofeedback as being within the scope of practice of psychologists who are properly trained. Based on general consistency among researchers, the QEEG method is evolving into a tool that may aid in the prediction of the clinical course of a disorder as well as predict a client's response to certain medications (Prichep & John, 1992; Chabot, 1998).

Research on the QEEG has demonstrated that it is highly reliable. Hughes and John (1999) reported:

Of all the imaging modalities, [the QEEG has provided] the greatest body of replicated evidence regarding pathophysiological concomitants of psychiatric and developmental disorders. [It] will: 1) Distinguish between dementia and depression, 2) Distinguish schizophrenia and mood disorders, 3) Assess cognitive, attentional, and developmental disorders, 4) Evaluate alcohol or substance abuse, and 5) Evaluate post concussion syndrome (as cited in Kaiser, 1999, p. 1).

There are now over 2,000 research publications on the use of the QEEG. For example, Townsend (2001) found that an adult outpatient group showed lower alpha relative power in 17 of the 19 sites measured. On a QEEG, some clients with borderline characteristics of extreme reactivity and rage show epileptiform activity (Schmidt, 1989). Young et al. (1995) described clients misdiagnosed with anxiety disorders when they were in fact having temporal lobe seizures. Ito et al. (1993) found that individuals with a history of child abuse showed EEG abnormalities in the frontal, temporal, and anterior regions. Another study compared the Minnesota Multiphasic Personality Inventory–2 (MMPI-2) and the QEEG for individuals who reported childhood sexual abuse. Researchers found that early abuse may result in temporal and frontal lobe abnormalities, particularly in the left hemisphere. This finding further implied that potential problems with depression and relationship difficulties might persist throughout life if left untreated (Townsend, 2001). Some clients keep secret the fact that they were abused; results on the QEEG can point the clinician toward asking for this information so that it may be gently and therapeutically addressed.

We have been trained to administer the QEEG test in our office; however, when we are unsure about what the results indicate, we ask our consulting neurologist to review the data. With his assistance, over the years, we have discovered a brain tumor in one client and the beginning of dementia in several. Upon finding abnormal activity, the clinician should make an appropriate medical referral.

rEEG

For those clients who may need medication, we suggest using the referenced EEG (rEEG), a patented system that uses the data from the EEG and compares it to a large clinical database of diverse medication responses that are age- and gender-normed. The rEEG can predict how people ages 6–90 will respond to certain medications before they are taken. By comparing the client's brain profile to people who have similar profiles and who have responded positively to certain medications, a more accurate selection of medication can be made (Emory, Schiller, & Suffin, 2004; Suffin & Emory, 1996; Suffin, Emory, & Proler, 1997; Suffin et al., 2007).

Markers for Improvement

We suggest to clients that they have the capacity not only to recover, but to move to a higher level of functioning than ever before. They have the ability to increase their level of happiness, to thrive, and to experience joy. As part of this evaluation, we ask each client to help us develop markers for improvement. We start by asking what exactly is keeping the client, as far as he or she knows, from not only functioning well, but from thriving. We ask the client to be specific about what would change if he or she started to function better. Together we create a list of concrete markers of improvement. These might include a more stable mood, better sleep, improved focus and concentration, better follow-through on plans or tasks that the client would like to accomplish, less reactivity to stressful events, more creative pursuits or ideas, and target states such as "more relaxed," "more joyful," or "more confident."

Therapeutic hypotheses and treatment objectives can be developed for each marker, and the clinician can decide when to intervene to address those objectives. For example, the clinician may hypothesize which circuit(s) is being triggered and which states the client most often finds him- or herself in. Treatment objectives may include preferred states and may involve a choice of change modalities to access those states. The issue that seems to have the most emotional charge is usually the best place to begin. Over time, we can transform psychobiological resistance to change into calm, focused attention using one or more of several brain technologies, including therapeutic hypnosis. With focused attention, the client's perception, emotion, and cognition are altered. Ultimately, the client's set point may shift and his or her default state may be changed.

Evaluation and Treatment Flowchart

Having determined which emotional circuits are too readily activated (Panksepp, 1998) and what dysfunctional neural imprints or life patterns are often governing behavior, we can create an evaluation and treatment flowchart to direct therapeutic interventions. Table 3.6 presents the evaluation process as a flowchart. Although this process is complex and certainly not unidirectionally linear, it can be helpful in determining a working therapeutic hypothesis and planning initial interventions. (Some arrows go in both directions because the sequence of the tasks may be in either direction.)

An important component of the treatment process is client education. When clients themselves understand which brain systems and life patterns are being triggered, they can learn a variety of therapeutic tools in order to manage the maladaptive states and shift to more positive ones.

One young man with whom we worked suffered terribly from stress headaches. His parents took him to several physicians, and extensive testing ruled out physical causes. We suggested a fairly new treatment called hemoencephalography (HEG). HEG provides functional near-infrared imaging of the level of neuronal activity in the brain, which can then be used as a biofeedback tool (Carmen, 2005). One feedback method simply involves placing an infrared sensor on the scalp to detect the amount of heat radiation at that spot. To give the client a very concrete demonstration of the links between thoughts, states, and migraine headaches, we asked him to focus on a pleasant thought and then on a negative thought. While thinking pleasant thoughts, his temperature regulated. When thinking a stressful thought, his frontal temperature fluctuated wildly. Understanding the connection, he began to make internal adjustments to his own stressful ideas. In the process, he discov-

Table 3.6. Evaluation and Treatment Flowchart

Identify client's habitually used emotional circuits ↔ Name common states ↔ Identify dysfunctional neural imprints/life patterns ↔ Notice filters ↔ Informally test for state flexibility ↔ Inquire about family system ↔ Assess available inner resources → Consider head trauma → Evaluate neurobiological conditions (QEEG, rEEG, etc.) if appropriate → Develop markers for improvement → Generate therapeutic hypotheses → At a macro level, plan initial therapeutic interventions

---

ered that he could willfully attend to a more pleasant state, which greatly reduced his migraine headaches.

The Evaluation Process: A Case Study

In despair, Nancy called for an appointment. She told the clinician that, after 8 years of marriage, she was on the verge of leaving her husband, Rick, who got drunk frequently and kept losing jobs. She complained that he was always depressed and yelled at her and the children. Additionally, she said that she had lost interest in having intimate relations with him. However, she had some interest, albeit mild, in seeing if they could reawaken positive feelings.

During the first meeting, Nancy described the problem states she experienced most as being anxious and distant (Table 3.2, Question 1). On further inquiry, she said that she perceived Rick as being "no fun" and "never being there for her," and that he was "different from when she married him." She mentioned that she tried to delay coming home from her office because spending time with him caused her to feel depressed (Table 3.2, Questions 2 and 3). She was aware that it now took much less of a negative response from him for her to run the inner movie of leaving (Table 3.2, Question 4) than it had even 6 months previously.

In giving the history of the problem, she reported having enjoyed the first year of marriage. The problems began when their first child was born (Table 3.2, Question 5). Rick wanted to stay out late and would never change a diaper. She felt abandoned, left to do most of the child care and housework, and was resentful of the time her husband spent going out with his friends (Table 3.2, Question 3).

Nancy told the therapist that she wanted to feel alive and in love again (Table 3.2, Question 6) but wasn't sure she could do that with Rick. She reported that she felt great at work, where she was highly competent (Table 3.2, Question 7). It was only around her husband that she felt unhappy. We also asked her if there were any times she felt close to her husband (another angle on Question 6); she was unable to remember any.

We observed the following flow for her patterned states (*neural imprint*): A lack of emotional connection (*emotional system: CARE*) and constant bickering led her to feel despair and anxiety, with a desire to flee the situation (*emotional system: FEAR*). She could switch on the fear circuit in an instant; at this point, all it took was seeing Rick's facial expression of anger when he was drunk.

She identified a life pattern of needing to be outstanding before she could feel comfortably competent. She had originally experienced this need with her father (*family system*). She wanted to be able to lean on her husband but no longer trusted that he could support her financially or, by extension, emotionally, so she fired herself up to be super competent. We inferred potential neurobiological imbalances, since she was insomniac (Table 3.4, Question 5) and pushed herself constantly. The family system from which she came was highly critical, and she noticed that similar dynamics had formed in her marriage. Both Nancy and Rick employed derogatory ways of speaking to each other; their comments were heavy with sarcasm and barely-masked anger. Originally, the major filter that both had used was distortion: Each had imputed a maliciousness in the other's intentions. Over time, that had become a self-fulfilling prophecy: There was a maliciousness, an intent to wound, in the sarcasm on both sides.

Nancy reported that she could relax with friends and did enjoy going on a date with her husband if there were no other stressors. We hypothesized that she wanted to be nurtured and gently cared for, but had developed such a hard shell that it was difficult for Rick to sense that she wanted to be with him. Our first intervention with her was to ask her to soften her tone of voice, causing her to change states and access feelings that came to the surface once her anger subsided.

We suggested that she begin to notice when she felt emotionally connected (*target state*) with her husband and the circumstances surrounding that occurrence. We had her practice not saying every negative comment that occurred to her, but rather attempting to notice Rick's states as they might be informing his behavior.

We asked Nancy if she would be comfortable bringing her husband with her for a few sessions. She agreed. From Rick, we learned how surprised he was that his marriage was in such bad shape. We realized he had no idea how despairing his wife felt. He had been so caught up in trying to find a satisfying career that he had paid little attention to the frequent negative states the couple experienced with each other.

Rick had been a successful real estate agent until the local housing market crashed four years earlier, when the area's major employer downsized by closing the entire production facility. With little chance of replacing a comfortable, commission-based income, and with the family increasingly dependent on Nancy's salary, he spent many evenings getting drunk.

He reported that he went out one night and blacked out. The car accident that resulted threw him into the front windshield, and he had sustained a severe head injury (Table 3.5, Question 1). Bouts of depression followed this incident for years (Table 3.5, Question 3). In fact, he reported that his moods seemed darker each year and that he could no longer find a way out of them (*minimal state flexibility*). He had tried a number of antidepressants, but none had been effective (Table 3.4, Question 3). Rick found himself dreading each day and frequently experienced what he referred to as "black moods." When he was in the depressed state, he had no access to any positive internal resources (Table 3.2, Question 3). He noticed, upon inquiry, that the only thing he looked forward to was the weekend. This pattern of feeling depressed and anticipating the worst each week became the usual expectation (Table 3.2, Question 4). Feeling less status and less self-confidence each year, the dark moods grew worse (Table 3.2, Questions 2 and 5). His vision of the future was still marginally positive in that he hoped that some external event would "fix things" and lead to a happier state of mind (Table 3.2, Question 6).

Rick could switch on the FEAR and ANGER circuits (Table 3.4, Question 1) easily and would then retreat to medicate them with alcohol (Table 3.4, Question 3). He lacked status with his wife (and with himself) and realized that he had recreated a pattern from childhood (*life pattern from family system*) of being unable to please his family. The communication style he had grown up with was apparently replicated in the harshness of the communication between himself and Nancy. Rick came to understand that because he felt so hurt, he had wanted to wound her. He became aware that what he needed was to feel acknowledged as a worthwhile person and as someone who could make a contribution (Table 3.2, Question 6; *markers for improvement*).

We wondered if Rick's head injury might be contributing to his dark mood and suggested that a brain map be done (QEEG). Indeed, the map showed evidence of a significant head injury, and we therefore recommended neurofeedback training in addition to marital therapy.

Rick also reported that he enjoyed spending time with his wife away from the children. This positive feeling provided a foundation from which it was possible to rebuild the marriage. We hypothesized that if Rick could improve his depression with neurofeedback work, his alcohol consumption would decrease, and he would be more emotionally available to Nancy. In that case, she might begin to feel that she could lean on him safely again.

As we worked with Nancy and Rick, both independently and jointly, on managing their states of overarousal and the consequent distressing behavior, they each began to access more of the emotional resources that previously had been "held hostage" by overarousal. Rick began to feel more of a sense of self-worth and, with Nancy's support, landed a sales position at a local car dealership, where his skills with real estate clients were immediately applicable. Gradually they became closer and found that they were spending more time in shared states of happiness.

Chapter 3 has covered the many aspects of client evaluation, with particular attention to assessing a client's habitually activated emotional circuits, neural imprints, state flexibility, level of arousal, and any relevant neurobiological conditions.

Chapter 4 describes the components of the BCT model, after first providing an overview of stress and its chemistry, brain involvement, and impact on memory. Case examples are used to illustrate various aspects of BCT.

Brain Change Therapy Model

Stress and State Change Interventions and Strategies

How a client presents in psychotherapy is indicative of his or her psychoneurological development. If there has been good-enough parenting, the adult has learned how to self-regulate emotional states and to be aware of others' feelings (Wake, 2008). If there are developmental delays, however, the therapist must work with the perceptions of the client and access "resources within the therapeutic relationship to enable . . . learning for the client while at the same time containing the process in a way that is safe and ecological for the client and therapist" (Wake, 2008, p. 78). BCT is a therapeutic approach based on neurological research demonstrating that learning alters the brain by changing the number and strength of synapses and that people have the ability to turn brain circuits on and off in a way that changes their psychophysiological states. In order for change to be more than temporary and for the client to learn how to manage state changes, the client must engage in neurological repatterning. At the most commonly shared level, what clients are reprogramming is their stress reaction—*stress* is the underpinning to most (if not all) clients' problems.

Almost without exception, by the time someone phones a therapist to schedule an initial session, the person is in emotional distress. Some aspect of the person's life isn't working; the individual has already done as much as he or she could to address the situation, and whatever the person tried was not adequate. The person turns to a therapist hoping someone else will have the insight and wisdom to help.

Reflecting the person's emotional distress, the individual's brain–body experiences the chemistry of stress. Because clients arrive in a state of stress, it is important for therapists to understand the neurochemistry of stress, the patterns of brain activation that typically occur during stress, and the effects of stress on memory, learning, and emotional stability. Based on the recognition that stress is the starting point, BCT focuses on therapeutic interventions that can create ultimately longstanding changes in clients' brain–mind–body states.

In this chapter we first provide an overview of stress and its chemistry, brain involvement, and impact on memory, and then explore the components of the BCT approach, with case examples as illustrations.

The Many Facets of Stress

Most people tend to think of stress in terms of *stressors*—causative factors—but the two are not synonymous. Stress is the *response* to stressors—we feel stressed by the erratic driving of a nearby motorist, a job loss, or a schedule filled with too many commitments, all of which are stressors. We can categorize the vast domain of possible stressors—the events or situations that lead to the body's stress response—into four broad categories: physical, physiological, psychological, and psychosocial.

• *Physical stressors* include situations of physical danger and environmental factors such as extreme temperatures, constant noise, a high pollen count, compromised air quality, or lack of sunshine.

• *Physiological stressors* include hunger, exhaustion, and injury or illness that changes a person's quality of life and ability to perform normal, everyday tasks. Surgery of any kind, particularly with full anesthesia, can be a significant stressor. In addition, an inadequate supply of oxygen or impaired breathing, which many people have because they do not breathe deeply enough, can stress the whole system.

• *Psychological stressors* are any events that are perceived as overwhelmingly stressful, such as the death of a loved one, financial hardship, the possibility of losing employment, or a move to a new community. Psychological stress can foreshadow cardiac events such as heart attack, cardiovascular disease, and stroke. In the months after the attack on the World Trade Center, there was a large increase in incidents of abnormal heart rhythms in cardiac patients living in New York City (Mahr, 2007).

• *Psychosocial stressors* are events that affect a family system's overall functioning. For example, juggling the needs of children, a part-ner's substance abuse, the care of a special-needs child, or even some-thing as seemingly minor as restrictions on topics of discussion, can be perceived as sources of stress. One client told the quasi-humorous story of her mother, who always asked, "What three things about this difficulty are good?" even when the problem was quite devastating. When people in the family needed to speak about difficult things, the mother would abruptly respond, "I don't want to hear anything negative."

The Chemistry of Stress

According to Hans Selye (1978), the "father" of stress research, the stress response is initiated when a threat is perceived by the brain. At this point, an alarm goes off in the body that begins a chain reaction. The hypothalamus activates the pituitary, which releases adrenocortico-tropic hormone (ACTH) into the bloodstream. The brain also produces glucocorticoids, which are chemicals triggered by stressors that flow along the hypothalamic–pituitary–adrenal (HPA) axis. ACTH travels in the bloodstream to the adrenal glands, causing them to secrete various hormones including adrenaline and cortisol. These hormones travel throughout the body and cause the changes that produce the fight–flight–freeze response: (1) blood is diverted from internal organs to the brain and skeletal muscles; (2) pupils dilate; (3) heart rate increases and blood pressure elevates; (4) metabolism and stomach acidity increase; (5) the brain shifts to a higher beta frequency; and (6) cortisol is re-leased to reduce swelling and inflammation. All of these physiological changes are accompanied by one or more emotions (e.g., fear, anger, anxiety, depression).

Because most of today's stressful situations do not require the body's engagement in a physical response, these chemicals are not efficiently eliminated from the system. In particular, the prolonged elevation of cor-tisol levels can damage the adrenal glands and impair the body's ability to deal with infection. In 1991, a group of British and American scientists published a study in the *New England Journal of Medicine* that con-cluded that people under stress were more likely to catch colds (Cohen, Tyrell, & Smith, 1991). In the study, 394 volunteers took nasal drops containing cold viruses. Those who described themselves on a question-naire as under a great deal of stress were five times as likely to become infected (as measured by viral replication) as those who were under less stress, and twice as likely to develop clinical cold symptoms.

A constant activation of the stress response causes wear and tear on numerous body organs and will eventually hasten death. Cortisol directly influences metabolism and insulin levels; by increasing insulin, it also plays an indirect role in chronic inflammation. Chronic illnesses such as cardiovascular disease, immune deficiency, or gastrointestinal problems may develop. Crucial in minimizing inflammation, a factor in many chronic diseases, is learning how to manage the mind.

Brain Involvement During Stress

Researcher Richard Davidson used fMRI (functional MRI) and advanced EEG analysis to identify the brain activity of people in certain moods. His studies indicated that when the subjects were anxious, depressed, or angry, the most active sites in the brain were the amygdala, part of the emotional center, and the right prefrontal cortex. These areas are strongly implicated in the hypervigilance of people who are chronically stressed, suffer from anxiety, or who have posttraumatic stress disorder (PTSD). When people feel happy and positive, these brain areas are quiet, and there is more activity in the left prefrontal cortex (Davidson, Scherer, & Goldsmith, 2002).

Stress tends to detract from a person's ability to change brain–mind states and use more effective strategies in problem resolution. In fact, when normal coping abilities do not seem adequate, chronically stressed individuals tend to fall back on older—and even less effective—strategies that put them in a rut (Dias-Ferreira et al., 2009). Badenoch (2008) identified four adaptations to stress: anxiety, addiction, depression, and dissociation. These dysfunctional states may develop as a result of "a soup of genetic vulnerability, alterations in neurotransmitters and hormones, certain deficits in brain structure and function, inner community disruption based on internalized patterns of relating, and social networks that often reinforce engrained neural circuits, rather than changing them" (p. 120). Badenoch defined the inner community as "multiple states of mind we all experience within ourselves" (p. 271).

The internalization of important figures throughout life, and especially at birth, often results in a tendency to favor the emotional circuits of a primary caregiver or significant other, even if they are physiologically damaging and psychologically dysfunctional. Prenatal research has discovered that newborns' nervous systems are shaped by the mother's mental state during the pregnancy. In fact, if the mother is depressed during the pregnancy, the newborn shows the same biochemical markers of an adult experiencing a depressive episode, including higher cortisol and lower dopamine and serotonin levels (Field, Diego, & Hernandez-Reif, 2006).

Stress as a Disruptor of Memory

Stress can contribute to brain dysfunction and erode memory in three ways. First, with the release of cortisol, the hippocampus is inhibited from utilizing blood sugar. The shortage of blood sugar inhibits the storage of memory; this is why people often have difficulty remembering accurately what happened in a stressful situation. Secondly, if a memory is recorded, it can be difficult to access because cortisol interferes with neurotransmitters and reduces the brain's ability to communicate with itself. Finally, cortisol actually kills brain cells by disrupting cell metabolism so that excessive calcium enters brain cells and produces harmful molecules called free radicals.

This process has been confirmed in animal studies, and there is evidence that it also occurs in human brains. Indeed, this may be the process that leads to the development of Alzheimer's disease (Khalsa, 1997). Cancer survivors who have the posttraumatic stress symptom of intrusive recollections of the experience have smaller amygdalas (Matsuoka et al., 2003). Over time, energy storage is compromised, and hypertension, myopathy, fatigue, and increased risk of adult-onset diabetes can occur. Suppression of digestion in this chronic state can lead to ulceration, and a lowered immune system response can lead to increased risk of death (Sapolsky, 2003).

Stress Is Not Inevitable

External stressors need not inevitably lead to physiological states of stress. Herbert Benson, pioneer of stress management, suggested that a relaxed state of mind should be the ordinary state. Unfortunately, for most of us, it is an extraordinary state. Benson described the relaxed state as intuitive, vibrant, and magical, and suggested that this state could be achieved with practice (Benson, 1997). In support of that idea, Davidson and Jon Kabat-Zinn trained workers in a high-stress job to meditate 3 hours a week over 2 months. Their internal experience shifted to a feeling of less stress and more happiness, and measurements of their immune systems also indicated improvement over this period. The study, among others, (1) demonstrated the ability of a person to significantly change the emotional circuitry of the brain, (2) confirmed earlier evidence of the plasticity of the brain, and (3) reinforced the idea that no one is necessarily a prisoner of either his or her early conditioning or physiology (Goleman, 2003).

States of low stress, safety, and peacefulness help clients reflect and allow them to integrate and resolve emotional issues. When these states are difficult for clients to access or maintain, brain technologies may be useful. If clients have experienced trauma, it may be dealt with best by teaching them how to increase their state flexibility safely through the use of brain-training devices (Chapter 6). Clients' problems need to be framed as having a variety of solutions, as long as clients can access and sustain an appropriate brain–mind state. The mind can create many ways to resolve a situation; it can generate ideas, author empowering visualizations, and imagine possibilities; and it can form new emotional patterns—if brain functioning is stable. At that point, new perspectives and ways of assigning meaning become possible. Particularly in the context of stressors, an essential element of psychological health is brain stability: the "proper balance of activation, inhibition, and integration of systems biased toward left-and-right-hemisphere control" (Cozolino, 2002, p. 123). The result of brain stability is psychological flexibility— that is, the successful management of the basic emotions of happiness, surprise, fear, sadness, anger, and disgust.

Overview of the Brain Change Therapy Approach

BCT uses brain–mind state change as a focus of treatment. As noted in Chapter 1, the therapeutic approach is based on the working assumption that effective therapeutic change must inevitably include a repatterning of neural pathways. We emphasize the necessity of changing states of consciousness and conditioning the changed state, through repetition, to access or build internal resources. When appropriate as an adjunct and support to brain-mind state change, BCT helps clients create new, empowering life experiences that can serve as the basis for new neural patterns. For positive state *stability*, however, attention training may be necessary. Whatever a person focuses on—a fear or an insight, a dear friend or a personal nemesis—tends to maintain the brain–mind state associated with the experience (Rock & Schwartz, 2007a). Learning to hold a focused attention will contribute to stabilizing brain circuits and improving the brain–mind's ability to maintain a state associated with a particular positive experience.

Table 4.1 summarizes the BCT approach from the perspectives of both the client and the therapist. The sections that follow amplify the points and processes noted in this table.

The Presenting Client

As noted, each person has an emotional set point of arousal falling somewhere along a continuum stretching from underaroused through balanced to overaroused. Under chronic stress, this set point moves further from the balanced middle such that increasingly softer stimuli can *names* set off a full-blown emotional reaction. Brain studies have found that it takes less than one second for a word or statement to trigger an emotional reaction (LeDoux, 1996). By the time someone says, "Don't get me started!" it's too late. When an individual is overwhelmed by an emotional reaction, access to rational thinking, memory, and the ability to be objective are greatly reduced. At that point, an individual is no longer regulated or in charge of his or her brain–mind states.

The hippocampus stores that negative experience, and the person's neural and emotional reaction to it, in long-term emotional memory. Elements of the original event can then become sensory triggers that reignite the same chains of neural firing—and the concomitant emotional reactions. These triggers can include actual images, internal images, or visual cues, such as a particular color. One man became overaroused and ill at ease whenever he was in a room that was any shade of green. Eventually we learned that his mother, with whom he had attachment issues, had had dark red hair and had dressed extensively in greens. Because she favored the color, she had also decorated the family home in the same shades.

Power words, particular words or phrases that have come to have an

Table 4.1. Brain Change Therapy Approach

Client	*Therapist*
Develops habituated emotional set point of arousal. ↓ When overwhelmed by sensation—including images/visual cues, power words, sounds, tastes, smells, touch, events, or textures—sensory gates are turned on, engendering intense emotions involving: • Problematic states of consciousness • Overarousal *or* • Underarousal *or* • Arousal instability (combines aspects of under- and overarousal) ↓ Emotional systems (neural circuits) generally activated: fear, panic, rage ↓ Person creates a negative narrative and/or internal movie accompanied by one or more of the following emotions: frustration, anger, fear, malaise, chronic disappointment, depression ↓ Attempts to reduce these unpleasant states often involve problematic behavior and, as a systemic pattern, can stimulate similar problematic behavior in others. ↓ Individual determines that his or her attempts have not been adequate. ↓ Person seeks therapeutic assistance. ↓	 Conduct initial evaluation of client while establishing therapeutic rapport (Chapter 3). ↓ Develop therapeutic hypotheses and an initial treatment plan ↓ Accept the client's reality. Acknowledge client's presenting state: its content and underlying issues. ↓ Articulate the positive intention behind the dysfunctional behavior. ↓

Table 4.1. Continued

Client	Therapist
Learn to reduce or increase level of arousal to more functional degree.	Define markers for improvement, generate a therapeutic hypothesis, and devise initial treatment plan. ↓ Define the problem as solvable. ↓ Utilize a variety of interventions to effect state change: • Facilitate a shift in physiology. • Use humor. • Expand vision from foveal/tunnel vision to peripheral, particularly with anxiety/panic states. • Engage motivation. • Use therapeutic hypnosis, including voice tone of empathy and hypnotic conversation (Chapter 5). • Use brain change technologies/ equipment, e.g., alpha–theta training (Chapter 6). • Facilitate deep state work using hypnosis or brain training equipment (Chapter 7). ↓ Implement therapeutic strategies as appropriate: • Utilize state progression. • Employ neural talk. • Assist client in becoming aware of and activating inner resources. • Identify where client's self-regulation already occurs; teach client to expand when and where it occurs. • Use therapeutic metaphor.
↓ Learn to identify current state and how changing that state enables client to move toward the target state with focused attention (deconstructing emotional reactivity, mind shifting). ↓	Teach client to self-initiate state change by: • Understanding the process of the mind. • Deconstructing emotional reactivity. • Using mind shifting. ↓ Encourage a belief in the "impossible"

Table 4.1. Continued

Client	Therapist
Resolution of problem behavior and activation of new neural pathways characterized by: • Brain stability: increased ability to maintain desired state and level of arousal • Mood stability • Motivation to accomplish goals • Sleep-cycle stability ↓	↓ Condition and reinforce the new state(s). ↓ Establish the new state as a means of resolving the underlying issues.
Increase activation of emotional systems of seeking, care/nurturance, and play. ↓	
Create workable alternatives to previously intractable issues. ↓	↓ Assist the client in creating workable alternatives or responses. ↓
Implement newly identified courses of action and ways to resolve life situations.	Encourage client to take action and follow up. ↓ Link the action to the client's social context so that new behaviors are generalized and practiced in the client's wider environment

emotional charge, whether positive or negative, can trigger a nearly instantaneous emotional response. One husband called his wife "cute," much to her dismay. From her childhood experience of being teased by boys in school who called her cute, she had a strong negative reaction to the word, such that her association to it carried the feeling of being demeaned. For another woman, the phrase "I'm sorry" carried a highly positive valance. As a child, she had never received an apology for anything from her parents, who had assumed that adults never needed to apologize to children. Thus, in later life whenever someone sincerely said "I'm sorry," she felt "treated like an equal" and found it immediately easy to access a gracious largesse.

A particular sound may be troublesome for a client (see below). Some people develop an oversensitivity to certain noises and may react physically to them with headaches, anger, or irritation. Certain music may be annoying to some people. The volume alone of an auditory stimulus can stimulate emotional circuits to create negative states.

Tastes, smells, even textures, can trigger highly negative reactions. One client with an eastern European background had a father who often made what she referred to as "peasant soups." In her experience, soup came to symbolize, and reevoke, all the trauma she had experienced growing up in a household that was not fully "Americanized," and, in later life, she never ate soup. Soup is a small thing and it's not particularly difficult to skip. But other clients may have triggers that are unavoidable and thus cause far more dismay.

Internal images of a parent disregarding a child or being emotionally or physically abusive can haunt clients, and the emotions connected to these images may easily trigger similar feelings in the present time. When this happens, the fight–flight–freeze response is activated, breathing is inhibited, and more intense upset may follow. When such situations are recounted in the therapeutic interaction, what often follows is a narrative, either spoken or internal. An explanation will be found to express states of overarousal, underarousal, or arousal instabilities that may involve fear, anger, frustration, or chronic disappointment. The narrative may be an attempt to alleviate emotional suffering as well as an explanation for a person's behavior, but it may in fact make the problem worse. When the story or explanation involves some malicious or pathological intent on the part of another, where none may actually exist, we can use what Carol called "siding descriptions" in *The Couple's Hypnotic Dance* (Kershaw, 1992). These are side-by-side interpretations of the same event from two perspectives: the client's negative interpretation and the therapist's suggestion of a more open and workable frame of the situation. Thus the therapist might ask: "Does your husband have a *adult* temper tantrum when things do not go his way [per the wife's description], or is he overcome with fear and panic and having difficulty knowing how to manage these feelings that therapy can help him master?" (p. 175).

adult temper tantrums & self regulation

The neural activation patterns that clients experience in the form of repetitive feelings and problems can change only when they have been activated. When such activation does occur, it is useful to guide it toward mastery experiences; negative feelings can then become pathways toward success (Grawe, 2004). For example, consider the following case.

Case Example: Appropriate Level of Arousal Facilitates Access to Creative Solutions

Caroline, a successful commercial real estate broker whom we had previously seen, called in a quandary over how to handle her business partner. As their firm began to have more difficulty finding commercial tenants, her partner started to complain that Caroline was not working hard enough to line up prospective tenants. Ostensibly to help her, he began attempting to micromanage her schedule and requested detailed reports of her efforts to secure new business. She was alternately anxious and depressed. Her husband showed little patience with her situation and told her to dissolve the partnership. However, because of legal and contractual obligations, she felt she could not just walk out.

Since they were on her managed care plan, Caroline had been to other therapists recently. All of them had encouraged her to take medication for depression. Bill listened to her, then validated her feelings of frustration and concern over the stability of the business partner. He reassured her that she was not crazy: Anxiety and depression would be understandable responses, given her situation. He also observed that although an antidepressant would treat her symptoms, she might not need medication. What she did need was to find a solution to the stressful situation in which she found herself.

Since Caroline had been an executive in a major corporation and was well-connected in the city prior to marrying and having children, Bill wondered aloud to her whether she was as backed into a corner as she thought, and he suggested that the problem had solutions. Bill used this intervention only after being sure that her level of arousal had decreased. He began to talk about strategies with which she could begin to make changes, dissolve contractual obligations, and end the business relationship. She told Bill that no other therapist had been as pragmatic with her. Pleased with his approach, she began to access states of self-empowerment. By the next session, Caroline had begun to take steps to terminate the contractual obligations, and both her anxiety and depression were noticeably improved. The addition of alpha–theta training (Chapter 7) helped her maintain a lowered arousal state and be more creative in her problem-solving efforts as she moved through the process of dissolving her business partnership. All Caroline needed was access to a calmer state, which then allowed her to marshal her own considerable abilities and resources.

The Therapist's Role in BCT

The BCT therapist proceeds organically, though with an underlying structure in mind. None of us lives in the linear world that analysis and description convey; nevertheless, some linearity can be useful in early learning stages, and so we provide a linear structure here. As noted in Table 4.1, the therapist begins with a comprehensive evaluation focused around the problematic state. We use the following questions to help clients become conscious of their habituated stress response patterns:

1. What are you feeling?" [State and emotional circuit]
2. "What is your focus of attention—how and where are you focusing?" [Develop conscious awareness]
3. "How do you explain this state? What led you to develop it?" [Life pattern]
4. "How are you breathing? Do you feel that you are in the middle of an emergency response or can you slow your breathing and create a calm response?" [Sympathetic vs. parasympathetic breathing; see Chapter 6]
5. "Do you find yourself frequently in this state?" [Default state or new state]
6. "Are you aware of the trigger(s) that set it off?"

A formal evaluation, however, is not always appropriate. In some cases the initial evaluation will need to be conducted slowly and much more casually while a stable therapeutic relationship is being developed. The following case demonstrates the use of accepting the client's reality and using empathic attunement as a means of creating a working relationship. The client evaluation was carefully integrated into the early stages of treatment.

Case Example: Accepting the Client's Reality, Using Empathic Attunement

Kevin, now in his early 20s, had a history of paranoid schizophrenia with a fixed delusional system. At the time he was referred to Bill, Kevin believed that he was an artist and that people were trying to keep him from a career in the arts. He had constructed an imaginary life that included being married and having a son. He was also convinced that Bill had cameras in the office and was taking pictures of him. Bill told him that he was correct about the camera in the office: It was in his cell phone.

Kevin had stopped taking antipsychotic medications and, although quite intelligent, was unable to hold a job. He was living at home and had physically attacked his parents. Although he did not look like a street person, he was disheveled and unkempt. During the first few visits, Bill mirrored his behavior; since Kevin would not look at him, Bill avoided eye contact.

Suspecting that Bill was part of the plot to derail his career in the arts, Kevin wondered aloud if Bill were colluding with his parents. Bill confirmed that he had spoken with his parents and added that they were concerned about the amount of time he spent drawing. Bill asked to see some of his drawings and said that he liked them. As an aside, he commented that it was difficult to make a living as an artist.

Since Kevin was clearly in distress, Bill told him that he did not know how he managed to handle the fear and stress and said to him, "I could not go through what you experience. I would need to take the medication." Kevin began to shift states with this intervention and open up to the therapy. He became curious about what therapy might be able to do for him. Bill found that Kevin could tolerate only a short session of 20–30 minutes. Most of the early sessions ended abruptly when Kevin would say it was enough.

Because Kevin talked about his delusions, such as the delusion of having a son, and could identify them as imaginary, Bill discussed these with him. Bill reflected his feelings and suggested that it must be horrible to have a son you cannot see and to believe that people are trying to ruin your career. The empathic comments that conveyed acceptance of Kevin's reality helped him begin to move into states of comfort and trust. Gradually, Kevin became less agitated, and Bill asked what it was like to be on medication. Kevin acknowledged that he felt much better on medication. Bill encouraged him to take the medicine in order to alleviate his distress. As Kevin continued to experience feelings of comfort with Bill, he resumed taking his medication on a regular basis.

Kevin was able to access his own ability for self-comfort by attuning to Bill's nurturing. Eventually, the medications cleared the delusions, and therapy took the path of helping him begin to socialize with others and hold a job.

Identify Appropriate States of Arousal

Next the clinician considers what states need to be activated to help this client. Arousal states for learning include anticipation, curiosity, urgency, or confusion and may be thought of simply as a range of beta frequencies. Other states, such as well-being or what Thayer (2001) called "calm energy," need to be activated when a client is anxious; these reside in the alpha range of frequencies. We can stimulate states of well-being by evoking positive memories, describing social connectedness (Panksepp & Burgdorf, 1999), or describing experiences of success. Helping a client have these experiences will build access to these states.

States of low stress, safety, and peacefulness help clients self-reflect and allow them to integrate and resolve emotional issues. When these states are difficult for a client to maintain, brain technologies may be useful. If clients have trauma, it may be dealt with best by teaching them how to increase state flexibility safely through the use of brain training devices (Chapter 6) and view what happened in the past from a witness perspective without blaming themselves.

The client's problem needs to be framed as having a variety of solutions once the client learns to access and maintain an appropriate brain–mind state. The mind can create many ways to resolve a situation; it can generate ideas, author empowering visualizations, and imagine possibilities; and it can form new emotional patterns—if the brain is stable. At that point, new perspectives and ways of assigning meaning become possible. Particularly in the context of stressors, an essential element of psychological health is brain stability: the "proper balance of activation, inhibition, and integration of systems biased toward left-and-right-hemisphere control" (Cozolino, 2002, p. 123). The result of brain stability is psychological flexibility, that is, the successful management of the basic emotions of happiness, surprise, fear, sadness, anger, and disgust.

Utilize Interventions to Effect State Change

Grigsby and Stevens noted: "Physiological state can be conceptualized as a complex, multidimensional control parameter influencing behavior by affecting the probabilities associated with the activation of specific neural networks" (2000, p. 362). Clients frequently become stuck in a particular negative state and do not know how to shift into a more functional state without the help of a guide. Since all clients have had the experience of shifting states of consciousness, this natural process can be made more deliberate as a means of facilitating transformational learning (Lankton, 2003).

In common with all defense mechanisms, a sustained focus on symptoms often has aspects of trance phenomena. Every psychological symptom has an element of dissociation with concomitant brain frequency ratios; every physiological symptom can be interpreted as an indication of being out of control—although, in another context, the same physical sensations may be interpreted as completely safe. For example, rapid heart rate and perspiration in a gym are to be expected. The same response while climbing the steps to a stage may be interpreted as anxiety. The issue is not the physiological sensations per se; rather it is always the meaning a person attributes to them. If a person becomes overly focused on symptomatic expression, he or she often begins to play internal mind movies of the worst possible future (Kershaw, 1992). In essence, this mental rumination is preparation for handling a negative outcome and may be seen as a survival mechanism. By helping the client to change states, a negative trance can be depotentiated. From the resulting more open state, the client may discover a new perspective or even an internal resource that had been previously overlooked.

State change can be accomplished in a matter of seconds and through a variety of ways: by altering physiology, using humor, focusing attention, and/or engaging motivation (Grigsby & Stevens, 2000; Fehmi & Robbins, 2007; Lane & Nadel, 2002). We discuss each in turn.

Altering Physiology

Physiology can be changed with a simple adjustment in the way a client stands, sits, looks, eats, or breathes. For example, with a depressive client who is slouched in a chair, create some reason for the person to get up out of the chair and walk a few feet. Such a reason might be to look at a diagram the therapist has quickly sketched on a piece of paper to illustrate a situation the client is describing (a few circles and arrows with a verbal description will do). The therapist can show the sketch and ask, "Do I have this right?" As well as engaging the client's curiosity, having him or her stand up, take three or four steps, look at a piece of paper, and sit back down will change his or her physiology, focus of attention, and state. In addition, changes in sensory stimulation from the external environment (e.g., opening a window for fresh air or changing the lighting) can change a client's physiology and result in a reduced anxiety level.

Using Humor

Humor is an effective way to change states. It turns on the play circuit and fosters attachment to others. In the context of psychotherapy, humor can provide relief from tension and stress and can shift a client's state from anxiety or depression to playfulness (Fredrickson, 2001). Sharing humorous experiences or stories encourages people to spend more time in social connection (Buckman, 1994; Driscoll, 1987).

Parents who were disturbed by their son's latest habit of ripping books out of frustration brought him to see Bill. After connecting with the family, Bill turned to the son and said with a twinkle, "Do you rip up telephone books? You need to be careful. I just tore my rotator cuff by gripping weights too tightly. If you grip too tightly, you may give yourself tendonitis." This intervention shifted a tense and fearful atmosphere to one of curiosity and play while still suggesting that the behavior had negative consequences. However, it was said in such a kind and funny way that it was clear there was no judgment, and the young man opened to therapy. On another occasion, after listening to a client recount the harrowing details of a weekend with her teenage sons, Carol smiled and said, "Well, I guess it comes down to this: How much life can you stand?" Suddenly the client broke into laughter and wryly commented, "How much indeed? I'm already having as much fun as I can stand."

Shifting Focus of Attention

One's focus of attention can either narrow—for example, in anxiety— or broaden to facilitate a shift from the problematic stimulus. Fehmi and Robbins (2008) suggested that high arousal states can result in a narrowed and inflexible style of attending that can lead to mental and physical distress. An example would be an individual who is attuned to a partner's negative behaviors and constantly holds them as a mental list, ready for immediate critical review.

When it accompanies anxiety, tunnel vision (extreme foveal vision) can provoke an extreme sympathetic response. If that state remains un-relieved for a sufficiently long time, the person may begin to feel helpless and hopeless—and that can trigger an extreme parasympathetic re-sponse. In the therapeutic setting, it may be important to assist the cli-ent in bridging from a highly parasympathetic response to a more balanced one by having the person get in touch with his or her anger over the matter in question. The anger in this case need not be seen as rage but simply as energy. If the therapist not only validates the client's hopelessness but also, given the situation, the legitimacy of his or her anger and frustration, the client may feel safe enough to consciously per-ceive the underlying anger. From there, the client can be assisted in us-ing the liberated energy to shift into a problem-solving mode. With that shift, the client's vision will broaden to include elements in his or her peripheral vision, and his or her state will become calmer. As a means of reinforcing this broader vision, we then suggest that the person notice what specifically is in his or her peripheral vision and describe it.

Engaging Motivation

Prochaska and DiClemente (1982) developed a model of motivational change that was accepted as a therapeutic standard for many years. They conceived of the process of change as proceeding in several stages: precontemplation (not having given thought to any change), contempla-tion (ambivalent about a possible change), preparation (experimenting with a change), action (practicing a new behavior for at least 3 months), maintenance (the new behavior becomes habitual and is continued be-yond 6 months), and possible relapse. About the same time, Miller (1983) developed an approach of motivational interviewing wherein cli-ents were persuaded to resolve ambivalence about changing behaviors using cognitive strategies. Taken together, the work of Prochaska and DiClemente and Miller provided an excellent framework for structuring the therapeutic alteration of dysfunctional behavioral patterns.

Recent neuroscience discoveries have suggested that motivation can be increased by specifically engaging certain neural circuits (Panksepp, 1998). When we can activate the SEEKING/CURIOSITY circuit for any problem, clients are more open to treatment. Curiosity leads to motiva-tion and is reinforced when it is followed by success. Furthermore, see-ing success in one area can give a client "leverage" with which to attempt other therapeutic goals. For example, one client who'd had severe neck pain had a surprising experience of pain reduction when she went into deep hypnosis. After this gratifying success, she became highly curious about what else she could accomplish and began a food management program that she had put off for years for fear of failure. A state of anger can be swiftly shifted into motivation, and the SEEKING circuit turned on, if the therapist asks an open-ended, judgment-free question that poses a plausible but radically different interpretation of an event. An example would be a parent complaining furiously about a teenage daughter who "doesn't hear" or "forgets" things said to her. *"Would you consider conducting an experiment?* It's possible that Sally is literally so focused on her own thoughts that she doesn't mentally process your words. When you need her to hear you, would you be willing to stand directly in front of her *and make eye contact* before you speak in a quiet conversational tone? Why don't you try that experiment at home and then keep track: How many times does she hear—or not hear—the things you say to her when you do it that way?"

Implement Therapeutic Strategies

An individual intervention may be thought of as a building block. To help move the client from a problematic state of consciousness to an integrated, desired state and ultimately to experience more time in a state of thriving, interventions can be built into effective strategies. Such strategies—structured groupings or sequences of interventions—should be focused on activating the client's resources rather than on the client's problem. Research has shown that a focus on resource activation is a common characteristic of the most successful therapists (Gallmann & Grawe, 2006).

In addition to correcting the neural foundations of dysfunction, an important therapeutic focus will be to help shape the client's life experiences such that the person's life is more congruent with his or her goals. Grawe noted, "Greater positive changes will be attained when one concentrates on the positive goals of the patient than when one focuses predominantly on fears and anxieties" (2007, p. 327). This does not mean that we should avoid talking about what is painful, but rather, that it should not be the emphasis in therapy. Here we describe state progression, neural talk, and resource activation as examples of BCT strategies.

State Progression

The purpose of the therapeutic interaction is to help clients learn to move from dysfunctional—or unresourceful—states to resourceful ones. In some cases, this will require a process of *state progression*: the gradual transition from an unresourceful state to a less unresourceful state to a neutral state to a mildly resourceful state and finally to a more effectively resourceful state. When a person achieves an optimal state and level of arousal for a task, he or she unlocks the possibility for healthy emotions, attitudes, and behaviors in relation to that task.

The first step is to identify the unresourceful state the person experiences (Hall, 2009). In discussion with the client, the second step is to identify a desired or target state conducive to achieving the client's therapeutic goals. The third step is to depotentiate the dysfunctional pattern and, in stages, activate state change toward the target state. As the level of arousal is increased or decreased while moving toward a balanced state, one or more state shifts will occur. If the presenting dysfunctional state is one of overarousal, it will be necessary to facilitate movement into a more relaxed and calm state of mind where a potential reorganization of perspective can more easily occur. If the brain is underaroused, as in depression, a therapeutic process that activates the person is a better approach. Activating anger or action of some sort can help the client change states.

State progression can be used as a strategy either within the confines of the therapeutic hour or as a series of exercises/assignments that the client does between sessions. Within the clinical setting, the therapist participates with the client in shifting states through changes in voice tone, timing, gaze, and focus of attention to begin to move toward more positive states. With this gradual shift the client loosens the rigidity of a previously held mindset, softens the energy directed toward the therapist, and begins to open to a new perspective and set of emotional experiences. Within the therapeutic encounter, the target state is an "access state" (Goleman, 1988) in which the client is more receptive to what the therapist has to offer. As "homework assignments," state progression can slowly dismantle a dysfunctional emotional response and its entrenched neural pattern.

The Case of the Sticky Mouth

We use our work with Melissa and her husband as an example of state progression accomplished through a series of homework assignments. Melissa came in with the complaint that her husband Brad made the worst sounds with his mouth when he was having sinus problems. Her very description caused her to curl up on the couch as she remembered how the sound made her feel. The state she entered was obviously uncomfortable (disgust is never pleasant) and intense. We asked her to bring her husband in and when she did, she pointed out the terrible, disgusting sound he made. We made every attempt to hear this sound, but our ears lacked Melissa's attunement.

Learning more about her history, we discovered that her mother used to scream in her face. As a young girl, Melissa had learned to use extreme tunnel vision to focus only on her mother's mouth so she could survive the ordeal. In doing so, she developed a sensitivity to sound that caused her to be overly sensitive to her husband's "sticky mouth."

We talked with her about this trauma and how painful it must have been to be screamed at so often by such a central figure in her early life. As she told her story, we noticed that she began to focus on our mouths and our mouths became a little dry. It can be easy to share the client's negative trance state and pick up a "mental virus."

As a way to help her begin to shift her negative state and "spread the symptom" (Kershaw, 1992) away from her husband, we suggested that she view certain newscasters to determine if any of them made this horrible noise (engaging her seeking circuit through curiosity). She discovered several who had "sticky mouth syndrome." We then suggested that she might notice if the newscasters did anything else that was annoying—for example, wiggle ears, raise eyebrows, or make other odd movements.

When she accomplished this task, we suggested that she begin to notice other movements with hands, feet, eyes, etc. Melissa reported that she had discovered other interesting and quirky movements that people make habitually; in fact, she was beginning to have fun with the assignments (engaging the play circuit). We asked her to continue to "spread the symptom"; as she paid more attention to total body language, the less she was emotionally assaulted by incidences of "sticky mouth." Finally she began to gain some control over her irritation.

Later in the therapy, Melissa finally acknowledged how upset she was with her husband. She felt that Brad was not helping her with their new-born son, but could not bring herself to complain about it directly. Instead, she hyperfocused on his mouth. We encouraged her to share this insight with her husband in a marital session and suggested that she had practiced the state-specific ability to hear sound so well that the next time she was disturbed by her husband's mouth noises, she should notice whether she was keeping her "voice" to herself when she needed to talk to him. Ultimately, this reframed symptom became a resource: It became a warning sign that she needed to share her feelings. In the process, she had rewired longstanding neurological circuits, calmed her hyperresponsive amygdala, and turned on circuits of curiosity, play, and self-nurture. As LeDoux (2002) wrote: "Psychotherapy is fundamentally a learning process for its patients, and as such is a way to rewire the brain. In this sense, psychotherapy ultimately uses biological mechanisms to treat mental illness" (p. 299).

Neural Talk

Neural talk is a strategy that makes intentional use of words, metaphors, phrasing, and tone of voice to access appropriate brain circuits for change and to inhibit neural connections that lead to dysfunction. Acting as a bridge from one state to another, neural talk may shift a client's state only in a small way, but so effectively that the person cannot continue to feel and behave in the same way. Neural talk uses empathy to come into an emotional alignment with the client and then, carrying the client along, it takes off in a new direction. We use this method to move people from states of stress, anxiety, depression, or other problem states to states of calm, cheerfulness, and affiliation (Porges, 2007). For example, with a client struggling with insomnia, we might say, "This situation has really been difficult for you, and while you feel terrible, and would certainly like to feel better, you managed this fatigue and have been doing amazingly well these last few weeks." Neural talk is often used to shift the client's attention from problems to resources.

The following case shows the use of neural talk in an initial therapeutic session. Because Carol had been given substantial background information from the referring physician, she did not begin with a formal client assessment but opened the conversation to establish rapport. Evelyn, age 86, was referred for therapy for help with anxiety about using her CPAP (continuous positive airway pressure) machine. She needed to learn how to accommodate this method of respiratory ventilation to ameliorate the oxygen deprivation caused by her sleep apnea.

Of an independent nature and embarrassed that she needed help, Evelyn had been resistant to seeing a psychologist and was initially quite ill at ease. As Carol began working with her, she complimented Evelyn's independence and told her that this was a wonderful resource that had helped her throughout her life (empathic pacing). The client began to relax visibly and nod her head in agreement. Carol told her she had many abilities and might even discover some things she could do that she hadn't known previously (moving the conversation in a new direction). Then Carol explained that practically everyone has trouble getting used to sleeping with a breathing machine but that, as with any other learned skill, the brain can adapt with practice. Carol noted as Evelyn's breathing slowed and she became more attentive and curious. Carol alluded to the client's independence again (maintain pacing). At that point, feeling secure enough to be more open, Evelyn admitted that she at times felt frightened when alone, especially at night. Carol suspected that, to some extent, Evelyn's general nighttime anxiety had become focused on using the CPAP machine. She suggested that Evelyn allow her "deep mind" to give her an image or symbol of something in her house that made her feel safe and secure. The client began to smile; she had a collection of crosses on the wall. Carol nodded and suggested that there is an energy that radiates from sacred symbols, that if you are quiet, you can almost feel it (reinforce new state of security). Carol suggested that that energy can fill an entire space so that when Evelyn looked at her collection, she could feel safe and secure. The client began to look even more comfortable (further reinforcement). By the end of the session, when Carol asked her to come back and said that together they would work on Evelyn's unease with the CPAP equipment, Evelyn's anxiety regarding being in a psychologist's office was reduced significantly, and she was amazed at what she had already accomplished.

Resource Activation

We want to identify how and in what context a client has experienced past success and, when appropriate, we want to refer to the success. Those areas in which the client is already motivated can clue us in on the client's intrinsic sources of motivation and strengths to make change (Grawe, 2007, p. 328). To notice where clients have acted in courageous and confident ways is to suggest that the resource is available to them in other contexts. For example, Bill asked the boy who ripped up books to tell him how he felt when he played tennis. The young man shifted states and described feeling calm and powerful. Bill suggested this was a solution state he could access more frequently at school. The young man was intrigued by the comment, and that curiosity led him to explore other empowering states.

We had one client who identified himself as a "loser" but who happened to mention early on that he'd had a successful experience of skydiving. He had disregarded this example of courage, risk taking, and confidence that he could accomplish the goal. As he began to appreciate these aspects in himself, he became increasingly less apt to think of himself in such a negative manner.

The clinician can also facilitate change and access highly resourceful states by altering the cognitive or perceptual frame that a client places around a particular problem. Questions such as "What are the possibilities we have not thought of?" or "What else could work in this situation?" or "What can you learn from this situation?" are better questions than asking "What is wrong?" Open-ended frames lead a client toward generative states and support growth and healing. For example, when a husband complains that his wife is uncooperative in a particular situation, we might respond: "Is she doing this on purpose or might there be some other motivation behind her behavior? What might her reasons be? When she behaves that way, how do you feel? What is stirred up in you? Is there anything you do in response that escalates the situation?" When we ask such questions in a warm and inquiring way, we engage the client's curiosity (the emotional circuit of seeking) rather than defensiveness. What then goes on at the client's unconscious level is quite a different conversation and may lead to a reconnection with the partner.

Therapeutic Metaphor

We are always reworking the past by the way we remember it. Life experiences affect memory, and the more we understand life's difficulties, the more we are inclined to view the past (both our own and that of others) compassionately. As clinicians, we hear stories of heartbreak and despair, madness and destruction, accomplishment and love. Sometimes the narratives people share are painful childhood memories; sometimes they are explanations of current pain; at times they are frozen narratives that provide no clear way out of a dilemma. Joan Didion (1979) remarked: "We tell ourselves stories in order to live. . . . We live entirely . . . by the 'ideas' by which we have learned to freeze the shifting phantasmagoria which is our actual experience" (p. 11). Clients' stories often reflect narrow and rigidly maintained beliefs that fail to account for much of the complexity of life and that keep them on a barren path, with certain emotional circuits and states chronically turned on. At other times, the stories express resiliency and abilities that even the narrators themselves fail to recognize.

We suggest to clients that giving a mental state a metaphorical name can be useful in managing the responses of their autonomic nervous system. Mental imagery can rewire the brain and have a therapeutic effect (MacIver, Lloyd, Kelly, & Nurmikko, 2008; Ganisa, 2004). One of our patients called his state of upset "trigger happy"; another person used the phrase "red-lined" (as when a car engine is so wound that the tachometer is in the red section) when she was overwhelmed to the point of "seizing up" and being unable to function. Both of these metaphorical descriptions helped the person to observe a brain state and subsequently to shift the emotional circuit to one of increased calm and self-nurturance.

To use metaphor in the session, the clinician merely needs to review his or her own learning during some adventure, trip, conversation, or experience. The object is to assist the client in focusing on positive possibilities that open a life, rather than on negative frames that close potential portals. Sharing a brief vignette with the client can shift the neural circuit and the frame the individual has been using to order his or her life. Carol tells the following favorite anecdote:

"A few years ago when I was in New York on business, I took the time to stroll through Central Park. It was a pleasant day with a slight breeze, and the park was full of interesting sights. I saw one man who had trained his cat to balance on his shoulder while he took a walk. Winding around the paths, I came upon the merry-go-round. The calliope was playing and the children's voices sounded so excited as they stood in line for a ride. Then I saw the sign: TWENTY-FIVE CENTS FOR A RIDE.

"Twenty-five cents—that's all it takes for the ride of a lifetime when you are a little child. Just twenty-five cents, a quarter of a dollar, just a little change to experience a new adventure. So when you go on your trip, perhaps you will discover something wonderful that will offer you an interesting perspective, or you could just have a great time."

The story suggests that "a little change" is all it takes to begin having more fun. A person may make only a slight state shift, and yet this can open up new vistas, new options, and new potential solutions to old problems. The suggestions, embedded within the story, speak to the unconscious mind. A metaphor does not need to be elaborate. Something simple can be very effective. The skeleton of Carol's anecdote above is: I took a walk; I saw something; it made me reflect.

To create a metaphor, the therapist starts at the end (the point to be conveyed) and works backward to the beginning. Holding the point of the metaphor in mind, think of something that exemplifies the point. It may be an event, a single fact, or just an object. For example, we had a Scottish client who grew up drinking tea. With her, we used the process of letting tea leaves steep in a teapot as a metaphor for the idea that once something has been set in motion (e.g., the client has begun therapy), there will be a good outcome—if the client is patient and allows the process to unfold. Create the minimum number of characters needed to interact in the event. An implied "you," the client, may be the only character. For example, the therapist might introduce the tea metaphor by saying, "When you make tea. . . ." If the metaphor is centered on an event, place the event in an appropriate locale. At the end of the metaphor, create a sense of closure: "And when the tea is ready, you pour it into your favorite cup, add two sugars, and sit down to relax with a lovely hot cup of tea." To make the story more engaging, use details that appeal to as many of the five senses as possible; elements of smell and touch are particularly effective. The crucial element is the therapeutic message; it will suggest all the rest of the metaphor. After telling the metaphoric anecdote, it is important to allude to the point. The allusion should be overt enough that the client understands it unconsciously, as evidenced by ideomotor indications (e.g., a slight change in facial expression or posture), and yet subtle enough that it does not ruffle the conscious mind and possibly create resistance. Figure 4.1 summarizes the process of constructing a simple metaphor.

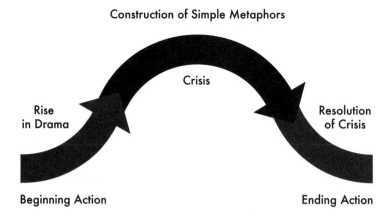

Construction of Simple Metaphors

Crisis

Rise
in Drama

Resolution
of Crisis

Beginning Action   Ending Action

Figure 4.1. Construction of Simple Metaphors

mind and possibly create resistance. Figure 4.1 summarizes the process of constructing a simple metaphor.

Therapeutic metaphors can also be used to activate potential resources by tapping into the unconscious and retrieving memories of past learning, as well as to teach skills a person needs. In listening to a story, a client will make certain associations and may be able to grasp a different perspective. Personal shifts in feeling and attitude can happen. By helping to contain a client's feelings about an experience, metaphoric stories can have a healing power.

Chapter 7 contains a section on how to create lengthier, more involved therapeutic metaphors, which may be used in the context of deep hypnosis. We find that, over time, each therapist develops a unique repertoire of stories that fits the therapist's personal style of working with clients and is consistently useful in similarly recurring therapeutic situations.

The following is another story that we have repeatedly found meaningful to clients who need to overcome some adversity or who may have been kept from realizing their own potential through a kind of negative hypnosis. Our hope is that the story will encourage the client to access his or her deeper self to problem-solve, build confidence, and create opportunities. The story also is an example of how seemingly negative emotional states (e.g., feeling like the family black sheep) can provide the impetus to accomplish personal goals (e.g., becoming an artist and finding a place where one does fit). As we explain to our clients, "If you

"Several years ago, when we were in San Antonio for a conference, we spent an afternoon walking along the river and browsing through a variety of shops. One gallery featuring wood sculpture especially caught our attention. Its shelves held all kinds of animals from mythical to real. Each of the hand-carved animals had exceptionally long legs, and the underside of one foot was stamped with the image of a black sheep. We asked the gallery owner about these creatures.

"He told us the artist was a young woman who grew up in a poor family and, although she yearned to attend art school, her parents told her that her dream was completely impractical. They were worried about having enough money for the family and knew art was a difficult way to make a living. The young woman kept her dream to herself and read as much as she could on her own. Because her siblings teased her and discounted her dream whenever they saw her reading an art book, she felt ostracized from her family and retreated further. When she was old enough to move out on her own, she worked and put herself through art school. She began to carve these beautiful animals and eventually became a successful artist. She gives all her animals long legs to symbolize the ability to rise above difficulty, and she stamps a black sheep on one foot of each. In her family, she said she felt like the 'black sheep' and wanted to remember the challenges she needed to overcome to be successful."

We can also help clients see that their own life experiences can be understood as metaphors. Rose Marie was a musician who entered therapy for neurofeedback training to stimulate brain functioning after having brain surgery in the frontal lobe area to remove a benign but invasive growth. Although her cognitive processing was quite slow afterward, she still maintained the ability to play the violin. We asked her to bring her violin and play something for us. She tenderly removed the instrument from the case, tuned it, and began a lovely interpretation of Ave Maria. Tears came to our eyes and, with them, hope for continued improvement.

When she finished playing, Rose Marie told us a story that was, to us, a living metaphor of future possibility. While in the north of France and shopping in a small village antique shop, a friend called her over to see a dusty, old, unstrung violin tucked among other things in a back corner of the shop. The shopkeeper said that she had kept the violin a long time, but that what she did in life was bring the past into the present, so she would sell it for the equivalent of $20. Our client picked it up, looked it over, and saw a dark indentation of inlaid wood around the edge. In turning the instrument over, she saw written at the very top a violin maker's name. From that, she guessed the instrument was over 100 years old and might be quite valuable. She bought it, brought it home, and had it refurbished and restrung. The violin had a richness of tone that only a handmade instrument crafted by an artist can produce. In fact, the violin was worth thousands of dollars. Touched to be a part of her recovery journey, we said to her, "Perhaps you don't realize just how alike you and this beautiful instrument are." Eventually, Rose Marie regained much, though not all, of her functioning and went on to play more expertly and artistically than before her surgery.

Teach the Client to Self-Initiate State Change

Ultimately, the client needs to take personal responsibility for the process of self-regulation. Dysfunctional emotional states and their concomitant neural patterns tend to fall into two broad categories: Either they are responses to immediate, external events (e.g., a partner's behavior) that trigger well-worn neural circuits, or they are responses to immediate internal events—the brain's activation of neural circuits, which are then often consciously rationalized by internally generated scenarios (e.g., a state of anxiety or depression can always be justified on some basis). The state may actually have been triggered by a fleeting thought, which may not even be remembered a few seconds later; it may have been triggered by an unconscious resonance with someone else in that state (transference); or it may simply be one of a person's default states of neural patterning.

Here we discuss three approaches to state change that clients can learn to self-initiate: understanding the process of the mind, deconstructing emotional reactivity, and using mind shifting.

The Process of the Mind

Before a client can learn to shift states, often the person must learn to perceive the process through which he or she stepped into the negative state. In explaining the process of the mind to a client, we describe a common progression of thoughts that leads from registering a physical sensation or experiencing an event to an internally held, and frequently negative, state. The following is a example of what we might say as we teach clients to become consciously aware of this process in their daily lives:

"The human mind is constantly chattering; over the course of each day, it entertains thousands of thoughts. Frequently, a person will notice a physical sensation, such as pain or warmth, and then label it—that is, give it words such as 'warmth on the back of my neck.' This is almost immediately followed by a judgment as to whether that warmth is good or bad. The judgment commonly leads to an internal response: turning on one of the emotional circuits or states [as identified by Panksepp, 2003].

"The state is followed by developing a story about the feeling. 'It feels good to get out and get some sunshine. What a great afternoon for a hike with the kids [play].' Or: 'I forgot to bring sunscreen [irritation]; I'm worried about the kids getting sunburned [anxiety].' Double-binds are frequently part of the judgment, the state, and the story: 'I want to be a good parent and spend more time with my sons, but I wish I hadn't promised to take them on a hike this afternoon because I need to be working on a presentation that I'm scheduled to give next week.' With the story in place, often the ability to shift states, particularly to shift from a negative state to a positive one, becomes difficult.

"Any negative experience, whether it is an occurrence of physical pain or an emotionally painful situation, has many elements. There is the sensation of pain, memories of past painful experiences, certain associations to the pain, and future projections on what might occur [Salmon & Maslow, 2007]. However, being attentive to what occurs *without any judgment* begins to initiate a change. When all of these elements are simply observed, the mind becomes calmer and the sense of discomfort lessens. Also, in the process of observing, it is possible to notice thoughts and emotions without acting on them. And you may catch sight of reactive patterns that would otherwise be well underway. Over time, the simple act of observation helps you develop a non-reactive mind and stay focused in the present rather than the past or the future. The worries we carry or conversations we replay are the mind's way of recalling a past or rehearsing for a future, but in fact they only serve to maintain internal states of stress.

"The process of the mind can be interrupted at any point by becoming curious about a sensation, exploring the feeling for its texture, color, or trigger, rather than analyzing it. Another way to interrupt the process of the mind is simply to drop the judgment and the story. Becoming aware of the mind patterns that were probably learned in your family of origin creates an opportunity to understand something that may have been hidden from your awareness for most of a lifetime.

"The mind senses the world in habitual ways, and its patterns can easily develop into rigidities. Too often, these patterns become lenses through which we view our experiences. The patterns cause us to make assumptions about 'how things are' that may be incorrect. For example, to try to make sense of events, we tend to make a story about all that transpired. Storytelling is particularly likely when we try to understand someone else's behavior. But our stories are not always accurate. However, if we can hold our interpretations lightly and know that things may be more complex than we had presumed, we may be able to have an interaction or resolve a conflict in a way that we feel good about. If we calm the mind chatter, put aside our habitual or learned interpretations, and give up believing the sole 'truth,' we are more likely to be able to resolve conflicts and solve problems. Clutching tightly to a particular meaning puts us in negative states. Being aware of the process of the mind allows you to interrupt the negative state and replace it with a more functional and flexible one."

Deconstructing Emotional Reactivity

When an emotional trigger is external, typically a person is aware of the immediate triggering event, the emotional reaction, and the consequent behavior, but will not know how to alter the pattern. To begin to change it, the client must learn to recognize and name the reactivated state into which he or she has fallen. The process of identifying a state when it occurs and naming it gives it a visibility that it may not have had previously. The next step is to be able to refrain from responding with a habitual behavior even when flooded with the emotional state. Eventually the individual needs to learn to "step aside" internally and detach from the emotion. Without reacting to the feeling, he or she needs to shift into a stance of curiosity and attempt to understand it.

One method for deconstructing an emotional reaction is to have the client observe the feeling state as though from a position outside the self and identify which life pattern has been activated. The client may even be able to identify an early triggering event that shaped the life pattern. Next we ask the client to observe and evaluate his or her usual reactive response from this external perspective. Another way to frame the notion of detachment is to ask the client to imagine being a cultural anthropologist gathering data about members of a newly discovered indigenous society. Observing from a distance calms a reactive response. In either case, the client activates a seeking state characterized by a distanced curiosity; the key is being "warmly aloof" in order to remain centered. For example, with a client who has conflicted relationships with family members, we may suggest the following: "Go and visit your family. When you are there, I want you to take mental field notes just as an anthropologist might do. If, during the visit, you find that you have become caught up in the family drama, just internally step back and silently return to talking mental notes." The process creates a detachment that tends to lessen potential reactivity to comments that family members may make.

This process is also particularly important for therapists who may feel an internal negative charge when working with certain clients. For example, some clients adopt a dismissive style of interacting with the therapist. This subtle aggression and mixed message ("I want you to help me, but I don't want the help you are offering") can be frustrating and hurtful. To avoid becoming entangled by the client's style of interaction, the clinician can mentally move his or her personal boundary closer and stay focused on his or her curiosity as to what led the client to adopt this way of interacting with people.

Applying Mind Shifting

When the trigger for a dysfunctional state is internal, we suggest that clients learn to shift states quickly by identifying the present state and its content and the desired state and its object of focus. They can practice "mind shifting" by changing breathing rate, body posture, and/or object of attention, or remembering a time when they experienced the preferred state. Since overfocusing on a sensation or problem can lead to tunnel vision, they may also find it helpful to expand their field of vision. They can use the term *mind shift* as a cue to themselves to practice changing states more quickly. In addition, clients may use music, thoughts of a beautiful place, or a relaxed activity such as sipping tea or lying in a hammock to change to peaceful states. In this case, it is the act of altering the mental focus that shifts the brain state.

One client was a successful portrait painter, but she greatly feared throwing up in public and would often overfocus on the sensation of anxiety in her stomach to the point that she did throw up. We explored her original family system, in which violent eruptions occurred frequently. She had developed a hypersensitive stomach in response to stress and carried this symptom into adulthood. By having her become aware of what was on either side of her ("Focus on what is directly on your left and name the exact color of the closest left object. If you wanted to mix that shade in oils, what paints would you use? Focus on what is on your right and name the exact color of the closest right object. If you wanted to mix that shade in oils, what paints would you use?") and breathe more deeply, she developed the ability to control her stress symptoms and keep her state managed.

The following case exemplifies the process of assisting a client to identify preexisting self-regulation skills and inner resources in order to self-initiate state change.

Case Example: Fear of Flying Becomes a Laughing Matter

This therapeutic process involved retrieving the memories, sensations, and emotions of childhood play and turning them into resources. Elaine could board airplanes but, when her husband was with her, she would dig her fingernails into his arm so firmly that, on occasion, she had even drawn blood as the plane was taking off or when it encountered turbulence. If he was not flying with her, she would grab the arm rest and experience a panic attack. She was an interior designer and began therapy because she knew that she needed to make a multilegged trip from the United States to Singapore and then to Hong Kong and back.

Bill had Elaine focus her attention and go into a trance with an accompanying arm levitation. He reassured her she would adapt to the feeling of having her hand float in the air. Bill then had her revisit memories of bouncing up and down as a child. These included memories of bouncing on her father's knee and jumping up and down on the bed, a sofa, a hobby horse, and a trampoline. Bill did this by telling stories about Tiffany, our daughter; as he talked he would switch the pronouns from the third to the second person. For example: "Tiffany knew that when you jump up and down on your bed, not only is it fun, but you are doing something mischievous." Bill would watch for ideo-motor signaling, such as rapid eye movement or a slight smile on her face. Then Bill asked her to memorize the good feelings.

Continuing to tell stories, ostensibly about Tiffany, Bill next asked Elaine to remember riding a bicycle down a hill, over a bumpy road. Bill did this in order to identify the sensation as if she were watching a movie, without alerting her consciously that the process was intended to ad-dress her issue. Bill had her experience an arousal of adrenaline by tell-ing stories of Tiffany and him going through a haunted house and of children playing telephone games, like calling people up and asking them silly questions such as, "Is your refrigerator running? You should go and catch it." In telling the stories, he mentioned the physiological symptoms of increased adrenaline, such as a racing heart, fast breathing, and sweaty palms—followed by simple childhood laughter.

At each step, Bill asked Elaine to memorize the sensations and corre-sponding emotions, and told her she would use these later in a directed fashion. This process was repeated a few times. All of these suggestions were designed to stimulate the play circuit (curiosity) and to connect fear and play so that if she became frightened, it could be exciting and fun rather than anxiety-inducing. Bill also suggested that while her con-scious mind did not know what he was saying, her unconscious under-stood quite well.

Between some of the stories, Bill brought her partially out of trance to look at her hand. He asked her how it felt to see it floating. She was amused by it. At the end of each session, Bill would suggest that her hand could come down and "land safely." After four or five sessions, Elaine asked if she could just imagine her hand floating up on the plane. Bill understood, although Elaine may not have, that her unconscious was prompting her to create a way to reconnect with Bill and remember the playful safety of the trance experiences while in the stressful situation. Bill nodded, "Yes."

After Bill was certain that she could experience these emotions, he had her relive these early experiences more quickly (jumping up and down and riding a bicycle down a hill). Bill was preparing her to make the connection between these experiences and similar sensations en-countered in flying. He would say, "Your unconscious mind knows where you are going to experience these sensations and emotions." She looked confused (turning on curiosity), and Bill would say, "You are going to feel these sensations, and it is alright to feel them on an airplane. You are certainly entitled to have a good time and laugh. Every time the airplane bounces, you can remember bouncing on your daddy's knee and all the other wonderful times from childhood." Bill had her feel an adrenaline rush by remembering the haunted house or the telephone pranks and connected this to the adrenaline rush she would feel when the plane would drop suddenly.

There is a fine line between experiencing a surge of adrenaline as fear and experiencing it as excitement. In their later sessions, Bill reduced the negative connotations of fear by directly pairing it with excitement. He suggested that both stem from encounters with novelty and surprise—and that both are cures for boredom.

When Elaine returned for a session after the trip, Bill learned that three significant things had taken place. First, she had flown from Houston to Los Angeles and Singapore without trouble. As she was leaving Singapore, an airplane crash was on all television monitors, but she had experienced little fear. And finally, as the plane was descending into Hong Kong, there was substantial air turbulence, because the mountain ranges create uneven heating of the atmosphere. During the landing, a number of people were shouting and upset, but Elaine burst out laughing. People around her wondered what she'd had to drink, but she had drunk no alcohol. One passenger even said, "I want what she had."

She learned to pair the experience of bumpiness or a sudden drop in altitude with the fun of those sensations in an earlier context. In doing so, Elaine shifted the "meaning" of adrenaline rushes from fear to excitement and bridged the excitement of childhood events to the experience of commercial flight.

Encourage a Belief in the "Impossible"

We suggest to clients that we have all been told that our dreams are impossible—and too often we have accepted that dictate as true. Almost everyone has dreams of something that he or she secretly wishes to accomplish but has been told is impossible. Instead of believing in the impossible, we learn to imagine that the possible is much smaller than it really is. When Alice in Wonderland said she did not believe in impossible things, the Queen of Hearts replied, "I dare say you haven't had much practice. When I was your age, I always did it for half an hour a day. Why, sometimes, I've believed in as many as six impossible things before breakfast" (Carroll, 1872, pp. 220–221).

As a homework assignment, we encourage the client: "Write down six 'impossible' but desired life achievements. Then set these impossible goals aside for a while. The power of the unconscious mind is tremendous; it will work on solutions to accomplish goals while the conscious mind is thinking about other matters."

Conditioning and Reinforcing Brain Change

Changes in brain state, like changes in behavior, are not usually a one-shot accomplishment. Only with time do the changes become familiar and feel "natural." When a client has successfully achieved a target state, we have the person practice the new state in the office by reviewing it repetitively or by moving slowly into it and enjoying the feeling of the target state. As the therapeutic interaction progresses, target states shift from being states that the therapist has identified as resourceful to being goals that the client has identified. When the client becomes more capable of entering into and sustaining the target state outside the therapeutic container, we suggest that the client very consciously begin to take note of when he or she achieves the target state. This effort effectively reinforces and conditions it. Each time the client experiences the new state and reports it to us, we congratulate him or her for experiencing the desired target state.

In the process of conditioning and reinforcing new states, it is important for therapists to do two things: (1) Wait for an opening created by the client, when he or she asks the therapist for assistance, and (2) model appropriate states for the client. Much of what we do will be processed at an unconscious level by the client—for example, modeling an ability to laugh at life's paradoxical situations. The therapist also needs to use humor at appropriate times to keep pleasant states going and link them to him- or herself. When the therapist is confident, respectful, and uses him- or herself as the target of humor, it teaches the client not to take him- or herself so seriously. The new state of calmness and humor is linked to the resolution of underlying issues, and the client begins to develop new alternatives (plans) to move toward the future he or she most wants.

In her first session, Trish said that she no longer loved her husband. She explained that following back surgery, George had been out of work for the last year; he still suffered from chronic pain and was depressed. Bill worked with each of them separately, first validating Trish's emotional state and her stress over having her husband at home 24 hours a day, 7 days a week. She felt that running the house was up to her and resented the fact that because George was now at home all the time, he frequently wanted to have a say in how things should be done. By going through her e-mails, George had also discovered that she was having an affair with a boyfriend from her college days who lived in a different city. George was extremely angry, and Bill's work with him included providing initial emotional support. George defined the problem as one of uncertainty over whether the marriage would last.

As Bill worked with Trish, he continued to validate her stress but called into question the reality of her love for her college flame and his love for her. Whether the love affair was a fantasy and a break from the stress of her marriage was a question Trish needed to consider. As it turned out, she discovered from her boyfriend that he did not want to leave his wife or children and that he had done the same thing with other women. She realized that her husband was not so bad and decided to stay.

Bill's work with George shifted from validating his anger to helping him overcome that anger and drop his obsessive tracking of his wife's every electronic move. George began to realize that he did not want to spend the rest of his life being angry with his wife. Bill suggested that that this problem could be solved and that there were approaches that could help him resolve his anger. Bill suggested that he read Thich Nhat Hanh's *Miracle of Mindfulness*, as well as *The Joy of Living*, by Yongey Mingyur Rinpoche. Through these books, George learned the basics of meditation.

Trish soon dropped out of therapy, but George continued and, through his meditation practice, became able to change his state of mind more easily. He learned more about how to live in the moment and how to allow his thoughts to pass through his mind without fighting with them. This was the target state George had yearned to discover. As Bill reflected in an approving way that George was making progress, he was helping George condition and maintain the target state of calmness for increasingly longer periods of time.

With the marital situation much improved, Bill turned his attention to the background issue and suggested to George that this period of unemployment might be an opportunity to pursue some skills retraining, make a career shift, and do what he had always wanted to do professionally. In suggesting this, Bill was fostering George's activation of curiosity and his play circuits. When Bill acted in a nurturing way, he was not only modeling the nurture circuit but encouraging George to turn it on. Bill was also supporting George to take action (investigate job retraining programs and local community college credentialing programs) and linking those actions to his social context.

Support the Client in Taking Action and Follow Up

It is not generally enough for a client to learn to adopt more resourceful states. Frequently, the client also needs to utilize those inner resources to make some changes in his or her situation. However, often we find that clients are "frozen" or immobilized and have difficulty taking action to make a difference in their lives. To overcome this tendency, we have to help the client discover the motivation to make changes. This may occur in therapeutic assignments or by stimulating motivating anxiety (see Chapter 9).

Bob grew up with a neglectful father who failed to provide adequate warmth and shelter, both literally and emotionally. Bob's father had been so depressed that he spent a lot of money on a stereo system and then sat for years in a house in which the interior walls had been framed but lacked sheetrock and drywall finishing. Construction debris and miscellaneous junk were piled in the front yard, and, as a teenager, Bob had been acutely embarrassed by his home.

Bob had not filed an income tax return for several years because he was overwhelmed by the task. He could build anything and was expert at computer work, but he was terrified of facing the IRS. The task was to help him reframe what or whom he feared and access a feeling of courage. Bill put him in trance and, as a metaphor, told him a brief history of the Buddha's life. In Buddhist mythology, a character named Mara, the personification of evil or the Buddhist version of Satan, shows up several times. When the Buddha was meditating, Mara came at him as a herd of elephants and warriors to frighten him. He then sent his most beautiful daughters to seduce the Buddha. At each encounter, the Buddha said,

"Ah, old friend, I know you" (Bachelor, 2002). Bachelor suggested that Mara is part of the Buddha's own self, and the encounter between the two is played out as a psychodrama. Mara leaves when the Buddha acknowledges his awareness of this part of himself.

Bill told the story to move Bob out of his spiral of shame and panic and to encourage him to accomplish the goal through curiosity and competence. In truth, Bob was afraid not of the IRS, but of his own psychological dynamics, and this led to procrastination. He needed to face his fears and walk through them. Bill helped him differentiate between the capable adult that he currently was and the child who had needed care so long ago. Bill then assigned him the task of downloading the appropriate forms and instructed him that whenever he encountered any fear, he was to say, "Ah, old friend, I recognize you." In using therapeutic metaphor (the story of the Buddha conquering his own weaknesses), Bill helped Bob mobilize his own motivation and adult capabilities to take action.

Link the Action to the Client's Social Context

New states leading to new behaviors need to be attached to and practiced in the client's wider environment. The more a person does something, the more it becomes a habit. For example, we might initially ask the client to perform a low-risk behavior, such as talking to the checkout clerk at the grocery store in order to establish social contact if the issue is overcoming a fear of interaction. We might precede our request with a metaphor or story.

Anna was a person who took everything personally and wound up quarreling with everyone with whom she had contact. After a trance induction, Bill began to recount some of the history of the United States during the 19th century, years filled with episodes of national conflict and resolution. For example, during the War of 1812, the battle of New Orleans and particularly the earlier successful defense of the city of Baltimore (which inspired our national anthem) engendered a wave of nationalistic exuberance over winning a "second war of independence" against Britain. That in turn led to the "Era of Good Feelings," and England became our ally. Less than 50 years later, the "War Between the States" broke out. But eventually the Civil War was over, and resolution took place. Again we became one nation. In another hypnotic session, Bill used as a metaphor all the different local ethnic restaurants and talked about how the world would be poorer if everyone were the same. He suggested that perhaps Anna had forgotten that there is beauty in diversity.

With hypnotic work, one must wait to see how a client responds to the seeds that have been planted. We look for indications that the unconscious mind has understood that, in this case, conflict and resolution are two parts of a process of working things out. The link to Anna's social context was implied, along with the suggestion that she needed to be more open to different opinions (different restaurants). At that point, Bill assessed the degree to which behavioral change was beginning to occur. Had it been necessary, he would have worked further around issues of conflict. From there, the focus of the work moved to encouraging Anna to learn to consider things from the other person's point of view and then to forgive people. Bill tackled these issues both through the use of metaphor and by finding instances in Anna's past where she had forgiven others. We later heard that she had begun connecting with her peers in a more positive way.

This chapter has examined the brain chemistry of stress and its effects on memory, functioning, and well-being. Stress, however, is not inevitable. By learning how to change habitual brain–mind states, a client can reduce stress, access previously unavailable internal resources, and take action to make positive life changes. The chapter then outlined the BCT model both from the perspective of the person entering therapy and from the perspective of the therapist. Following that, each aspect of the BCT model was elaborated.

In the next chapter we explore how Ericksonian hypnosis facilitates state change by utilizing clients' already existing resources and the multiple levels of communication that are possible in trance states.

CHAPTER 5

Brain Change Techniques Using Ericksonian Hypnosis

Language has extraordinary power: Just as "mere" words can precipitate wars, the right words can heal wounds that nothing else can touch. In a keynote address to the 16th International Congress on Hypnosis and Hypnotherapy, Peter Bloom (2004) noted that words can alter brain states and exclaimed, "We now have proof: Words change physiology." Hypnotic suggestion creates changes in brain activation that are similar to actual experiences (Raz & Shapiro, 2002; Raz, Fan, & Posner, 2005). It can also override automatic processes such as implicit memory (a type of memory based on previous unconscious learning), pain perception, and attention processes (Egner & Hirsch, 2005). Additionally, the hypnotic process appears to activate brain areas involved with memory and self-imagery.

This chapter explores the nature and use of hypnosis as part of the BCT model of facilitating long-lasting state changes in clients that result in greater state flexibility and more enjoyment and confidence in daily life endeavors. We provide overviews of the neurophysiology of hypnosis, the basics of Ericksonian hypnosis, trance phenomena and their therapeutic uses, conversational hypnosis, and using hypnosis to access the wisdom of the unconscious mind—all in the context of applying the BCT approach.

All therapists know that, as with infants who have anxious attachments, some clients are harder to soothe. Frequently, the following intervention, used with a soothing tone of voice, can change the patient's state from one of severe emotional pain to a calmer and more open state: "Tell me if I have this right and tell me if I have left anything out. . . ." A summary of the emotional process the client is experiencing then follows. There are times, however, when listening and reflecting what a patient says or offering soothing comments seems to be less than what the client needs. The client still may be unable to shift to a more productive state. It is at this point that hypnosis becomes a particularly valuable tool. With hypnosis, the therapist gains another avenue by which to directly and indirectly teach clients the process of *changing states of consciousness, modulating affects,* and *learning to solve problems*—the three skill domains essential for healthy living.

In this context, BCT is a process wherein clients learn to utilize their own associations; where failure is understood as an occasion for learning; where memories of success become resources; and where imagined possibilities presage actualized future success. The earliest paradigm of the hypnotic process was that change occurred by *implanting* suggestions in the mind. The more recently developed Ericksonian hypnosis focuses on *eliciting* resourceful states and abilities that the client already possesses in other contexts and applying them to the current problem area. For example, one client froze when it came to making sales calls. Upon reminding him of the courage he had demonstrated as a soldier in the Iraq war, he began to remember the state he had mustered to get through the difficult experience and to revivify it.

Through the use of formal hypnosis, a client can experience the empowering ability of changing his or her body sensation—for example, by watching an arm levitate seemingly of its own volition, by sensing numbness in one part of the body, or by raising the temperature in the hands. Any one of these can act to stimulate the curiosity circuit and lead a client to shift into a state of anticipation that life satisfaction might be a possibility. This process demonstrates to clients that not only can they control their own physiology, but, with the guidance of the therapist, there is the possibility of mastering life's circumstances.

Neural change involves the processes of organization, disorganization, and reorganization. Prigogine (1983) suggested that systems are always moving into chaos and reorganizing into new systems. This idea can be applied to hypnosis and to psychotherapy in general. Each person's neural patterns are organized in a particular way that predisposes him or her to a certain outlook on life and to certain emotional–physiological experiences. What becomes troubling to the client are not really external events—although they may be the triggers—but the state the person chronically experiences. Potentially even more troubling, the person's brain may organize information in ways that may make it too painful to accomplish important goals.

As a psychotherapeutic intervention, hypnosis intentionally disrupts or disorganizes patterns of neural activity that underlie problematic states and utilizes prior experiences that have nothing to do with the perceived goal but have similar desired state experiences. Hypnotic reframing, the process of suggesting other perspectives or meanings, can assist in breaking up personal constructs that otherwise maintain problematic states. Chen (2002) suggested that since language is a product of neural activity, when neurological repatterning occurs, the client responds to situations with different verbal and nonverbal responses.

Bill worked with one client who was phobic toward tarantula spiders. Merely thinking about them would make Angie shake, sweat, and cry. She had just landed a contract for some work in Arizona; unfortunately, some species of tarantulas are native to Arizona. These spiders can become quite large, but they do not leap and their preferred defense is to retreat. If that does not work, a tarantula will pull hairs from its abdomen and fling them at an attacker. Only in an extreme case will a tarantula bite—and, for a person, the bite is no more serious than a bee sting. Nonetheless, Angie was terrified of them. However, she liked Superman and happened to be interested in learning to skydive. So Bill hypnotized her and had her remember the Superman movie. He suggested that she visualize flying in the air with Superman. He also had her imagine how small things look from up in the sky (a dissociative review). Bill then had her focus on how much bigger she was than a tarantula. Next he suggested that she imagined Superman flying down and stomping on the spider. Following that, she imagined Superman carrying a woman down who stomped on the tarantula. After that, she envisioned the tarantula morphing into the clay character from *Saturday Night Live* who says "Oh, no, Mr. Bill" while it is being smashed. Finally, Bill had Angie imagine wearing cowboy boots and squashing a tarantula herself. Angie's fear was entirely resolved in two sessions. Of course, no real tarantulas were harmed in the creation of this metaphor, nor did the client feel a need to kill them after this intervention. In a follow-up conversation, Bill learned that at one point while she was in Arizona, Angie had been able to allow one to cross the road in front of her without screaming or running away. What she had needed was to be in touch with her sense of power and her ability to take care of herself, which the metaphor stimulated.

The Neurophysiology of Hypnosis

In a review of the neurobiological research on hypnosis, Gruzelier (2006) suggested a three-stage process of the neurological response in hypnosis: (1) the sensory fixation and concentration evoked by induction activates the thalamic–cortical attentional network, which in turn engages the frontal limbic system; (2) anterior executive functions are suspended and directed by the stimulation of the frontal limbic inhibitory systems via suggestions of tiredness and relaxation; and (3) engagement of the right posterior temporal functions results in passive imagery and dreaming. What this physiology tells us is that specific brain processes and pathways are indeed altered by hypnotic states. In addition, Kosslyn, Thompson, Costantini-Ferrando, Alpert, and Spiegel discovered that hypnotic suggestions create blood flow changes and concluded that "hypnosis is a psychological state with distinct neural correlates and is not just the result of adopting a role" (Kosslyn, Thompson, Costantini-Ferrando, Alpert, & Spiegel, 2000, p. 1297). There are, in fact, neurophysiological correlates of state changes (Crawford, 1998).

Other researchers have added to our understanding of the neuromechanics of hypnosis. Rainville et al. (1999) reported that hypnosis activated the occipital region of the brain as well as the anterior cingulate cortex, the thalamus, and the brainstem. Overall, there was a decrease in cortical arousal and an increase in attention during hypnosis. Maquet et al. (1999) concluded that "hypnosis is a particular cerebral waking state where the subject, seemingly somnolent, experiences a vivid, multimodal, coherent, memory-based mental imagery that invades and fills the subject's consciousness" (p. 332). Crawford and Gruzelier (1992) found that the theta frequency is active during hypnosis and trance phenomena. We notice that when a client enters a state of trance, anxiety often disappears and is replaced by an inner flexibility in which the person can experience a range of emotions differing from the problematic ones associated with a stuck state.

Through neuroimaging techniques, researchers have determined that hypnosis is probably a special state in which normal patterns of communication between separate cognitive systems are disturbed and the normal relationship between conflict monitoring and cognitive control is disrupted. In fact, a study done at the University of Geneva suggests that hypnosis alters neural activity by rerouting some of the connections in the brain (Oakley & Halligan, 2008). In addition, because the brain exhibits activity-dependent plasticity, and the hypnotic experience interfaces with the limbic and neocortical systems (Rossi, 2002), hypnosis can facilitate the turning on and off of gene expression (Lipton, 2005; Rossi, 2003).

Rainville (2002) compared a nonhypnotic condition with a hypnotic condition that produced brain activity involving the brainstem, thalamus, anterior cingulate cortex, right inferior frontal gyrus, and right inferior parietal lobe. The research suggested that these activations were evidence that hypnotic absorption involves executive attentional networks and is central to the hypnotic experience. Further, it pointed in the direction of a "neural signature associated with hypnosis together with increases in mental absorption and reduction in spontaneous conceptual thought commonly reported by hypnotized individuals" (Oakley & Halligan, 2008, p. 265).

Current research on the neuroscience of hypnosis is moving in two directions. The first includes studies that explore the cognitive and neural nature of hypnosis itself. For example, brain scans show that the control mechanisms for deciding what to do in the face of conflict become uncoupled when people are hypnotized. Some studies using fMRI have demonstrated specific areas of the brain that are activated with hypnosis (Jamieson, 2007; Oakley & Halligan, 2008).

The second direction explores specific hypnotic suggestions and their impact on the brain. In highly hypnotizable subjects, when suggestions were given for decreased fibromyalgia pain, certain brain areas that register discomfort "lit up" (Derbyshire, Whalley, Stenger, & Oakley, 2009). Raz, Fan, and Posner (2005) used neuroimaging techniques to determine the effect of hypnotic suggestion on the brain. They discovered that subjects who were given a string of words could block their meaning with a hypnotic suggestion to do so, and that specific brain areas, including the visual areas, modulated activity and altered information processing during hypnosis. In other experiments, in which researchers instructed subjects to avoid thinking about word associations, long-term memory was reduced (Anderson, Barr, Owall, & Jacobbson, 2004). A study using brain scans demonstrated that posthypnotic suggestion, in this case an amnesia, was reflected in the suppression of certain brain activity (Mendelsohn, Chalamish, Solomonovich, & Dudai, 2008). This capacity to suppress mental activity under hypnosis has been used to help trauma clients dampen the emotion surrounding a traumatic event while they review the memory for mastery of it (Bryant & Mallard, 2002). What then occurs is a reconsolidation of the memory without the intense emotion connected to it.

Neuroscientists have discovered that the process by which we make decisions is influenced by the amygdala, a part of the limbic system (Goleman, 2003; Shibata, 2001). To do this, the limbic system constantly monitors an individual's circumstances. Based on a prediction of the likely outcome of any impending decision, the limbic system produces a presumed emotional response. Armed with that response, the cortex immediately and unconsciously refines the decision. Thus, stimulating appropriate affect with hypnosis can influence state and behavior change (Lankton & Lankton, personal communication, June 18, 1989).

Due to the brain's neuroplasticity, suggestion, imagination (metaphor), and mental rehearsal can stimulate brain growth and the development of neural pathways. Each of these acts of attention causes neurons to connect in specific patterns and sequences of firing. A new idea or suggestion turns on different groups of neurons, and, when reinforced by the clinician in indirect communication, different areas of the brain light up. This implies that although it may not be easy, change is always possible.

Ericksonian Hypnosis

Milton Erickson blurred the line between hypnotic and ordinary states. He suggested that everyone commonly experiences trance states, from being "lost in thought" while driving and missing a freeway exit to being so absorbed in reading a novel that hours vanish. Erickson conceived of hypnosis differently from the ways in which it had been understood historically:

> Psychologists are beginning to discard the old belief that hypnosis transforms a person into some strange, passive, dominated new creature. Instead they are beginning to realize that hypnosis can be used

and should be used to elicit the natural and innate behavior and reactions of the subject, and that through such a measure human behavior can be studied in a controlled and scientific manner. (Erickson, Vol. 3, p. 18)

Ultimately, Erickson defined hypnosis simply as a "focused attention" that leads to an alteration in the way a person experiences the world. The Greens suggested that at the level of brain physiology, hypnosis functions as a method of speaking directly to the limbic system (Green & Green, 1977). We would add that *focused attention facilitates changes in states.*

Erickson's unique style involved strategies, multilevel communication, relationship connection, suggestion, and overt and covert persuasion. Also diverging from the mainstream psychological perspective of his day, Erickson saw the unconscious as a vast storehouse of experiences, memories, and learning—in fact, as a repository of resources that every person possesses and which can be engaged to help a client overcome some difficulty (Lankton & Lankton, 1988). For instance, under hypnotic suggestion, a client recovering from serious burns can remember the cooling sensation of holding an ice cube. He or she can then begin to imagine that coolness in the area of the burn. In response to hypnotic suggestion, the client's physiology will shift, thereby reducing the inflammation and promoting a more rapid healing.

Erickson pointed out that the line between ordinary consciousness and trance is very fine, and that it is important to note that there are many types of trance. For example, a baseball pitcher often will be so focused that he or she sees only the catcher's glove and shin guards, but not the batter (who is irrelevant). Neither will the pitcher hear the crowd. Good pitchers seldom remember what happens from pitch to pitch because they are so focused in the moment.

When we view a film, we step into its reality through imagination. We laugh, cry, and "suffer the slings and arrows of outrageous fortune"; we can become terrified, righteously angry, or sexually aroused. One part of the brain realizes that we are in the movie theater, but another part of the brain has identified with one or more of the characters in the film based on analogous events in our own lives. For the duration of the film, unconscious memory and imagination have been used to change states.

Reading a book, watching a movie, or simply having a daydream can not only generate an emotional response as intense as would be the case if a person were physically experiencing those events, it can also generate similar physiological responses. An individual can unconsciously change blood flow, heart rate, and blood pressure just by thinking of an arousing scene. For example, this is what happens when a person has a sexual fantasy. Similarly, using consciously focused attention, a person can engage different neural processes and turn on (or off) various physiological systems: One can raise skin temperature, lower heart rate, alter blood pressure, or redirect blood flow in his or her body. An individual can also imagine future goals and, through mental rehearsal, practice and accomplish them.

During periods of highly focused attention or trance, dissociation, a sense of automatic or unconscious motoric behavior, and an altering of sensory perceptions characteristically occur. Dissociation leads to an experience of something happening automatically, outside of one's volition. A cellist might say, "I didn't play the concerto; *it played me*." Excellent golfers experience automatic motoric behavior as they tee off. They don't think about their swing or their form; they simply step out of the way and let the body do what it knows so well how to do. Many athletes have had the experience of suddenly finding that the ball seems to be traveling in slow motion, such that it's practically effortless to be at exactly the right place at the right moment to intercept it. All of these experiences are common when athletes or musicians are performing at their peak or are "in the zone," but they are also common in everyday life.

Practically everyone has had the dissociative experience of hearing words coming out of their mouth that they had no intention of saying— for example, at a community meeting, suddenly volunteering to take on a task and immediately wondering, "Who said that?!" Anyone who drives a vehicle with a standard transmission knows a great deal about unconscious motoric behavior. When taking off uphill from a red light, it's not possible to consciously direct two feet to manipulate three pedals with the right timing; to do it smoothly, it has to be done without conscious interference. And everyone has come to the end of an important conversation and found that much less (or more) time has elapsed than one expected.

All of these are actually trance experiences occurring without a formal trance induction. In fact, Erickson utilized a formal trance induction only about 10–20% of the time (Zeig, personal communication, January

19, 1988). He was a master of inducing trance through a casual conversation. Then he would subtly introduce a suggestion and elicit unconscious resources to help a person. In using conversational hypnosis, a clinician might comment: "It is really difficult for you to remember feeling better because right now, having that particular feeling that you have, it is hard to notice when that feeling ends; kind of like a wave that comes and then it goes." This comment is designed to turn on the curiosity and nurturing circuits. Erickson taught, through word and example, that where we focus the client's attention is critical in stimulating emotional states; it can facilitate or hinder the healing process. Changes in the client's facial expression or tone of voice and a more positive energy indicate that these goals are being accomplished.

Therapeutic Uses of Trance Phenomena

Together, Milton Erickson and Ernest Rossi detailed a number of common trance phenomena that have therapeutic applications (Erickson, 1980; Erickson & Rossi, 1981). Understanding these allows a therapist to use hypnotic words more consciously and effectively in a healing manner.

1. *Dissociation* is the psychological phenomenon of experiencing an event as if it were happening to someone else. In trance, dissociation can be used strategically to review something that is emotionally or physically painful. A therapist may suggest, either directly or indirectly, that a client view a particular scene on a screen, through a window, or in a mirror. Dissociation helps a client to gain emotional or physical distance from an event.

2. *Age regression* occurs when a person in trance revivifies, or experiences intensely, some event from the past. In an age-regressed state, a client may learn or relearn psychological traits such as spontaneity, curiosity, playfulness, vulnerability, persistence, or the ability to take initiative. For example, using indirect techniques, a therapist may tell a story about a child to assist the client in identifying with the character and vividly reexperiencing a childhood event.

3. *Amnesia* is the innate ability to forget. Although most of us think of forgetting as an annoyance, forgetting a painful experience can be useful

in a client's recovery from trauma. Therapists may directly suggest that a client forget something or tell anecdotes about forgetting in order to assist a client in forgetting something.

4. *Time distortion* is a naturally occurring phenomenon, in or out of trance. If a person is absorbed in something interesting, a long period of time may seem quite short. The reverse is also true. A client may need to be able to shorten time to endure a physically or emotionally painful experience or expand it to complete a task. Time distortion can be suggested through an embedded suggestion or through a story about an occasion when a person lost track of time. The therapist may suggest that a client can do this out of trance.

5. *Pseudo-orientation in time* allows a client in trance to go into the future mentally, discover psychological resources, and then bring these abilities back into the present. A therapist may have a client picture a screen with an older self in the scene. Then the therapist may have the older, wiser, more successful self tell the younger self how he or she solved certain problems or accomplished certain tasks or goals.

6. *Automatic writing* is the process of writing or doodling unconsciously. Often done with the nondominant hand, automatic writing can be used to deepen trance or recover forgotten material.

7. *Positive hallucinations*, although often associated with mental illnesses such as schizophrenia, can be created for useful reasons by every person to some degree. Auditory hallucinations are most common, but olfactory, gustatory, kinesthetic, and visual hallucinations do occur for many people in trance. Erickson created a kinesthetic hallucination of an itch with a man suffering from phantom limb pain. He did this because he intuited that it would be difficult for his client to experience a complete lack of pain when previously the pain had been so intense. Erickson rightly thought it would be possible for his client to accept, psychologically, an irritating itch for a few days in a limb that was not present. Angered at Erickson for causing this annoying sensation, the client was ready to accept the loss of his leg and the physical comfort that accompanied the cessation of the itch.

8. *Negative hallucination* is the inability to perceive something that is right in front of a person. People can fail to see what is right before their eyes or to hear a person's voice from just a few feet away. In moments of intense concentration, particularly in emergencies, a person may have no sensation of pain. Any period of intense concentration is, by

definition, a trance state. A therapist might suggest that a client *not* experience something—for example, chronic pain—and then bring the lack of experience with him or her out of trance through a posthypnotic suggestion.

9. *Posthypnotic suggestion* allows skills learned in trance to become available to a client in a more common state of awareness. A therapist may suggest that a client recreate some experience he or she had during trance at a later point in time; for example, the client might find him- or herself feeling uncharacteristically relaxed while giving a presentation at work.

10. *Anesthesia*, the experience of a total numbness of some body part, is sometimes suggested hypnotically when a person is unable to tolerate chemical anesthesia during surgery. Since most people have had the experience of sleeping on an arm or hand and feeling a complete lack of feeling in that limb, this anecdote is frequently mentioned to a client in order to aid in the experience of numbness.

11. *Analgesia* allows the client to tolerate the sensation of pain while remaining mindful of the injured part of the body. Pain is important because it is protective of an injured or sick part of the body. However, pain that is too intense is counterproductive. The therapist may suggest a lessening of pain through the experience of analgesia. The pain is still present but to a lesser extent, and the client is in a better frame of mind.

12. *Hypermnesia* is an ability to remember in great detail events from the past. This is the opposite resource from amnesia (Lankton & Lankton, 1988). Remembering the lyrics of a song that you haven't heard in years is a common instance of hypermnesia. A person may need to remember information for an exam or to report a crime to the police. An actor, athlete, or musician may need to recall the right lines, moves, or notes for a performance. Hypermnesia can be enhanced by linking memory to the appropriate state.

In the BCT approach we make use of trance phenomena in a highly integrated way because our therapeutic focus seeks to facilitate, engage, and shape state change. We now know that specific neural circuits can be activated or deactivated using words. While Milton Erickson was intuitively able to target a client's particular circuits, the use of BCT techniques allows the clinician to do so intentionally. For example, telling a story or using a confusion technique can trigger the curiosity circuit and function as a bridge to another state. Telling a story that includes parental approval of a child's mastery of a new skill can deactivate anxiety in the face of newness.

Deep Rapport Established Through Hypnotic Empathy

The most powerful tool in psychotherapy, no matter the approach, is empathy (Hutterer & Liss, 2006). Empathy turns on the nurturing circuit in the client and facilitates a state shift. An alignment between therapist and client occurs where there is a shared state of connection. Heinz Kohut felt that within the context of the empathic treatment bond, his clients were experiencing him as a needed extension of themselves (Rowe & Mac Isaac, 1991, p. 30). Clients record at an unconscious level the tone of voice, gaze, respiration, and posture of the therapist, and the clinician can use these subtle means to help shift the client's state (Meares, 2005). Whenever two people have established deep rapport, each is affecting the other at a neurobiological level.

Mirror neurons enable people to synchronize with each other. Sensing a supportive environment, the client is likely to come into unconscious synchrony with the hypnotherapist. When this is not the case, the therapist can consciously come into synchrony with the client and then gradually shift the client by shifting him- or herself. Empathic suggestion, metaphor, and guided mental rehearsal may create a shared state that can be healing for the client. The combination of encouraging state entrainment through the use of empathy and then inquiring what changes a client would need to make to live in accordance with his or her own values is a powerful influence for change (Miller & Rollnick, 2002). To facilitate this process, appropriately pacing the client in terms of affect and mental focus is critical. The following experience Bill had as a boy illustrates this point.

When Bill was 8 years old, his family made a trip to Bristol, Oklahoma, where his parents had grown up. One of Bill's great-uncles had a ranch and told the family that he had a horse for his nephew. The horse was a beautiful black-and-white paint pony—but it had never had a rider on its back. When Bill arrived at the ranch, he had visions of riding a bucking bronco and taming the horse, as he'd seen in the movies. His uncle had a different plan.

Uncle John asked Bill to name the horse. Bill chose the name "Cherokee." His uncle silently nodded. When they entered the corral, Uncle John had Bill sit in the opposite area from where the horse stood. And then Bill's uncle began to tell him stories of his Cherokee ancestors—a part of Bill's heritage of which he had had no conscious knowledge—all the while repositioning Bill in relation to the horse.

In fact, Uncle John was a horse whisperer who had observed mustangs in the wild and knew how to stimulate their curiosity. After they had spent a couple days just sitting at one edge of the corral, Uncle John placed a lump of sugar and an apple in Bill's shirt pocket. After a while, the horse came up to Bill and nudged him to get a bite of the tasty treats. Uncle John told Bill to sit quietly and let the horse get to know him slowly. Eventually, he placed the apple in Bill's hand and told him to hold it and allow the horse to eat. Then he showed Bill how to stroke the horse's face and neck so that the two could get to know each other without fear and anxiety. The next day, Uncle John placed an apple in Bill's hip pocket, and they walked around the corral with the pony following and every now and then nudging Bill's behind, trying to eat the apple. Pretty soon, the horse had walked around the entire corral with Bill. The following day, Bill's uncle placed a blanket on the horse, lifted his nephew up, and told him to just rub the pony's neck and face, and whisper his name in his ear. Bill's uncle walked the horse around the corral with Bill on his back. Cherokee and Bill developed a bond and, despite both the horse's and the boy's natural hesitation and fear, they became great friends.

This story illustrates the tools of verbal pacing and leading that Milton Erickson used when he aligned himself with a client and made a small change that he slowly expanded upon as the client solved problems. It is also an example of Erickson's utilization principle, which states that we can acknowledge the reality of the client (the pony or young Bill) and then disorganize it (horse moved from tendency to flee, Bill moved from idea of "breaking the bronco") by turning on the client's curiosity. Any time we alter neural patterns, we are disorganizing them. Subsequent to that, they can be reorganized: By mirroring the horse's behavior of staying distant but indirectly suggesting that a closer relationship would result in a food reward, curiosity was stimulated and helped the horse overcome fear. By the time the blanket was on the horse's back, both the horse and Bill felt a sense of safety with each other, and a new behavior was in place.

Most of the time, when a therapist is warmly empathic, the client's state shifts unconsciously in the direction of the desired and integrated state, and the clinician can follow this movement by reinforcing the state with positive comments. To disrupt the client's rigidly held construct of reality and loosen neural connections, the therapist can intentionally use empathy in the form of conversational hypnosis, which is the use of suggestion and indirect association without a formal trance induction. However, the use of empathy is likely to miss the mark if a client is dismissive. In that case, empathy may even serve to elicit hostility. A better approach, then, is simply to mirror back what the client is saying until an opening occurs for the therapist to provide an interruption in the pattern.

Empathy has a subtle hypnotic effect in that the empathic voice tone is soothing and helps gently shift the focus of attention off the problem and on to the voice of the therapist, ultimately shifting the client's emotional state. Hypnotic empathy spoken in genuine and caring tones also has subtle age regressive tendencies, evoking earlier times, when a person was cuddled and nurtured by a caregiver. When the gentle cooing of the therapist's voice is allowed in, the client's pain seems to diminish. Through empathy, the therapist intentionally facilitates the client's brain shift to a state that is less conflicted and more flexible. This state shift in turn allows a person to open up to possibilities he or she may not have considered previously.

Conversational Hypnosis (without Formal Induction)

All psychotherapies are suggestive. Where we focus the client's attention in therapy can lead the individual to experience positive or negative states. Carl Rogers, who contributed the idea of person-centered therapy and used unconditional positive regard, could be compared to an excellent hypnotherapist. He had the ability to use deep empathy, and while he never described his work in this way, he used suggestions in conversations. He would say, "You feel this and you feel that, and you really want to do this and that." Because people bonded deeply to him, he was able to move people through their issues with a soothing voice tone and effect state change using positive regard, which implied that the client had the ability to work through the problem.

Conversational hypnosis is a technique within the larger body of Ericksonian hypnosis. In a conversation, not only can we embed suggestion in the dialogue, but intentionally turn on certain emotional circuits. We might say, "It is really difficult for you to remember feeling better because right now, having that particular feeling that you have, it is hard to notice when that feeling ends; kind of like a wave that comes and then it goes." This comment is designed to turn on the curiosity and nurturing circuits. Where we focus the client's attention is critical in stimulating emotional states; it can facilitate or hinder the healing process. Changes in the client's facial expression or tone of voice and a more positive energy allows us to know that these goals are being accomplished.

Linguistic Forms for Eliciting Change (Indirect Suggestions)

Erickson used language adeptly in hypnosis. Understanding that hypnosis elicits resources and allows people to connect with abilities they already possess, he subtly crafted suggestions that would awaken certain psychological processes or states that an individual could use for problem resolution. For example, everyone—even those from severely deprived backgrounds—has experienced a sense of confidence, feelings of security, the ability to persevere, instances of facing a fear, etc., in some childhood setting. Erickson could find a way to elicit even a remnant of such a resource by using language with great care, circumventing the normal resistances that are evoked when we are simply told what to do. Instead, he would create a story containing a veiled reference to a client's situation. Then, through indirect suggestion, he would offer the client a new perspective or new means by which to address it. Erickson, Rossi, and Rossi (1976) codified Erickson's linguistic techniques as a means to influence the brain–mind–body. We have summarized them here with an example of each technique:

1. *Embedded suggestion.* This is a suggestion that is placed within a statement or question. The speaker shifts his or her voice tone slightly to emphasize the suggestion and indirectly lead the trance subject toward a specific goal.

   EXAMPLE: I wonder just how *comfortable you can feel.*

2. *Implication.* This is a statement or question that leads another person to think of an unstated thought and to behave in accord with that unstated thought.

EXAMPLE: "I do not know exactly how *your feelings will change.*" [There is the implication that the individual's feelings will change.]

3. *Illusion of choice.* This is a statement or question that offers only two alternatives, both leading to the same outcome.

EXAMPLE: "Do you want to go into trance, or would you prefer to just sit there quietly and focus on the sound of my voice?"

4. *Truism.* This is a statement that expresses something about which everyone generally agrees. The linguistic device is used to create a "yes set," or an attitude of openness to suggestions. Therapists can lessen resistance to the introduction of a new idea or behavior more easily after a person has been in agreement about a number of things.

EXAMPLE: "Everyone knows what it is like to sleep on your arm. It gets tingly and eventually becomes numb." [This suggestion is used to reduce resistance and elicit a yes set as the clinician teaches a person how to create a glove anesthesia (loss of sensation in the hand), which can then be generalized to another part of the body as needed for use in pain control.]

5. *Suggestions covering all possible alternatives.* When a therapist makes a suggestion so as to cover all possible experiences, he or she lets the client decide unconsciously just what the experience will be. Thus, there is less chance that rapport will be broken and the trance experience interrupted or ended.

EXAMPLE: "As you look at your hand, I do not know whether you will feel a tingling in your hand, or if that hand will start to feel numb. You might begin to feel lightness in one of your hands. It might be your right or your left hand. Or you might feel a heaviness, or nothing at all. I would like you to be curious about what is going to happen." [The therapist covers all possible experiences, embedding suggestions that imply that something is going to happen.]

6. *Apposition of opposites.* This is a statement that describes one experience and implies that the more it happens, the more something else, seemingly the opposite, will then happen.

   EXAMPLE: "The longer it takes for you to go into trance, the more surprised you will be when you finally go into trance." [These statements are counterintuitive. Clients who are being induced to go into trance often think that when something does not happen immediately, hypnosis is not working. Alternatively, they may think that they cannot be hypnotized. When a therapist uses an apposition of opposites, he or she diffuses resistance and confuses the conscious mind with a logical though counterintuitive statement.]

   EXAMPLE: "This may deepen your trance. Or it may heighten your trance experience." [Although *deepening* and *heightening* appear to be opposites, in this case they are functionally the same.]

7. *Open-ended suggestions.* When a therapist suggests a means by which to respond to a situation, but does not offer any type of solution, the client has a more difficult time resisting the suggestion.

   EXAMPLE: "Your mind can review all the ideas related to this situation. You don't yet know consciously which will be the most useful for coming up with a new solution but, as you look at the ideas, you may see new possibilities." [By making a suggestion in this manner, the client must take responsibility for the outcome, and he or she is more likely to look for more creative solutions. In addition, the therapist fosters curiosity and independence in the patient.]

8. *Conscious–unconscious binds.* This is a suggestion that separates the conscious and unconscious mind. There is an implication that the two are different entities and will respond differently to suggestions and to the trance experience as a whole. This bind creates a type of dissociation, where the patient begins to feel that what is occurring is doing so without his or her volition. People come to therapy because they feel stuck and in pain; they cannot figure their way out. When something seems to be occurring that the client is not consciously responsible for, he or she may have an easier time believing that change is possible.

EXAMPLE: "Your conscious mind may be distracted while I speak, while your unconscious mind can hear what I say."

9. *Double dissociative double-binds.* In this case, the therapist splits the conscious and unconscious mind in a manner similar to the conscious–unconscious bind. However, the therapist continues speaking and then reverses the alternatives. This technique adds more confusion and makes it more difficult for the client to follow the therapist's suggestions consciously. Dissociation eventually happens, and the patient experiences a trance-like state of consciousness.

EXAMPLE: "Your conscious mind may be distracted while your unconscious mind can hear what I say. Or your unconscious mind can pay attention to irrelevant things, while your conscious mind listens to what I say and develops a nice trance." [The patient is in a bit of a quandary. If she feels distracted, is her unconscious mind listening to what is being said, but outside of her awareness? Or, if she feels distracted by irrelevant things, is that her unconscious? If she hears what the therapist is saying, is she not going into trance because she feels consciously aware of what is happening, or is this just proof that her mind has become so focused that she is indeed going into trance?]

10. *Misspeaking.* This technique uses phrasing such that the therapist's words are intentionally open to multiple interpretations. The therapist may misstate something, use homonyms, or employ *double entendres* so that the client can hear what is being said in more than one way. Often, the client's conscious mind will perceive an overt communication while his or her unconscious hears the intent of the therapist.

EXAMPLE: "As you sit there and listen to me, I do not know if your unconscious is going to lead you deeper into trance." [In this case, the therapist embeds a suggestion by misspeaking. The covert suggestion, "you're unconscious," can be perceived as well as the overt message, "I don't know if your unconscious . . . " Another example would be, "You can sit there, can you nod?" The conscious mind will hear ". . . can you not?", but the question also elicits unconscious agreement in the form of a nod of the head.]

11. *Confusion using direction, time, and condition.* When a therapist induces trance or attempts to help a client maintain trance, he

or she may need to overload the client's conscious or habitual way of thinking or perceiving the world. Every person has habitual ways of thinking, feeling and perceiving. These habituated perspectives act as maps that guide a person through life, helping him or her to understand, interpret, and give meaning to events and experiences. However, these maps also limit what is experienced. Psychotherapy, and particularly hypnosis, broadens a person's internal maps so that life becomes richer with more possibilities or choices. This therapeutic process often alleviates pain that has occurred as a result of limited perception, cognition, or behavior.

EXAMPLE: "You seem to be stomping your left foot, which I thought was your right foot, and indeed was the right foot to stomp, when indeed you were stomping your left foot. What I wonder is why you are not stomping your right foot, which I thought was your left foot, and indeed was the foot you left out. Isn't that right?" [In this situation, Carol confused her then-4-year-old daughter to help her stop a temper tantrum which was taking place in the middle of a department store.]

EXAMPLE "As I sit here, which is your there, your here is my there, and my there is your here. You can hear deeply what I say to your unconscious." [The therapist is using directional confusion and embedded suggestions.]

12. *Confusion using multiple negatives.* A person can track only so many changes in a sentence. When a therapist uses multiple negatives in a sentence, it is difficult for the client to consciously follow what the therapist is saying. Multiple negatives overload the conscious tracking of what the therapist is communicating and thereby help the client move into trance. When the therapist has developed trust and rapport, confusion techniques can be a powerful way to help induce or deepen trance. It is important to note, however, that not all clients are comfortable with being confused. Betty Alice Erickson, one of Erickson's daughters and his primary demonstration subject for over 30 years, has said that she never liked her father's confusion techniques (Betty Alice Erickson, personal communication, May 18, 1990). For clients who have a difficult time letting go of conscious thought and attempt to analyze what is being said, confusion techniques may hinder the development of a trance.

EXAMPLE: "You don't need to do anything with your conscious mind not to discover what state is not useful for you to communicate something meaningful."

13. *Shifting pronouns.* During trance, a therapist may tell a story about a particular character. If the therapist wants the client to identify with this character for some therapeutic reason, she may begin telling the story in the third person and then, at strategic times, shift to the second person.

EXAMPLE: "I was watching a young boy kicking a soccer ball. He was kicking the ball between his two feet as he was running down the field. When you learn to kick a ball you first have to think about the action. Eventually, your unconscious mind takes over, and you don't have to think about the activity, just the goal." [In this case, the therapist is also embedding suggestions by changing voice tone and further underscoring the suggestion by changing the personal pronoun from third person to the second person. By delivering a suggestion in such a manner, the therapist invites the client to identify with the little child, but does so in a manner that reduces resistance. The unconscious mind is more likely to hear the reference as personal, while the conscious mind merely follows the story. The activity of kicking a soccer ball is a metaphor for pursuing any personal goal; the therapist's intent in this scenario is to help the client realize that by staying focused on the "goal," the activities needed to reach the goal will automatically be handled.]

14. *Characters in a story.* When a therapist tells a story about a child, father, mother, or some other character with whom a client has had an encounter, the client will normally think about his or her own experiences. In choosing stories, however, the therapist should be mindful of whether the client has had any unusually painful experiences with a parent, such as physical or sexual abuse (Kershaw, 1992; Lankton & Lankton, 1988).

EXAMPLE: "Once there was a little girl who wanted to make some cookies for her dolls' tea party, but she didn't know how to make cookies by herself. She knew how to make mud-pie cookies. But she didn't want mud-pie cookies. She wanted real cookies. So she asked her mother to help her . . ." [Here the therapist is beginning to tell a story in which the main character wants something that is more authentic than what she knows how to create for herself and is therefore asking for help. Through the story, the therapist is embedding suggestions about the greater value of authenticity and implying that asking for assistance can be an acceptable behavior.]

Ideomotor Cues

Because we do not look directly into the client's brain during a session (unless the person is hooked up to an EEG or other brain imaging equipment), we must rely on other means to track his or her experience. One of the best ways is by noticing the client's ideomotor behavior—that is, the unconscious muscular movements that are the basis of "body language," such as a slight change in facial expression, a shift in posture, suddenly watery eyes, dilation of the pupils, etc. (Rossi & Cheek, 1994). BCT makes extensive use of such cues because they usually accompany and reflect a change in brain state, as well as giving an indication of subjective experience. For example, if a person shifts from being identified with his or her emotional pain to being curious about it, the facial expression may change from a frown to a widening of the eyes, and a shift in emotional energy may be observed. If a therapist reframes a problem as one that may have entailed life adventures and valuable lessons, angst reflected in watery eyes may change to a surprised or excited look. The client's unconscious communication can be understood as an ongoing reflection of his or her internal experience and brain states.

On rare occasions, we work with a client who does not exhibit any ideomotor signs, give any indication of state changes, or show evidence of being in a trance. Such individuals might be called nonexpressive. Although they may just sit quietly and not respond overtly, they can still be following along internally and may actually be quite involved. The person is still vividly experiencing mental events within the hypnotic state. In the complete absence of ideomotor cues, the therapist may elicit a physical response by inquiring, "Does this make sense to you?" or "Have you ever had an experience like that?" An indication as small as a client's slight shift forward is enough to confirm that the client is following the therapist. At other times, the client will say afterwards that the experience "seemed so real," or the client will report that what happened after the session was remarkably close to what was suggested. However, like most people, clients tend to be unconsciously expressive—often far more so than they imagine. The therapist need only be closely observant to use ideomotor cues to confirm underlying state changes.

The Hypnotic Experiment

The hypnotic experiment is a creative activity the therapist can use to demonstrate to clients that they have abilities they may not have discovered. We can use formal trance work or indirect suggestion in a conversational intervention. Before using this technique, it is important to have assessed how well the client can respond to hypnosis as well as his or her level of motivation. A client must have a compelling desire for behavior change. This is particularly true, for example, with individuals who enter therapy to deal with weight issues or to stop smoking. If the person does not have sufficient leverage with him- or herself, the result will be failure, perceived as either the therapist's failure or as one more instance of the client's failure. The person also needs to be somewhat cooperative. Any resistance should be understood as an indication of how much fear and trepidation the client is experiencing. In the case of resistance, the clinician should work to establish better rapport before suggesting that the client try a hypnotic experiment.

As clinicians, we need to communicate a sense of curiosity and positive certainty that the problem that brought the client to the office can be resolved. To engage the client's curiosity, we then ask if he or she would like to "conduct an experiment." If an individual says "yes," we can begin to teach trance phenomena as a means of facilitating state change. For example, we may do this by having a client experience the numbing of a hand or by having a hand float in the air. Through this type of experiential learning, the person develops the ability to process multiple levels of communication. To begin the experiment, we may use one of Erickson's indirect suggestions. We never definitively say that the hand will float; instead, we ask the client to focus on the sensation in his or her wrist and imagine that there was a balloon full of helium tied to it. Due to suggestibility, the hand is then likely to float—which validates the trance and can be used to create anesthesia (because it is difficult to move blood upward). It also creates curiosity and surprise, especially when the person recognizes that he or she does not feel his or her floating hand. To stimulate playfulness, we may add, "We would like you to enjoy seeing this hand in this position."

Experiencing a cataleptic hand engenders both curiosity and confusion: This is not part of a person's normal experience. If the person then begins to develop numbness or tingling (glove anesthesia), the sensation further ratifies the trance and leaves the person with an experience for which he or she may have no explanation. The hand levitation and the confusion/curiosity that it creates momentarily disrupt negative self-talk and a defeatist attitude. We also give the client credit by saying, "You didn't know you could do this, and your conscious mind does not know what I am talking about, but your unconscious mind does, and that part of your mind is already wondering how to use this in the future." Consciously or unconsciously, the person then learns to alter physiological sensations. This learning takes place in the context of an early learning set: It is gently suggested, through a series of metaphors and implications that reinforce curiosity and mastery of life tasks, that the client remember learning to walk, read, write, or put together puzzles. A person cannot learn these tasks as a child without also learning persistence, imagination, initiative, curiosity, and other positive states.

As the person gets better at the trance phenomena, an element of play comes into the process. "Hey, look what I can do!" becomes a common attitude. The client may even come up with connections to floating hands and glove anesthesia of which the clinician has not thought. We do not necessarily know how an individual will utilize trance phenomena or what his or her own resources may be. For example, one client who came in to stop smoking learned to levitate his hand and make it numb. He would come out of trance with his hand completely numb, as it was suggested. He enjoyed waking up a numb hand, as though he had slept on it. Fairly soon, he had stopped smoking. As it happened, he worked at a delicatessen. One day when he was chopping lettuce, he took off a chunk of his thumb, and, without missing a beat, he went into trance and stopped the bleeding. He needed no stitches and afterward barely had a scar. Ericksonian hypnosis leaves the client with a high degree of autonomy. What happens is second-order change: The client learns to learn on his or her own. While this further reinforces state change, we do not always know how the person will use the experience.

We have worked with many people who have had panic attacks and worry that they will throw up in a crowd. Stress seems to set off the nausea and panic when in public. To use the hypnotic experiment, we suggest that the person experience just a little nausea in the office and then send it away. Most clients are quite good at bringing on the symptom and just as good at sending it away. The important part of this learning experience is for the client to become more aware of the activation of a stress state, its triggers, and his or her ability to consciously direct the state.

Another hypnotic experiment is to use a blood pressure cuff and take a reading before and after a state change process. Unless the pressure is quite low normally, the client is often surprised in the change of pressure after changing states to one of lower arousal. This is particularly appropriate if a client believes that "nothing will ever change." When a client is stuck, one of a number of things is happening. The person may be depressed or despondent; often, as a result, he or she will not notice when external or internal events do change. On the other hand, the person may become overly eager, possibly even anxious, to change, which hampers the process. In that case, too, the client may conclude that change is impossible. But when a client can demonstrate to him- or herself an ability to lower his or her blood pressure, the new skill strongly undercuts the counterproductive belief that "nothing will change." Additionally, the shift to a more relaxed state facilitates the desired change.

Deconstructing Hypnotic Ambivalence or Resistance

As noted, gazing in a warm manner, speaking in a pleasant tone of voice, and mirroring empathic responses tend to activate resources in a client. The way we ask questions can help shift states as well. However, if the client does not have a sufficiently trusting relationship with his or her therapist, he or she may experience fear around maintaining his or her self-organization. For someone who has developed rigid states of mind, family-of-origin issues around healthy attachment frequently exist. To allow another point of view may result in having to let go of some previous way of experiencing the world.

A client who had entered therapy in order to "figure out how to live her own life" wanted to experience trance work but seemed convinced that she could not achieve a state of focused attention. She communicated this stance nonverbally through a brusque and distant manner that said, in essence, "Don't try this with me because it won't work." Her conflict stemmed from believing that either she or Bill would fail. As Bill began to inquire about her background and growing edge for change, she told him that she had done what she had always *not* wanted to do, which was return to her old work and marry her high school sweetheart upon returning to her hometown after active service duty.

Using hypnotic empathy, Bill mirrored back to her, "So the yearning in you to do something else with your life is still right there under the surface, and it is really difficult when you become aware of it. You really love your husband, and yet something inside you seems to be knocking at your door." Bill asked her about an experience where she felt fully comfortable and relaxed about all inner conflict. She reported that when she was at the beach, there was an expansive feeling of not being caged and feeling very free. She began to relax and soften as she described the experience of being by the water. Bill watched for the emotional shift into the access state, an openness that would allow her to work with him. When she softened, he was able to begin the deeper state work with her, and she responded positively.

Through hypnotic empathy, Bill had created a bridge from an unproductive state to a transition state, so that ultimately another intervention could be utilized. In the transition state, there is still something somewhat negative—but with less arousal, less confusion—and there is something somewhat positive that begins to open the curiosity circuit to what might be possible. It is at this point that the client demonstrates change readiness, and the rapport may become a shared state of positive trance. Within the shared state a true dialogue occurs, and the therapist may experience images or have associations that turn out to be remarkably accurate when expressed to the client. Often the client is amazed by how the therapist has "picked up" information that was not shared verbally.

Another example of diffusing resistance can be demonstrated through the case of a client who asked to be hypnotized, although he was not sure he could go into a trance. As Carol began to work with him, he slipped into a deeper state, but he refused to let himself stay there. Carol suggested that he could come out and go back inside, in whatever way felt comfortable to him. At the end of the experience, this young man reported that his mother had left him when he was young. Even though they had a better relationship now, he had not forgiven her, and in the trance experience, he had overlaid both his yearning for that relationship and his anger onto Carol. He had a revelation that he wanted to change this dynamic in order to better relate to women in general.

Case Example: Panic Disorder and Social Phobia

Stan was the vice president of finance in a publicly-held technology company. He was well educated, articulate, and excellent at his job. At our first meeting, we noted that Stan was well-dressed and that he had an athletic build and an open and friendly manner. As we talked, he revealed that he suffered from panic attacks, some of which seemed to happen for no apparent reason. He would break out in a sweat, his heart would start racing, and he would become short of breath and begin to experience dizziness. After an examination, Stan's cardiologist had assured him that he was not experiencing a heart attack and was, in fact, in excellent health and physical condition.

Stan also described how he had an extremely difficult time speaking in front of groups. Unfortunately, Stan's position required him to make frequent presentations to the board of directors and department heads of his company. "I lock up. I start to stutter; I can't remember what I was going to say; and then I start breaking out in all those symptoms. This is silly: I know these people. I play golf with some of them." Stan went on to say that his fear was becoming worse. It had recently extended to family gatherings and reunions.

We asked Stan how long the panic attacks had been going on. He said that he had experienced this anxiety before, but this time, it was more severe and had been getting progressively worse for more than a year. He went on to say that he had been in therapy before and had learned some relaxation techniques that had originally seemed to help. Now the anxiety had come back, and he could not make any of the guided imagery or relaxation techniques work. Stan was not taking medication for this problem.

As we explored his difficulty, Stan told us that he was in his late 40s and very athletic. He had played competitive soccer until just a couple years earlier and now coached his son's soccer team. He was an avid golfer with a very low handicap (especially for someone who only played a few times a month). Stan also liked to ski and was planning to combine snowboarding with skiing on his next trip. He had done that once before and, though he had fallen repeatedly, he had made a great deal of progress combining two very different downhill techniques. Despite his fear of public speaking, Stan had an adventuresome spirit.

The conversation led Stan to the discovery that in all the athletic activities he loved, he experienced the same physiological characteristics as in a panic attack: he sweated profusely, experienced an increased heart rate, became short of breath, and at times felt a little dizzy. Furthermore, to golf, ski, or play soccer, a person must be able to narrow his focus, particularly when hitting the golf ball or kicking the soccer ball. Then he must be able to open his focus to see the entire fairway or playing field. Each shift in focus accompanies a brain state change. This same skill is important in public speaking. A speaker must, on one hand, become absorbed and, hopefully, enjoy the topic, if he (or she) is to be an inspiring speaker. He must also open his focus so he does not lose his audience. This change in focus and state must happen repeatedly throughout a speech if the speaker is to do well.

Stan had become so narrowly focused on his audience's reactions that he was misreading people's behavior. A yawn or wiggling leg might mean any number of things; these behaviors did not mean necessarily that Stan was delivering a poor presentation. Being so focused on people's reactions made him more anxious to do well, and thus, it became increasingly difficult to lose himself in his topic and enjoy what he was doing. The more overfocused Stan became, the more the anticipated anxiety occurred. Ultimately, Stan's anticipation became a self-fulfilling prophesy, creating the very fear and panic he so desperately wanted to avoid. Consequently, Stan began to avoid making speeches, further reinforcing his belief that if he gave a speech, he would have a panic attack. The more Stan avoided the situation, the more anxious he became, and because he knew that success in his job was dependent upon his making formal presentations, the anxiety intensified and generalized to non-work-related settings.

The interventions we used made use of early learning and were focused on observing Stan's hypnotic responsiveness. The trance phenomena that Stan displayed—for example, a floating hand—were utilized to impress upon him that something was happening beyond what he expected and already understood. Because certain sports were of inherent interest to Stan, Bill created metaphors using skiing, golf, and soccer. Those topics would potentially deepen his focus and trance experience—and, more importantly, they contained the solutions to his panic and fear of public speaking.

The following excerpts are taken from hypnosis sessions with Stan. They demonstrate a trance induction, therapeutic work utilizing resources from life experiences, a number of Ericksonian linguistic maneuvers, and the use of metaphor to change states and elicit trance phenomena and unconscious resources. Italicized words connote a subtle shift in voice tone and indicate interspersed or embedded suggestions.

Trance Induction

Trance inductions are used to help a client focus attention and to ratify to the client that he or she is experiencing something different from his or her usual state. In the following example, Bill used mild dissociation and playfulness to disrupt the possible anticipation that nothing would happen or that hypnosis would not help the client's problem. Even though the floating hand had nothing to do with the symptom, it was an unaccustomed phenomenon for which the client had no category. The novelty led the client to become a participant–observer of his own process, just as a meditating monk might observe his thoughts even as he disidentifies with them. Such an experience, in and of itself, helps a client begin to realize that there are things outside his or her field of experience that may lead to a lessening, or even complete cessation, of the symptomatic states that brought him or her into therapy. Trance ratification and trance phenomena are used throughout the hypnotic experience. The initial trance induction with Stan, the client, took about 20 minutes. Subsequent inductions took increasingly less time as Stan became more proficient at going into trance.

> "Stan, as you *sit there* and I sit here, which is *you're there*, and *your there* is my here, I would like you to do nothing but *sit there* and just *hear* what I say to you [confusion technique and misspeaking to turn on curiosity and seeking]. I don't want you to *go into trance* just yet, but I would like you to *focus your attention* on your hands, which *rest comfortably* on your lap [bind of comparable alternatives]. And I don't know if your right hand will be the right hand to *experience something different*, and your left hand will be left out, or if your left hand

will experience something different, but I would like you to *be curious* which hand *will begin to experience a tingling, or a lightness or even a heaviness* [embedded suggestion for the curiosity circuit], and you don't know just yet what it is that *you're going to experience*, but I do hope you will *enjoy* what is going on [all possibilities of a class of behaviors]. And as I speak, I'm going to count from 10 to 1. . . . 10 . . . *that's right* (HAND BEGINS TO MOVE SLIGHTLY), 9 . . . *that's right* (HAND BEGINS TO LIFT UP OFF THE LAP), 8 . . . And you have a conscious mind and an unconscious mind. 7 . . . *that's right* (HAND CONTINUES TO LIFT) *that's right* 6 . . . and your unconscious mind controls *you're breathing . . . more slowly now.* . . . It controls your heart rate is slower . . . 5 . . . 4 . . . And you didn't know that it would *be this easy*, did you? But it is . . . 3 . . . *that's right* (HAND LIFTS EVEN MORE). And that hand can find its most comfortable place to float, just like it is not even a part of your body . . . 2 . . . 1. . . . And I don't know how well *you can remember* a time when your eyes became heavy, maybe you were up late studying *trying to keep your eyes open*, but finding that with every blink they became heavier (EYES BLINK, THEN CLOSE).

Early Learning Set

In this next segment of the transcript, Bill suggested that the client had already learned many resourceful states, such as how to get up when he falls down and how to deal with pain. In addition, Bill suggested that persistence and determination were states that Stan had experienced and could call upon now. Bill continued to speak about learning the alphabet in school, learning to read, and learning to write (a favorite that Erickson used repeatedly). He did so in the same way he had been throughout the trance. After Bill reoriented Stan to the outside world, they finished his first hypnosis session. Subsequent sessions began in much the same manner, with a trance induction and a shortened version of an early learning set.

Many young therapists think that therapy must be directed to induce unbridled catharsis. However, uncontrolled catharsis may do a client more harm than good. If there is some trauma that intrudes into a person's conscious awareness, then catharsis may be therapeutic with a safety net of positive resources, security, and trance phenomena. Having such a safety net in place is rare and should not become the primary goal of therapy. Bill used a mildly painful experience with Stan, but the focus was to remember that *pain abates*. This memory helped Stan relearn, from his own experience, that all people fail at tasks—but then they also recover, learn further, and then succeed. This experience was later linked more directly to his fear of public speaking. The suggestions offered were indirect. Bill used changes of tense, voice tone, and pronouns to cue the unconscious mind that a suggestion was being delivered. In each case, Bill observed Stan's ideomotor behavior to confirm that he was having the therapeutic experience that Bill intended. Although it appears that a monologue is occurring, in reality the therapist is in a dialogue with the client, who is responding with minimal cues.

"Now all my children, on a day *you could not go outside*, would go to the toy box, book shelf, or closet and pick out a puzzle. Now the first puzzle *you put together* has only a few pieces. And *you pick up the piece, and you turn it this way and that way. And you become so absorbed* in what you are doing that *you have no idea how much time is going by* [time distortion]. And when you put that first piece in *you feel a sense of pride* (STAN BEGINS TO SMILE IN TRANCE) . . . *that's right*, I want you to *remember that feeling of pride* (STAN CONTINUES TO SMILE) and I want you to *memorize that feeling*. Because you are going to use that feeling in the future in a directed fashion [posthypnotic suggestion]. Now you can talk in trance, and you can open your eyes in trance, so in a moment I am going to count to 3 and I want your eyes to open, but you can stay deeply in trance. Okay, 1 . . . 2 . . . 3 (STAN'S EYES OPEN AND HE LOOKS A BIT CONFUSED). I would like you to look at your hand (STAN LOOKS AT HIS HAND FLOATING IN MIDAIR AND BEGINS TO SMILE WHILE LOOKING A BIT CONFUSED). Have you ever seen your hand float like that before? (WITH SOME DIFFICULTY, STAN SAYS "No"). How does it feel to see your hand floating like that, or does it even feel like your hand? (STAN SHAKES HIS HEAD JUST A BIT, INDICATING "No") [trance ratification and maintenance]. Your eyes can close, and you can become even more absorbed in your inner world, as your unconscious mind continues to listen to what I say.

"Some time ago I took my oldest son to get his driver's license. And while he was taking his road test, there was this little boy in the waiting room learning to walk. Now when *you learn to walk*, you pull up on a sofa, a chair or a table, and *you start to stand on your own two feet*. This little boy stood there with his feet placed wide apart. He would pick up his foot, begin to place it down, and he would fall. *And you can't even count the number of times you fall down* when you learn to walk. Most of the time, you fall where it is padded. But sometimes *you fall down and bite your lip. And it hurts!* (STAN'S FACE BEGINS TO WINCE EVER SO SLIGHTLY). And you don't think the pain is going to stop, but it does. The child doesn't know that, but an adult does (STAN'S FACE BEGINS TO RELAX). I want you to remember that the *pain does go away.* Now when *you persist,* you *feel pride.* And I want you to *remember that feeling of persistence and determination* (STAN'S FACE TIGHTENS A BIT, AND HAS A LOOK OF DETERMINATION) because you are going to use those feelings later."

Metaphors Linking Resources

In this portion of the trance, Bill suggested that Stan increase his breathing, heart rate, and body temperature by using a metaphor about playing soccer. Implied in this section is the idea that Stan has felt the sensations of a panic attack before. Also implied is that by being able to create these physical sensations and then stop them by using just his imagination, he will be able to accomplish this goal at other times. Since this session was early in the hypnotherapy, Bill did not mention public speaking. Stan, being a moderately good hypnotic subject, was able to respond to the indirect suggestions. However, if he had not been able to do so, the rapport built in trance would not have been broken, because no direct suggestions were made concerning public speaking. The therapy was set up so that Stan could not fail to respond to the suggestions. Since he already used open and closed focus in playing golf, he had the necessary abilities to become absorbed in his speech and then return to connect with the audience.

"Stan, you told me that you have played soccer, you coach soccer, you play golf, and you ski (STAN BEGINS AN UNCONSCIOUS PRESERVATIVE NOD) [eliciting a yes set]. When you play soccer, you exert yourself, especially in the Texas heat. *Your heart rate increases, your breathing increases, and you begin to perspire* (IN TRANCE STAN BEGINS TO BREATHE MORE QUICKLY. HIS HEART RATE BEGINS TO INCREASE, AND HE BEGINS TO PERSPIRE SLIGHTLY). And when you exert yourself it *feels good.* I'd like you to *remember an exciting soccer match.* That's right! I'd like you to *really breathe hard, and feel the excitement* as you bring the ball down field, or pass it, or make a score. When the game is over, *you begin to breathe more slowly, your heart rate slows down, and you begin to feel cooler*. (STAN'S HEART RATE SLOWS DOWN, HIS BREATHING DE-CREASES, AND HE STOPS PERSPIRING). And I want you to *memorize this*, because you can *increase your breathing, and heart rate, and body temperature. And you can decrease them too* (STAN BEGINS TO NOD UNCONSCIOUSLY). And you didn't know you could do that just by thinking about it, did you? (STAN SHAKES HIS HEAD SLIGHTLY)."

Bill saw Stan a total of 13 times, and 10 of those sessions included hypnosis. Metaphors about playing golf were employed to help Stan use open and closed focus; metaphors about skiing and snowboarding were used to demonstrate that, in another context, Stan could fail, be uncon-cerned by the failure, get up, and try again. Each time, Bill watched Stan's face and observed minimal cues to learn whether he was following the metaphor and experiencing the emotions that would commonly be engendered by it. After using these metaphors, Stan was given a post-hypnotic suggestion that he could hold his hand as he would a golf club. This suggestion acted as a way to induce a light trance whenever Stan became nervous while speaking in public. He practiced this private cue during a number of sessions. Eventually he was able merely to put his thumb and forefinger together and achieve the same result of confidence and relaxation.

Stan's panic attacks ended almost immediately. However, he did not have a major presentation scheduled for some time and wanted to con-tinue therapy until he did. Prior to that, he attended a family reunion and experienced no discomfort. Each week Stan reported feeling more confident around his co-workers and was symptom-free in meetings where he had to discuss issues that had previously provoked discomfort. Eventually, Stan was scheduled to make a major presentation before his board of directors. His presentation went smoothly, without any signs of panic or anxiety. He told Bill that he actually enjoyed making the presen-tation, and they terminated therapy a couple weeks later. Bill contacted Stan 6 weeks after termination to check on him. Because of the distance he had to drive to come to the office, Bill interviewed him over the tele-phone. Stan was continuing to do well; he had had no panic attacks, and the fear of speaking before a large group had disappeared.

This case illustrates the disruption of a dysfunctional pattern of neu-ral activity, as evidenced by a state change. The hypnosis utilized prior experiences that had nothing to do with the goal but that had similar state occurrences. Bill intentionally elicited memories that were tied to particular brain states. This case is also an example of the fact that an individual may initially be unable to access what he or she already knows how to do. Everyone has experience in being curious, controlling pain, exercising persistence, being nurturing, managing anger, etc. Remembering how to elicit and use these states has been suppressed only because of learned limitations. Ericksonian hypnosis depotentiates these limitations by helping a person change states. By eliciting different states, we invite the person to make enduring brain state changes that he or she had not been able to do consciously. In trance, a person may also learn a needed new skill through a metaphorical intervention. Most metaphors suggest that life is a learning process. They tend to demonstrate that the more flexible a person is and the more a person can access needed states, the more he or she lives in states of thriving.

In the next chapter we consider the many ways in which brain technology equipment can help us teach our clients how to move to, and maintain, more comfortable, flexible, and enjoyable states of being.

CHAPTER 6

Utilizing Brain Technology Equipment

Even in the context of a warm and supportive environment, therapeutic words may not be powerful enough to surmount the effects of deep wounding and ingrained dysfunction. When the verbal interventions of BCT are insufficient to address symptomatic emotions and to effect needed neurological and behavioral change, we may supplement them with one or more of the new devices utilizing recent brain research. The following case demonstrates the introduction of brain technology with a person for whom verbal interventions were unable to sufficiently address her issue.

Leslie, a high school junior and already a promising harpist, experienced intense anxiety before every performance, at times becoming so extreme that she would shake uncontrollably. As Carol gently probed to learn more of her family situation, Leslie mentioned that her mother had abandoned an early career as a concert oboist when she married. "She never says anything, but I know she'd love it if I wound up in a major symphony." Regarding her performance anxiety, Leslie added, "Before each concert, all I can think of is that my mother will hear every mistake."

Carol's initial treatment plan included teaching Leslie to alter her state by slowing her breathing (inhaling to a count of 5 and exhaling to a count of 5) and by shifting her internal focus. In conversation with Carol, Leslie mentioned that as a child at her parents' beach house she had been fond of lying right at the edge of the ocean and letting the tide wash back and forth over her. This led to the practice of imaginary "ocean swinging" as a means for Leslie to shift states.

poly vagal would encourage an exhale longer than an inhale

Although Leslie's preperformance anxiety improved somewhat, it became clear that neither talking therapy nor client education would be able to do more than mitigate the anxiety. Because hypnosis was difficult for Leslie—she began to feel as if she were falling when she relaxed—Carol suggested alpha–theta training to divert attention away from the body and refocus it on the visual and auditory feedback. This type of training both reinforces the calm state and distracts the client from thoughts potentially leading to tension.

Alpha–theta training allowed Leslie to access a more relaxed and comfortable state (a taste of what was possible) and to experience several scenarios: breathing in tranquility, imagined as the scent of a beautiful flower; imagining her mother's face with her eyes closed and smiling as she feels the music; and looking for people in the audience who seem to be caught up in the music (at times when she was on stage but not playing). After approximately 15 sessions, Leslie reported that she had auditioned for a state-wide high school symphony—without any shaking. Beaming, she then said, "And I'm in!"

Using brain imaging to study the neural activity of Buddhist monks, yogis, and ordinary people, neuroscientists have developed a number of cutting-edge tools that can lead to a reduced stress threshold, better control of one's thoughts, and an increased ability to hold a selected brain-mind state. These include biofeedback, neurofeedback, and photic stimulation with binaural beats. In addition, a variety of specialized computer games are now available that help people develop particular psychocognitive skills, such as achieving and holding particular brain states, perceiving positive expressions, maintaining focus and concentration, enhancing memory functions, and relaxing.

Meditation

Sophisticated equipment is not necessarily required for sophisticated observation. Based on meticulously detailed observations, ancient Egyptian and Mayan astronomers were in possession of facts concerning the sun, planets, and other heavenly bodies that were only reconfirmed in the 20th century. Similarly, sophisticated exploration and training of human brain–mind capabilities has been going on for thousands of years, and only in the last 50 years has contemporary science begun to comprehend the abilities of those individuals long trained in various practices of meditation.

To facilitate state change, BCT makes use of simple meditation techniques such as slowing the breath and heart rate by focusing on a repetitive word or sound, breathing in to the count of 7 and out to the count of 7, and other methods that have proven to be powerful self-regulation strategies in dealing with stress-related issues. With training, the sympathetic nervous system can remain calm and the state of neural arousal remains low, even under potentially stressful experiences. Through meditation, individuals can develop the ability to reflect on their own feelings and behavior and overcome the tendency to react automatically to events. Self-awareness, mindfulness, or an attitude in line with what the great economist Adam Smith described as the "impartial spectator" helps a person observe events that would previously have engulfed him or her and led to reactive behavior (Rock & Schwartz, 2007b).

In studying happiness, Richard Davidson (2001) at the University of Wisconsin discovered that people had a happiness set point. That is, although external events might shift the level of happiness temporarily in one direction or another, people invariably returned to their default setting. As one would expect, people fell along a bell-shaped curve with respect to happiness; most were moderately happy most of the time. Changes in external circumstances would bump them in one direction or another, but they would return to the middle range. However, one person he measured was on the extreme end of the happiness scale. That was Matthieu Ricard, a Buddhist monk, who has been dubbed the "happiest person in the world" by popular media.

Richard Davidson wondered why Ricard was so happy and determined to study his brain with an fMRI. Davidson discovered that he could remain quite calm under experiences other people would typically find very stressful. Ricard's amygdala, which is the part of the brain that senses danger or anger, was quiet, as was the right prefrontal cortex. When there is significant activity in the amygdala, a person experiences anxiety or fear. Davidson posed the question: Was Ricard an anomaly or could other people experience the same calm neurological activity with meditation? That led Davidson to study other monks and, in them, he discovered a similar calm state.

Davidson then wondered if regular people in high-stress jobs could learn to change their brain activity with meditation. He worked with Jon Kabat-Zinn to design a program using Vipassana meditation (which emphasizes the observation of one's thoughts, sensations, and emotions without reactivity) for highly stressed employees at a chemical plant. The employees followed the program for 6 weeks and began to show neurological changes similar to those of the monks (Goleman, 2003).

Ricard suggested that it would be useful to study monks meditating on the themes of devotion and fearlessness. He described the meditation of fearlessness as "bringing to mind a fearless certainty, a deep confidence that nothing can unsettle—decisive and firm, without hesitating, where you're not adverse to anything. You enter into a state where you feel that, no matter what happens, 'I have nothing to gain, nothing to lose'" (Goleman, 2003, p. 6). Through this meditation, advanced practitioners achieve what Ricard called the "open state". He characterized it as "open, vast, and aware, with no intentional mental activity. The mind is not focused on anything, yet totally present—not in a focused way, just very open and undistracted. Thoughts may start to arise weakly, but they don't chain into longer thoughts—they just fade away" (p. 6). When an experiment was done to see if he could suppress the startle reflex, he was able to do so by being in the open state when a gun was fired next to his head.

Another study investigated the possible correlation between therapists who meditate and the therapeutic outcomes of their clients (Alvarez de Lorenzana, 2008). The study found that when a therapist has a quiet mind, he or she can notice more accurately what is happening, rather than overlaying a theory onto the client or reacting to what the client brings into the therapy session. As the therapist models better self-care, the client may replicate that behavior at home. Both of these factors contributed to improved outcomes.

If it is appropriate in terms of the therapeutic goals and a client is interested, Bill may teach a person how to meditate on compassion. This practice engenders a sense of connection and a feeling of safety while also promoting positive attachment and mental stability. One way of meditating on compassion, found in traditions of Tibetan Buddhism and mindfulness, is to sit quietly with closed eyes and direct a feeling of compassion first toward people whom you love, then toward neutral strangers, and finally toward people whom you do not like. The meditation is usually found to be calming and tends to reduce a person's judgmental attitudes. (Davidson & Lutz, 2008). Later, Bill might introduce meditating on a role model, such as a saint. If a person feels more comfortable using a style of meditation from his or her own tradition, Bill will teach that. For example, with a person who is at home in the Eastern Orthodox Christian tradition, Bill might encourage him or her to meditate on the Jesus prayer.

Along with meditation, it is also important to teach clients how to accept the impermanence of life and the inevitability of change. Some clients become depressed about being depressed. We suggest that depression or anxiety is not a static state and that it changes throughout the day. Learning to recognize more pleasant states as they occur is uplifting and encouraging for clients.

Bill worked with an attorney who had suffered for years from a debilitating obsessive–compulsive disorder. Bill encouraged him to meditate. As the client began to do so several times per week, his obsessive–compulsive symptoms were reduced in frequency and intensity. What he learned through meditation was not only to calm the brain but to allow thoughts to come and go without giving them any meaning. His state of tension reduced dramatically. When a person performs a compulsive act in order to reduce tension, the relief is only temporary. Using meditation, the obsessive thoughts driving the compulsion abate. We often explain to clients that thoughts are only electrical activity that often signify nothing unless a client gives them meaning. The more the attorney was able to observe his obsessive thoughts without giving them meaning, the less frequently they occurred. Through this practice he also became more insightful and self-aware.

Biofeedback

Biofeedback encompasses a variety of techniques for training the autonomic nervous system (part of the peripheral nervous system) by feeding back information regarding a client's physiological condition. For example, by watching a computer display showing a person's moment-to-moment skin temperature or heart rate, a client can learn to influence physiological processes that were previously unconscious, such as heart rate variability and skin temperature.

Using biofeedback, we teach clients to moderate the fight–flight–freeze response. When the thalamus perceives a threat, the endocrine and sympathetic nervous systems activate and concomitant physiological changes occur, which may include increased breathing, increased blood pressure, muscle tension, decreased skin temperature, and the elevation of slow or rapid brain frequencies. The adrenal glands begin pumping out adrenaline, epinephrine, and norepinephrine, which can impair immune function, digestion, and tissue repair (Demos, 2005).

Among the types of biofeedback are feedback of skin temperature, galvanic skin response (GSR), and muscle biofeedback. GSR measures changes in skin conductivity. Under threat, the sweat glands on the hands tend to produce saline perspiration; moisture increases electrical conductivity. Temperature biofeedback can be used to teach a client how to regulate finger temperature. Under threat, blood tends to pool in the center of the body, and the extremities become cold. Clients experiencing anxiety frequently have cold hands. By learning to increase the blood flow to his or her hands, the client not only interrupts the physiological pattern (constriction of blood flow to the extremities), but also quiets the internal feedback loop from the extremities back to the brain, instead of reinforcing it. Temperature training is also used for headaches, Raynaud's disease (decreased blood flow, especially to the hands and/or feet), and hypertension. Muscle biofeedback can be useful when patients are unconsciously tensing muscles and creating problems, as in temporal mandibular joint (TMJ) problems.

Whether clients are learning to relax specific muscles, regulate their heart rate variability, or alter the temperature of a finger, in most cases, the primary *state change* is from anxiety to calmness. Having achieved this shift in the office, the client can remember the physiological sensations of calmness, generalize the learning to other situations, and replicate the sensations. In family therapy, this is especially helpful for parents to learn, both to help calm them about their children and to encourage them, as role models, to exhibit calmness.

With continued practice, feedback that is given for the alteration of certain physiological functions can be generalized to the resolution or mastery of life issues. Using biofeedback, one young woman who entered therapy to deal with severe test anxiety learned how to raise her finger temperature. We explained to her that memory and learning are state dependent and suggested that, when taking an exam, in order to retrieve the information she had learned, she needed to return to the calm state she was normally in while studying. Having learned to control the temperature in her finger, she was able to envision mastering other, more encompassing physiological states, such as calmness even in a situation that had previously been highly stressful. By the end of the semester, she was capable of maintaining a calm state during her final exams, a significant shift from her original feeling that her brain "froze" due to anxiety.

Some clients, after having addressed the symptoms that brought them into therapy, terminate fairly soon; fixing the symptom seems adequate. But often, those clients will return later to deal with an underlying or related issue. Or, having experienced change and becoming curious about what further improvement might be possible, they will continue until they find themselves experiencing states of thriving for longer periods of time. For example, as one client's freeway driving phobia abated, he realized that he also wanted to overcome his fear of flying. So he continued in therapy and began to clear up many related problems; eventually he started to practice developing states of happiness during his sessions and then outside the office.

Neurofeedback

A subset of biofeedback is neurofeedback, also known as EEG biofeedback, which specifically trains the CNS. This is done using scalp electrodes (some instruments use a cap rather than individual electrodes; some are now wireless) and computer software that monitors brain waves and turns on a light, plays a sound, or runs a game as long as the client's brain continues to function within set parameters. Although the technology has existed for over 30 years, research is only now suggesting that this approach is a powerful alternative to medical avenues for eliminating anxiety, depression, attention disorders, sleep disorders, immune problems, and epileptic seizures (Othmer, 2009).

Dysfunctional neural patterns may be genetic, learned, acquired suddenly during trauma, or developed gradually under long periods of stress. Regardless of their origin, the purpose of neurofeedback is to effect rapid electrical and (as a corollary) chemical changes to an individual's brain in order to alter or extinguish the dysfunctional patterns and stabilize new ones. Changes in affect, attitude, and behavior occur through the stimulation of some frequencies and the suppression of others, a process that engenders brain stability with new neural configurations.

almost
(R)
brain tx

Most psychotherapeutic approaches work from the premise "Talk about it and you will feel better"; neurofeedback operates from the assumption "Feel better and you will talk about it." Because of this difference, neurofeedback is often able to help those for whom other mental health interventions have not been successful. When used in conjunction with learning how to change states outside the office setting, a person can experience more frequent and consistent states of thriving.

For example, beta training of the sensorimotor rhythm (SMR) between 12 and 15 Hz is a physiological intervention that strengthens sensorimotor activation in the cortex and inhibits patterns that may slow brain functioning. In the treatment of attention-deficit/hyperactivity disorder (ADHD), research has shown significant efficacy using beta training, as recorded near the sensorimotor cortex. More recently, neurofeedback has been expanded to include "deep states" or alpha–theta training in the treatment of anxiety, alcoholism, and other addictions. We have also found this useful for weight loss, anxiety reduction, and resolving traumatic memories.

Additionally, neurofeedback is a powerful tool for deeply exploring one's true self. For example, over time, a mind obsessively fretting and imagining "the worst" becomes conditioned, and then locked, into inflexible styles of thinking and chronic anxiety. These attentional or emotional states are narrow, habitual, and lead eventually to physical and mental stress and burnout (Fehmi & Robbins, 2007). Correlated with these habituated attentional styles and behavioral pathologies are particular EEG signatures. Once these signatures are recognized and the individual learns to change them through gradual reinforcement of more appropriate brain waves, a more flexible emotional state and range of satisfying behaviors can occur.

Most clients can benefit from brain training (although it is generally contraindicated for those who fall along the continuum of autistic disorders and may not be able to sit comfortably in front of a computer monitor with electrical leads on their heads). At times, neurofeedback can promote a dramatic turnaround in a client's life.

Rachel spent much of her time depressed and in tears. Beneath her depression was a smoldering anger directed at her husband, whom she was only steps away from divorcing. His primary fault, she reported, was that he spent too much time in the garage making golf clubs. Based on a QEEG evaluation, Bill worked with her using SMR training. After the first session, she noticed very little change. However, following the second session, Rachel was not as weepy the rest of the week. During the week after her third session, her mood lifted dramatically, and she was able to observe that her tears had nothing to do with her husband. In fact, during her next session, she began to recount all the good things her husband had done. After about 40 sessions of neurofeedback, Rachel's mood was consistently happy and she was again in love with her husband.

In tandem with a client's internist or neurologist, we can do brain training to ameliorate many medical issues. Strongly implicated in Rachel's distress were the hormonal imbalances related to menopause. The brain is involved not only in regulating hormone levels, but with a sudden shift in hormone levels will display a corresponding shift in brain waves. For example, a hot flash is reflected in an EEG, with the amplitudes becoming quite high during its course. We cannot stop the natural process of menopause itself, but we can significantly mitigate some of its symptoms. Hot flashes and night sweats have been reported to cease for weeks with a few sessions using Cygnet Neurofeedback Software (discussed later in this chapter). In another case, using SMR training, we treated a young girl with epileptic seizures to the extent that her seizures stopped.

By working to change brain wave patterns, neurofeedback can also assist clients in breaking through defenses, changing belief patterns, loosening inflexible perceptions, and allowing them to make better use of the therapeutic interaction. Neurofeedback can facilitate changes in many domains, including the quality of attention, motivation, affect, attitudes, behavior, and understanding of the client. Additionally, many clients report benefits such as less mental chatter, greater mood stabilization, less concern with "trying to achieve," and more focus on developing an improved quality of life.

One of the speculations coming out of neurofeedback research is that emotional and behavioral dysfunctions reflect brain disorganization in the domains of timing and frequency. Neurofeedback technology actually has the capacity to restructure brain functioning (which involves these two key elements of timing and frequency) through attention training. Farmer (2002) noted: "We are beginning to understand that brain rhythms, their synchronization and desynchronization, form an important and possibly fundamental part of the orchestration of perception, motor action, and conscious experience, and that disruption of oscillation and/or temporal synchronization may be a fundamental mechanism of neurological disease" (p. 1176). Based on this understanding, neurofeedback is also being used to help athletes and artists achieve peak performance. And more good news: Its use can contribute to optimal aging (Budzynski, Budzynski, & Tang, 2006).

Light Technologies

BCT makes use of recently developed equipment that combines light (photic) and sound (aural) stimulation. However, the therapeutic use of flickering light dates at least back to the early 20th century. Pierre Janet, a pioneering French psychotherapist, noted that when he had patients gaze at the light of a kerosene lantern, filtered through the spindles of a turning wheel, their symptoms of depression, tension, and hysteria were reduced (Pieron, 1982). In the 1920s and 1930s, Dr. Harry Spitler, a physician and optometrist, experimented with flashing colored light into the eyes to correct visual problems. In the 1940s, Dr. Gray Walker, a British physician, discovered that the brain's dominant frequency tends to become entrained by a flickering light.

More recently, flashing colored light has been shown to affect or "drive" the brain in specific ways. Komatsu (1987) found that there is a relationship between the color of the flickering lights and the evoked brain wave response. In a study of college students, flashing red light drove the 17–18 Hz band of brain waves, whereas green increased 15 Hz waves, and blue stimulated 10–13 Hz waves. Similar results were found with the Lumatron, a device that beams light directly to the brain through the eyes. Red light stimulated brain waves above 15 Hz, yellow drove 13 Hz, and green drove 10.5 Hz; blue light increased 9 Hz, and indigo/violet drove the theta and delta frequencies (Breiling, 1996). Amber light (between red and yellow) stimulated activation at 14 Hz and was found to be "warmer" and more pleasant than red (Austin, 1991). EEGs show that the brain also responds to steady colored light. Researchers found that the alpha amplitude is suppressed when subjects are exposed to red light as opposed to blue and concluded that red light tends to increase vigilance (Ali, 1972).

Frequency-specific flickering lights can also entrain brain waves. A light flickering at 8–12 Hz can induce an alpha state. Shealy (1990) reported that 88 of 92 patients with chronic pain experienced both pain relief and relaxation after 30-minute sessions during which the 10 Hz rhythm was stimulated. Budzynski (1999; Budzynski & Sherlin, 2002) and Fahrion (1995) reported that using 3–7 Hz in photic stimulation resulted in an extremely calm feeling that lasted 3–4 days after the session. In addition, migraine headaches have successfully been treated by Anderson (1989), who used red light-emitting diodes (LEDs) to stimulate the optic nerve with frequencies between 0.5 and 50 Hz.

EEG-driven stimulation is a type of neurofeedback that involves monitoring and analyzing EEG signals read through surface electrodes on the scalp and then using the EEG itself to guide low-intensity light stimulation. The EEG signals influence the stimulation, which in turn changes the EEG pattern. For example, the flashing lights are set either to lead or lag the dominant brain wave by some fixed amount—say, 5 Hz— meaning that the lights always flash 5 Hz faster (or slower) than the dominant brain frequency. This stimulation tends to prod the dominant frequency into a slightly higher or lower range.

Patrick (1996) reported on the effectiveness of using photic stimulation in just 15 sessions for attention problems. When the light stimulation is presented, there is a slight brain response in the EEG, where there is an event-related potential (ERP). This ERP is an indication of brain response to the stimulation. The research suggests that repetitive stimulation tends to improve attention and reduce pain (Kikuchi, 2002) as the EEG begins to respond at the same frequency as the stimulation (Trudeau, 1999).

Sound Therapy

Like light, rhythmic sound can also be used to entrain brain waves. For example, Tibetan Buddhist chanting entrains the brain in theta rhythm, in which people may experience rejuvenation, "flashes" of intuition, or suddenly grasp an understanding of relationships or ideas.

Binaural beat frequencies, first discovered in 1839 by the Prussian physicist and meteorologist Heinrich Wilhelm Dove, have been used for years to alter consciousness. Binaural beats are auditory brainstem responses that occur in the superior olivary nucleus of each hemisphere.

They result from the brain's integration of two auditory impulses, originating in opposite ears and differing just slightly in frequency. The human ability to "hear" binaural beats appears to be the result of evolutionary adaptation and is one mechanism used by the brain in audio direction finding.

The beat frequency is usually "carried" by another frequency of less than 1,000 Hz. For example, a 10 Hz alpha wave beat is caused by a difference of 10 Hz between two "pure" frequencies, one resonating at 400 Hz and another at 410 Hz. When auditory signals are presented to the brain with slight phase differences, the brain can detect the difference, although the listener does not consciously hear it.

Resonant entrainment of oscillating systems is well understood within the physical sciences. If a tuning fork that produces a frequency of, say, 800 Hz is struck (causing it to vibrate or oscillate) and then brought into the vicinity of another 800 Hz tuning fork, the second tuning fork will begin to oscillate. In this case, the first tuning fork has entrained the second. Entrainment can also occur in biosystems, including the entrainment of electromagnetic brain waves. Neural entrainment is defined as any instance in which an EEG reflects the brain wave frequency duplicating that of a stimulus, be it audio, visual, or tactile (Siever, 2004). Binaural beats can be used to entrain specific neural rhythms through the frequency-following response (FFR; Moushegian, 1978)—that is, the tendency for cortical potentials, as evidenced through brain waves recorded by EEG, to entrain to the frequency of an external stimulus. Based on this, it has been shown that a specific binaural beat frequency can be used to entrain the cortical rhythm to that frequency. Binaural beats can be readily perceived at frequencies below 30 Hz, which are characteristic of the EEG spectrum (Oster, 1973).

Binaural beats have also been found to synchronize the two hemispheres of the brain because both ears send neural signals to the olivary nuclei (sound-processing center) in both hemispheres of the brain. Therefore, when a binaural beat is perceived, there are actually two identical beats perceived, one in each of the two hemispheres. In this way, the binaural beats promote hemispheric synchronization similar to that observed in meditative and hypnogogic states of consciousness. Binaural beats have been used to enhance the learning process, promote relaxation, improve memory (Kennerly, 1994), stimulate creativity, and assist the onset of sleep (Hiew, 1995).

Combining Sound and Light Therapy

Any given frequency of stimulation that can be reflected in brain wave activity and is observable on an EEG or QEEG can be "driven" (meaning, the brain can be induced to entrain to that frequency) using flickering light, sound waves, or a combination of the two. The combination of photic and aural stimulation, now formally called audiovisual stimulation (AVS) or audiovisual entrainment (AVE), is the basis for the functionality of many neurofeedback devices used in BCT.

The use of AVS has been shown to effectively relax people who exhibit high sympathetic activation and/or traumatic states of mind by bringing a return to homeostasis. Siever (2000) suggests that AVS achieves its effects through several mechanisms simultaneously, including dissociation, an increase in neurotransmitters, possible increase in dendritic growth, altered cerebral blood flow, and normalized EEG activity. Particularly if the flickering occurs in the alpha–theta band, an individual is likely to go into a state of hypnosis. Subsequent research has shown that using photic and aural stimulation to effect brain entrainment, and thereby engender various states of consciousness, may have potential not only for a therapeutic goal of relaxation but also for healing certain mental and physical conditions (Siever, 2004).

Many AVS devices make therapeutic use of two physiological facts. One is that light is processed contralaterally: Light entering the right visual field of both eyes is transmitted as neural stimulation to the left side of the brain, and light entering the left visual field of both eyes is transmitted as neural stimulation to the right side of the brain. Signals move from rods and cones in the ganglion cells to the optic nerve and then to the brain. The network of nerves called the *optic chiasm* sends images from the left visual fields of both eyes to the right lateral geniculate and then to the cortex, and vice versa. The second fact is that the human brain naturally switches hemispheric dominance, on average, every few seconds. The tenor of the left hemisphere is more upbeat and expansive, more focused at the macro level; the tenor of the right hemisphere is more downbeat and contained, more involved with the details. Recent studies suggest a correlation between slower-than-average switching rates and bipolar disorder. One hypothesis is that, in bipolar swings, the brain tends to get "stuck" or linger in one state over the other (Pettigrew & Miller, 1998).

Harold Russell (1997a, 1997b) conducted a study using photic and aural stimulation with boys who had learning disabilities, ages 8–12. The pulsed light was varied every 2 minutes between 10 and 18 Hz. Aural stimulation at the same frequency accompanied the pulsed lights. The researchers reported significant increases in the boys' intelligence, as measured by the Raven IQ test, and increases in their ability to sustain attention and inhibit impulsive behaviors, as measured by the teacher-completed Attention Deficit Disorders Evaluation Scale. Russell (1997a) patented hardware and software for further work and conducted several studies with their equipment. All of the studies found an increase in intelligence measures and an improvement in behavior. Using the EEG, earlier studies had found hypoperfusion (lack of blood flow) and an associated increase in the theta band (4–8 Hz) at certain brain locations in individuals with attention-deficit disorder (ADD) as well as in elderly people (Alexander & Schneider, 1996; Celsis, 1997). Russell reported that auditory and photic stimulation, used repetitively, induced changes in EEG frequency, increases in glucose and oxygen metabolism, an increase in cerebral blood flow, and changes in brain chemistry (Russell, 1997a, 1997b).

The periodical *Alternative Therapies* published a systematic review and analysis by Huang and Charyton (2008) of 20 of the major studies done on brainwave entrainment using photic stimulation, aural stimulation, or a combination of the two to improve cognition or treat stress, anxiety, pain, headaches and migraines, mood, and premenstrual syndrome (PMS). The authors summarized:

> Preliminary evidence suggests that alpha stimulation was preferable for trigram recognition, short-term stress, and pain relief, whereas beta was used to enhance attention, increase overall intelligence, relieve short-term stress, and improve behavior. The alternating alpha and beta protocol was used successfully to improve behavior, verbal skills, and attention. A protocol that alternatively ascended and descended from beta to gamma enhanced arithmetic skills and attention. A protocol that alternated between 14 and 22 Hz increased overall intelligence. Several protocols, including a combination of theta and delta and a progressive slowing over 30 minutes to delta, were effective in relieving short-term stress. Migraines were prevented with a 30-Hz stimulus that alternated between left and right hemispheres, and a few studies that allowed the subject to choose the frequency of

stimulation were successful in alleviating long-term stress, pain, and migraines. However, this review concluded that research had yet to prove the effectiveness of brain wave entrainment for addressing mood issues. (Huang & Charyton, 2008, p. 48)

A pilot study reported by David Cantor (2007) at the annual conference of the EEG and Clinical Neuroscience Society suggested that the research to support such a conclusion may be forthcoming. The pilot study included 16 patients with a mean age of 45 years who had a long history of refractory depression that was minimally responsive to medication. Patients were required to stop all medications one month prior to the start of the study. Half of the group received 20 minutes of AVE therapy daily for 4 weeks at a frequency of 14 Hz. The other eight patients wore the AVE equipment for 4 weeks but did not get the stimulation treatment. After 4 weeks, testing revealed a significant decrease in self-reported depression scores in the treatment group and no change in the untreated group. QEEG testing also showed neurophysiological changes in the treated patients (but not the untreated group) that corresponded to their reports of improved mood. The groups were then reversed, so that the untreated group received treatment, and vice versa, for the next 4 weeks. Similar results were noted in the newly treated group, and the group that had received the first phase of treatment showed a sustained effect of treatment, both behaviorally and neurophysiologically, even 4 weeks after discontinuation (Cantor, 2007).

Devices Facilitating Brainwave Entrainment, Neurofeedback, and Biofeedback

Many companies now offer brainwave entrainment devices, biofeedback and neurofeedback equipment, and various software products suitable for professional use. Of those currently on the market, we discuss a few that we feel are representative of each general type of equipment and are among the "best of breed."

Neurofeedback certification and licensure requirements vary from state to state. The therapist who considers integrating any of these feedback devices into his or her practice may wish to look into the various professional societies, such as the Biofeedback Certification Institute of America, the International Society for Neurofeedback and Research

(ISNR) and the Association for Applied Psychophysiology and Biofeedback, which provide treatment standards for using these approaches.

The DAVID PAL Device

The DAVID PAL (Digital Audio-Visual Integration Device—Portable and Lightweight) equipment combines flashes of lights and tone pulses to effect brainwave entrainment. The manufacturer's specifications note that the equipment is about the size of a mobile phone, plus headphone and eyeset (wraparound "eyeshades"). It includes 18 preprogrammed protocols for a variety of brainwave stimulation sessions, including (1) a brain "brightener" (for ADD and cognition); (2) fractionation hypnosis (the process of moving in and out and then back into trance in order to deepen the trance state); (3) an alpha–beta mix (for depression); (4) Schumann resonances (specific very low frequencies) with dissociation and heart rate variability (for meditation); (5) a beta "perker"; and (6) theta (for improved sleeping).

To disperse the light evenly, the eyesets for the DAVID PAL use eight blue-tinted white LEDs mounted over a silver reflector behind a translucent screen. The eyesets allow the left and right visual fields of each eye to be stimulated separately. The lights flash alternately into the left visual fields of both eyes and then into the right visual fields of both eyes. This alternation makes it possible to stimulate the two visual cortices differentially. For example, a person who functions strongly from the left brain might receive 8 Hz in the right visual field (and therefore the left brain) to slow down left-brain function and receive 18 Hz in the left visual field to increase right-brain function.

The DAVID PAL has three types of sound output: isochronic pulsed tones, monaural beats, and binaural beats. To enhance the effectiveness of audio entrainment, the *isochronic pulsed tones* are evenly spaced, of equal pitch, and are turned on and off at a specified rate. The *monaural beats* are similar to the isochronic pulsed tones, but turn on and off more gently and therefore are smoother, fuller beats. This pattern is recommended for those who find the pulse tones too stimulating. The *binaural beats* are two pure tones (one in each ear) that are perceived as a beat.

The DAVID PAL has no input function. It does not track the user's brainwaves, heart rate variability, or other biological data. With only output functions (the various protocols), it has no capacity to modify its output based on such data; however, there is a version of the DAVID PAL that can be programmed to individual specifications. We have found it helpful for clients to take the DAVID PAL equipment home and use it in between formal neurofeedback sessions at the office. We have also used it with people to stop food and alcohol cravings while they work with us.

One client, deeply grieving after the death of her father, began to drink wine excessively. As her drinking grew increasingly serious, her husband became extremely upset and finally demanded that either she had to stop drinking or he would leave her. She did not want to put her marriage at risk, but she had great difficulty stopping and would deal with stress at the end of the day by sneaking a glass of wine. We suggested that she purchase the DAVID PAL and use it before she had any wine. Eventually, her desire to drink disappeared and her marriage remained intact.

Another woman, who had tried all kinds of diets in vain, still desperately wanted to lose weight. Strongly suspicious that this tool was just like all the other diet "tricks" she had tried, she purchased the DAVID PAL and began to use it at work before she ate junk food. Her desire for sugar and carbohydrates diminished significantly; she lost over 80 pounds and kept it off for many years.

The ROSHI Neurofeedback System

The ROSHI® combines photic and aural stimulation with a neurofeedback system. The device was created by Chuck Davis in conjunction with Ray Wolfe of Photosonix. Davis said that he was inspired to design this device by the state of healing and regeneration naturally achieved by meditating monks. Using the ROSHI, an individual can increase brain metabolism and blood flow, experience improved concentration, and stay in the "zone."

The ROSHI monitors how the brain is responding to the stimulation and modifies its output in response. For example, it can be set to follow the dominant frequency of the brain and change as the frequency changes. The unique aspect of the ROSHI is what Davis calls its "complex adaptive" visual stimulation (Olesen, 2004):

> The raw EEG is fed through an algorithm that treats the complex EEG as "chaos" and modulates the LEDs accordingly. Thus the intensities of the lights are constantly "adapting" to neuronal conditions in real-

time. What the user sees in the light goggles is a complex, constantly changing flicker, based on changes in his or her own brainwaves. It's like the brain "seeing" itself. (p. 4)

The ROSHI can both entrain brainwaves and disentrain them. For example, it can reduce certain frequencies, such as the slow frequencies associated with ADD, as well as increase desired frequencies. Davis suggested that this process encourages the brain to discard old patterns and develop flexibility (Davis, personal communication, September 18, 1999). The changes occur at an unconscious level, thereby circumventing any conscious resistance such as might occur in any other psychotherapeutic approach. Research by D. Corydon Hammond (2007) on the treatment of clients with depression has shown the ROSHI to be effective in cases that were resistant to more conventional treatments. Other applications for the ROSHI include the treatment of anxiety, strokes, headaches, bipolar disorder, age-related cognitive slowing, and brain injuries. The ROSHI is also used in training for peak performance, for example, by training the brain at 40 Hz. This frequency is being researched in terms of its relevance to experiences of transcendence in which people have reported feeling at one with the universe.

The LENS

The LENS (Low Energy Neurofeedback System), developed by Len Ochs in the early 1990s, is a neurofeedback system used to treat CNS problems. Different from traditional neurofeedback systems, the LENS equipment is designed to both map a client's brain (standard EEG) and to deliver minute electromagnetic impulses as short as one second to 19 different scalp locations simultaneously. Utilizing the same wires that carry the brainwaves to the amplifier and computer, the LENS software generates the feedback based on the EEG signals that it records. Feedback occurs in the form of a radio frequency carrier wave, administered at a positive offset frequency from the person's own dominant EEG frequency, or the one highest in amplitude, using a 19- or 21-site topographic brain map. The electromagnetic feedback is of such low intensity that, although the brain perceives it, it is not consciously perceived by the client. However, when exposed to this feedback frequency, the EEG amplitude distribution shifts in power and ultimately improves the brain's ability to regulate itself.

The system does not require the client to pay attention and is efficacious even if the client has difficulty sitting still. It can be used with other neurofeedback devices or alone as the case demands. Hammond (2007) said that the LENS has been shown "to produce rapid resolution of difficult cognitive, mood, anxiety, clarity, energy, movement, and pain problems when compared with more traditional forms of psychotherapy or medication treatment" (p. 8).

Cygnet Neurofeedback Software

Cygnet software is a suite of functionalities including EEG training, hemoencephalography training, and alpha–theta training. The software works with a digitizing device that measures EEG signals, performs real-time analysis of the signals, and controls feedback devices such as video, audio, games, and tactile systems based on rules defined by the therapist. Cygnet is a two-component training system, involving both a reward function focusing on a particular EEG frequency and an inhibit function that operates on the EEG broadly. The inhibit function is handled in the background entirely by the software. The clinician only selects the overall level of difficulty to match the client's needs and retains full control of the reward frequency. The system's basic configuration is that it runs on one computer with two screen displays. The main screen, (therapist screen) displays the Cygnet user interface and allows the therapist to access all the software functions. The second screen (client screen) shows the feedback via video display (i.e., video player, DVD player, or flash game). In essence, this software supports *multiuser feedback in real time*—both client and therapist simultaneously respond to feedback provided by the software and thereby "drive" the program. The Cygnet software is also capable of controlling a tactile feedback device (Cygnet, 2008).

emWAVE and Heart Rate Variability Training

The healthy heart speeds up with every in-breath and slows down with every out-breath. Plotted over time, the variation generates a pattern called heart rate variability (HRV). The degree of HRV is an important indicator of an individual's resiliency and flexibility under stress.

The research team at the Institute of HeartMath (IHM) has demonstrated that combining intentional heart focus with sustained positive feelings leads to what they have termed physiological coherence in HRV. This coherence is associated with a sine wave-like pattern in the heart rhythms, an increase in parasympathetic activity, greater heart–brain synchronization, and the entrainment of various physiological systems. In physiological coherence, the body's systems function with an efficient harmony, and healing processes are facilitated. When an individual experiences stress or negative emotions such as anxiety, despair, or frustration, HRV becomes less coherent or orderly (McCraty, 2002).

The IHM has developed the emWave device to train HRV by controlling the breath. The biofeedback training involves a shift in breathing to slow respiration and to generate steady and even heartbeats. Accompanying this practice is an emotional shift accomplished by attending to the heart and holding a positive feeling toward someone or something. This shift in focus is followed by having the user imagine breathing through the heart. What is achieved is a degree of coherence in which emotional stability, self-regulation, and states of well-being are better maintained (McCraty, 2008).

The emWave equipment comes in two versions: as software that can be loaded onto a desktop or laptop computer with a pulse sensor that plugs into a USB port and clips to the user's ear, or as a small stand-alone, handheld device with a thumb sensor or optional ear clip. The desktop version has greater capabilities in terms of graphic display, interactive exercises, and training games; the handheld version can be carried and used during potentially stressful situations. We use both versions of the equipment. The desktop version can serve as an important diagnostic tool during the initial assessment with clients who have rapid heart rates and are often anxious. In later sessions, we use it therapeutically for clients with anxiety issues. Once the person has a solid experiential sense of the calm state, it can be practiced outside the office. In marital therapy sessions, we may give one of the handheld models to each partner to assist them both in better managing their physiological arousal as we all work together. When both partners practice calming techniques, issues of conflicts often can be worked out without negative emotions taking over.

On our recommendation, the parents of an active 5-year-old daughter with serious discipline problems purchased an emWave device for her. Working with us, she learned to slow her breathing, and her family continued to help her practice with the device at home. She enjoyed the game quality of the emWave and began to generalize the breathing techniques to her everyday situations. As she learned how to calm herself, the dynamics of the entire family system began to shift. As a result, the tenor of the parent–child interactions evolved from often being somewhat adversarial to being generally cooperative.

Another client, having difficulty with high blood pressure, was highly motivated to use the emWave daily. By learning to control her level of arousal, she dropped her blood pressure from 147/100 to 110/80. We strongly suggested that she continue to check her pressure at least once daily and consult her physician if she noticed it starting to rise.

Relaxing Rhythms

Relaxing Rhythms (formerly called Healing Rhythms) is a biofeedback-based training program that teaches techniques of deep breathing and meditation using biofeedback. The software package includes a USB-based biofeedback reader, a device that attaches to three fingers and measures HRV and skin conductance. In this program, experts in the field of wellness, including medical doctors Deepak Chopra, Dean Ornish, and Andrew Weil, guide the user through 15 lessons designed to teach relaxation and stress management. The software allows the user to select either guided instruction or to go directly to interactive exercises, called "energy events," such as learning to juggle balls with laughter, build a stairway using breath, and meditate to open doors.

Journey to the Wild Divine

Journey to the Wild Divine is a biofeedback-based system in a computer game format suitable for adults but also for children as young as 5. It uses the same type of biofeedback device and covers the same content as the Relaxing Rhythms software. The first game, "The Journey to Wild Divine: The Passage," encourages the user to explore a fantasy landscape of gardens, cottages, and temples by learning the yogic breathing and meditation skills necessary to complete 40 biofeedback energy events, including levitating golden orbs and releasing a falcon from a cage. The visual confirmation of mastery provides effective reinforcement of newly learned behaviors.

The second title in the series, "The Journey to Wild Divine: Wisdom Quest," offers a deepening of the relaxation skills practiced in the earlier software. In the "Game Quest" mode, the user can travel through the "Sun Realm" in search of seven precious stones that promote inner peace in the "Realm" and in the user. The "Guided Activity" mode features 20 advanced interactive activities for mind–body training. Also, Wisdom Quest allows the user to select the difficulty level for each activity.

MindHabits Trainer

MindHabits Trainer is a suite of four video games designed to train states of self-esteem by limiting attention to social rejection and conditioning attention to social acceptance responses (Dandeneau & Baldwin, 2004; Dandeneau, Baldwin, Baccus, Sakellaropoulo, & Pruessner, 2007). Often, with social anxiety, clients unconsciously tend to search out cues that they construe as indicative of rejection. To maintain positive states, a person needs to develop a mind frame that ignores rejection and looks for acceptance.

Researchers at McGill University in Canada found that cortisol was reduced by 17% in people who played a game designed to have users notice smiling faces and ignore negative facial expressions for 5 minutes a day. Subjects also reported feeling happier and having a reduced tendency to scan the environment for negative responses to themselves. Stress reduction and self-confidence are achieved through accessing positive states and their accompanying automatic thought patterns. Although more studies are needed, the early research suggests that when clients play this game several minutes each day, their positive focus is conditioned throughout the day (Dandeneau & Baldwin, 2004; Dandeneau, Baldwin, Baccus, Sakellaropoulo, & Pruessner, 2007). The game can be a helpful training adjunct between therapeutic sessions.

Integrating Brain-Training Devices into Treatment with Adults

Only rarely are brain-training devices the primary therapeutic intervention, although we do occasionally have referrals for just neurofeedback when the client has another therapist. Usually, however, the devices are used as an adjunct to the more encompassing therapeutic relationship in which the clinician models both outward styles of behavior and patterns of positive neurobehavior for the client. Nonetheless, they can play an important role in the therapeutic encounter. The majority of brain training is done on the Cygnet device. This is used for ADD, depression, anxiety, and chronic pain when psychotherapy cannot fully address these issues. For mild anxiety and stress, we use the emWave device so that clients can literally see that they have the ability to be in charge of the body. We recommend the DAVID PAL and the MindHabits game for home training; these tools allow clients to practice changing states and reaching the target state. Beyond the fact that brain training devices are intrinsically functional in helping a client to shape brain behavior, they bring two other elements to the therapeutic process: They give the client a *visible* degree of control over the therapeutic outcome, and their sheer novelty activates the circuit of curiosity, which promotes learning.

As an example of a brain-training device functioning at a metalevel as well as fulfilling its intended application, we once worked with a young man who had inherited $13 million when he was 18 years old. Because of that, Roger lacked the motivation to go to school, study anything, or develop any employable skills; he had no life goals. However, he was quite depressed and suffered from frequent and severe headaches. As we explored the circumstances of Roger's life, initially the only motivations we could tap were in relation to reducing his depression and his headaches. Finding the motivation for change is imperative in being able to activate appropriate neural circuits. Because headaches are often successfully addressed with biofeedback, we started there. Roger became amazed that he could get rid of his worst migraine headaches using biofeedback equipment. That amazement then fueled a curiosity about what else he might be capable of doing, not only in terms of biofeedback but in other endeavors, and eventually he began to be more curious about the wider possibilities in his life.

The use of a brain-training device may also help create an emotional opening to further work with a client who is otherwise resistant to any self-examination. For example, some clients firmly believe that a relationship problem completely rests with the other person. The unconsciously conveyed message is a projection of blame without any evaluation of the client's potential part in a dysfunctional interaction. Frequently in such a case, the client needs someone outside him- or herself to lower his or her state of arousal before he or she will be able to "hear" any other perspective. For the client to change states of arousal, the therapist must help him or her feel understood and focus on the intent of the other person's behavior rather than on the effect. However, coaching this client to change states in a direct manner may have poor results.

Complicating this dynamic is the therapist's countertransference, which may be an accurate representation of how other people in the family respond to the client. The therapist needs to note his or her own reaction, calm his or her emotions, and step back to question whether there might be a positive or benign intent in the midst of the client's troublesome blaming behavior. Often, after hearing such an explanation, the client will calm down and be able to change states, because his or her feelings have been acknowledged. As an example, the therapist might say: "I am concerned about the amount of stress you are experiencing with your husband and daughter. I don't want to see you be eaten alive by this circumstance." If the client responds positively with signs of lowered arousal, then the therapist might say: "How can you protect yourself from these conflicts so that you do not become a scapegoat? And so that you do not end up so stressed, let me suggest a brain technology to help you manage your stress levels better." As the client's arousal levels come down, he or she may be open to looking at his or her part in the interactions.

Using Brain-Training Devices with Children

We have worked with several children who were diagnosed as having ADD and who have been able to either lower or eliminate medication. We have found the emWave especially effective for children who present with school anxiety. To help children learn state change, we also use the Journey to Wild Divine in its game mode in the office and recommend it for home use. When the family is relatively functional and does not overreact to the child's behavior, we can work primarily with the child to improve his or her neurological patterning. When the parents are reacting intensely because the child is inattentive, doing poorly in school, and perhaps lacking inhibitory ability, we may also find it necessary to "coach" the parents.

If parents simply want to drop a child off to be "fixed," we may introduce neurofeedback fairly early in the therapeutic work with the child—who usually enjoys the video game aspect of it. However, we attempt to engage the parents as much as possible. Lubar, Swartwood, Swartwood, and O'Donnell (1995) extensively studied the use of EEG biofeedback with children and adults who have ADD or ADHD and find that a child who has been doing well using neurofeedback that then goes home to a dysfunctional system will lose some ground by the next session. Our experience has been similar. Every child is part of a family system; changing any one element in it—the child, for example—does begin to shift the entire system. To the extent possible, addressing levels of arousal and resulting behaviors in the entire family system is far more effective.

Matthew, for example, had a severe reading disability and very poor academic performance. His parents had already taken him to every learning center in Houston, to no avail. An initial QEEG evaluation showed that Matthew had unusually high levels of delta and theta frequency waves in the prefrontal cortex and temporal lobes. However, after roughly 30 sessions of neurofeedback training rewarding SMR in both frontal lobes, his brain functioning had improved enough that his attention span increased noticeably. By the end of the school year, his grades had improved so greatly that the principal called to ask what we were doing.

This chapter has discussed a number of devices and software products that can be used to assist clients in learning how to change states and maintain a preferred state. Devices that range from relatively simple output-only ones to some of those that respond through biofeedback to the client's changing state can be used during the therapeutic interaction and may be suitable for home use by the client. Far more sophisticated software utilizing neurofeedback can pinpoint and reward target states as narrow as a particular EEG frequency. The use of such systems requires specialized training and is appropriate only in the clinical setting.

In the next chapter, we explore deeper states of alpha–theta, which, whether achieved via meditation, hypnosis, or biofeedback, have been found to lower stress and increase positive feelings.

CHAPTER 7

Deep State Work Using Hypnosis and Alpha–Theta Training

In Latin, the word *limen* means a literal threshold beneath a door, that place that is neither inside nor outside. *Liminal* has come to mean "the space between," the point or period of transition between one place, state, or thing and another. That neither–nor state is characterized by indeterminacy or ambiguity. Dawn and twilight; adolescence; sitting in an airplane, seeming to hang in the sky after having taken off from one place but not yet arrived at another: These are all examples of "the space between."

Psychologically, the liminal space encompasses the transitional states between full conscious awareness and a complete lack of consciousness; it is a space that slopes down gradually, starting just beneath the bright light of full consciousness and stopping just above the darkness of deep sleep. It encompasses the preconscious, the subconscious, and the upper reaches of the unconscious. Intuitions, creative ideas, perceptions, and impressions pop into consciousness from this level of the mind. In the upper levels of liminality, the mind exhibits alpha frequencies; in the lower levels it exhibits theta frequencies. And there, poised between waking and sleeping, deep states' work takes place.

This chapter takes us into the liminal realm of the alpha and theta states—deep states of change. We explore the characteristics and effects of these states, their biochemistry, and their use in BCT as it incorporates alpha–theta training to achieve these states.

We also provide a theta training protocol with a sample script, techniques, and exercises for cultivating deep state work.

The deeper states of alpha and theta, whether achieved by meditation, through hypnosis, or with biofeedback, have been found to lower stress and increase positive feelings. Modern life lived in states of stress tends to reduce the amount of waking alpha and theta waves that people produce. When clients can produce more of these frequencies, they are inclined to feel happier, have better access to motivation, be more creative, and relate to life events and family in better ways (Hardt, 2007). Fear seems to melt away. The research on meditative, trance, and alpha–theta states suggests that the use of deep therapeutic states leads to less self-criticism; in addition, there is less shame from childhood, state-bound guilt, and deautomatization (White, 1995; Travis, 2009; Gruzelier, 2006). In short, the deeper states seem to deactivate negativity.

Milton Erickson and Aldous Huxley explored states of deep trance together. Huxley found that in a state of dissociation he termed "Deep Reflection," he could go deeply inside his own psyche. This was a somnambulistic trance state where Huxley lost all awareness of external events and entered what he called "the Void." Here he experienced vivid color and images. Any questions he might ask in this state would be answered from his deeper mind. Huxley also experienced new perspectives in Deep Reflection that he found relevant to daily living. He reported that he achieved a state of "orderly mental arrangement permitting an orderly free flowing of his thoughts as he wrote." Huxley added:

> I use Deep Reflection to summon my memories, to put into order all of my thinking, to explore the range, the extent of my mental existence, but I do it solely to let those realizations, the thinking, the understandings, the memories seep into the work I'm planning to do without my conscious awareness of them. Fascinating . . . [I] never stopped to realize that my Deep Reflection always preceded a period of intensive work wherein I was completely absorbed. (Erickson, 1980, Vol. 1, p. 85)

While trance phenomena accompanied lighter states, extraordinary phenomena occurred in deep states—such as Huxley's ability, even with his eyes closed, to finish reading a sentence that Erickson had started in a verbal reading to Huxley. As Erickson explained:

> He now realized that he had developed a "deep trance," a psychological state far different from his state of Deep Reflection, that in Deep Reflection there was an attenuated but unconcerned and unimportant awareness of external reality, a feeling of being in a known sensed state of subjective awareness, of a feeling of control and a desire to

utilize capabilities and in which past memories, learnings, and experiences flowed freely and easily. Along with this flow there would be a continuing sense in the self that these memories, learnings, experiences, and understandings, however vivid, were no more than just such an orderly, meaningful alignment of psychological experiences out of which to form a foundation for a profound, pleasing, subjective, emotional state from which would flow comprehensive understandings to be utilized immediately and with little conscious effort.

The deep trance state, he asserted, he now knew to be another and entirely different category of experience. External reality could enter, but it acquired a new kind of subjective reality, a special reality of a new and different significance entirely. For example, while I had been included in part in his deep trance state, it was not as a specific person with a specific identity. Instead I was known only as someone whom he [Huxley] knew in some vague and unimportant and completely unidentified relationship. (Erickson, 1980, Vol. 1, p. 85)

As we began to explore the use of deep states in therapy, we recalled how frequently Milton Erickson worked with people in trance states for extended periods, often hours at a time. From our own experience, we came to realize that it was not only what Erickson said during this time but also simply the deep state itself that was curative.

Characteristics and Effects of the Alpha State

The alpha state occurs when the dominant brain waves range between 8 and 12 Hz. The subjective experience of the state is one of relaxed alertness or tranquility. In this state people are able to lower their autonomic arousal and achieve slower and deeper breathing. In addition, the alpha state is conducive to emotional flexibility, increased coherence of thinking, and increased quality of attention (Moore, 2000). Intuitive abilities may become enhanced. Hardt (2007) commented that "increased alpha wave activity brings increasing optimism, motivation, and a general state of happiness and well-being. These beneficial changes both extend life and improve the quality of life" (p. 115). Dean Ornish and his colleagues demonstrated that increasing alpha waves via meditation tended to dilate blood vessels in the brain, thereby increasing circulation, lowering blood pressure, and beginning to clear arteries. Meditation was coupled with diet and exercise in this study (Ornish, Weiner, & Fair, 2005).

Athletes who can deliberately keep their mind calm and focused tend to perform at or near their personal best. Developing the ability to "go into alpha" (our shorthand) at will is also a strategy for aging well. Whereas younger people tend to produce alpha waves easily, older individuals often show a decrease in alpha rhythms. However, seniors can be trained to increase their alpha wave production with neurofeedback.

Characteristics and Effects of the Theta State

Theta brain waves typically range between 4 to 7 Hz and produce an experience of deep relaxation characterized by hypnogogic images (as a person is falling asleep) and hypnopompic images (as a person is waking) from the unconscious mind. As mapped by neuroscientists (Davidson, 2003), theta states show less activation in the left hemisphere and more in the right, and this brain signature is seen in a corresponding blood flow. Because the critical mind is much less engaged, the theta state seems to engender hypersuggestibility.

Commonly, theta states are associated with reverie and with transitional or twilight states. From the theta state, people can access a depth of knowledge and wisdom beyond what most think they possess (Atwater, 2001). Each person's mental models are built from personal past experience. However, the perspectives encountered in the theta state suggest that reality, as we commonly experience it, has illusory aspects. By entering into a deep theta state, the client can reach a pool of knowing and clarity that transcends personal reality (Peniston & Kulkosky, 1989). Questions held lightly in a theta state can be answered from the larger impersonal mind or "collective unconscious" (Jung, 2006).

There are many anecdotes in which people dream about solutions to problems or have "waking dreams" filled with hypnogogic imagery. The images that occur as someone begins to awaken have been called products of the "transliminal mind" (Rugg, 1963) or the "transliminal experience" (MacKinnon, 1964). It is in the transliminal mind, a corollary of the brain in theta state, that sudden flashes of insight and creativity occur. By stimulating theta development, creativity can be trained or improved (Green & Green, 1977). As well as improved creative problem solving, theta state imagery can contain information and direction for specific strategies in healing an illness (Kershaw, 1980).

Elmer Green also thought of the theta state as one in which both psychological and spiritual development could take place. He noted: "Theta provides a way to walk through a doorway and gain access to the file of the unconscious—everything from the basement to the penthouse" (as cited in Schwartz, 1995, p. 154). Green believed that through the theta state, one could access the higher self or "True Self." He went on to say that using the theta state, a person could work toward developing greater compassion—or plan the perfect crime. Green found that the theta state led to awareness and objectivity, and noted, "you can feel all the mental, physical, and emotional things going on around you and in you and yet not be identified with the individual pieces. . . . We may think we are born to save ourselves. In truth, we are here to transform our nature in order to save the planet" (p. 155).

A kind of surrendering—a letting go of anxiety, depression, or stress—occurs in deep theta. There is an access to some new source within that moves a person into a different sense of self. In the liminal space, the client may discover a different way of being and a different quality of attention. Opening to deeper levels of awareness and inner resources may allow the client to develop a "psychological immune system" (Wallace, 2006, p. 3) so that he or she can begin to release the mind's baggage.

The therapeutic use of the theta state can help an individual alter negative programming and shift limiting beliefs. The return to a more resilient and vulnerable state, similar to returning to a younger age, can open the door to dramatic change. Centuries ago Lao Tzu observed, "The key to growth is the introduction of higher dimensions of consciousness into our awareness" (2008). As the client becomes a compassionate witness to his/her mind's thoughts, judgments, fears, and envies, it may be possible to let them go. Along these lines, Hardt (2007) commented, "When consciousness becomes the object of consciousness the change is so powerful that it goes beyond mere change and becomes *TRANSFORMATION*" (p. 216).

Characteristics of the theta state include the following (entries that do not include citations are based on our 30 years of clinical experience):

- Time distortion creates the impression that time has slowed down or disappeared.
- Mental activity slows and mind chatter disappears.

- Recovery from illness can be aided. Lewis Mehl-Madrona (2003) conducted research on identifying the moment that healing occurs in the brain of a recipient of prayer, positive thought, or ritual ceremony. He was interested in learning how intent and thought interacted with the human brain–body and at what point the interaction occurred within the brain's biofield. He reported that during a Native American ceremony, delta and theta increased in the left prefrontal cortex and the right temporal cortex, and alpha increased in the right occipital cortex. The largest changes in the EEG were observed during the point in the ceremony when the first sacred song was sung and at times when formal prayers occurred.

- Because attention is concentrated, all pain sensation can disappear, as well as any body awareness.

- Core beliefs about the limits of what is possible in one's life may be transcended. Perceived constraints may disappear, allowing an exploration of previously unavailable possibilities. Unique solutions may be discovered that would not have been found in other states of consciousness.

- Fear disappears and a state of flow ensues.

- Suddenly perceived insights may guide personal decision-making and the resolution of difficult issues. Problems that seemed insurmountable when viewed from the theta state may become interesting adventures.

- Creative ideas or information are stimulated from the "field of information" (Green & Green, 1977). Artists, musicians, writers, and others have used the theta state to engage their creativity. In the hypnogogic state, ideas are released as if from a hidden source. Einstein "received" his theory of relativity in a theta state, and he knew it was correct (Archer, 2005). In 1865, Frederick von Kekule knew from his dream of a snake eating its tail that the carbon atoms of benzene form a ring.

- Unresolved material can be addressed and cleared. Emotional issues that have been left unattended frequently float up to the surface, and the clinician can assist a person in dissolving their charge. This intervention does not involve abreaction but rather a gentle process of talking about the material and developing a new understanding before releasing it.

- Awareness of stress and the ability to reduce it, as well as the reducition of levels of medication used, can be achieved. Clients who practice achieving the theta state often report that they can tolerate life obstacles more easily.

- Qualities of compassion, detachment, and inner security develop more fully with theta practice.

The Biochemistry of Deep States

Wisneski and Anderson (2005) reviewed several studies that described receptor sites for a neuropeptide, anandamide (also known as the amide-of-bliss, an endogenous cannabinoid neurotransmitter with a chemical composition similar to that of marijuana), which produces a calm state (Devane & Axelrod, 1994; Axelrod & Felder, 1998) and is thought to be a major factor in systems regulation. Researchers found that the brain, heart, and spleen have ligands (chemicals that bind specifically and reversibly to another chemical entity to form a larger complex) with cannabinoid receptors for anandamide (Devane & Axelrod, 1994; Felder & Glass, 1998; Piomelli, Giuffrida, Calignano, & Rodriguez de Fonseca, 2000). They discovered that anandamide is able to diminish pain and to modulate the effects of stress. In addition, it influences the perception of time, decreases hypomobility, and produces transient feelings of well-being.

Brief periods of time in a theta state also reset sodium and potassium ratios, which are necessary for the osmotic processes that filter chemicals in and out of brain cells (Thompson, 2006; Peniston & Kulkolsky, 1989). Wisneski and Anderson (2005) suggested that there is a "theta healing system" and that the "cannabinoid ligands are potentially neuropeptides of deep relaxation" (p. 133). Expanding on that possibility, they proposed that the theta healing system "involves the integration of the physiological, mental/emotional, and even the spiritual aspects of our being" (p. 119). They wrote: "It is my contention that deep relaxation places humans within a 'target zone' for the endogenous release of any of the family of neuropeptides of relaxation. The target zone is a state of alpha brain resonance, while the interface, sometimes referred to as a state of hypnagogic reverie (theta resonance), is the bull's eye of the deep healing process" (p. 132). Budzynski (1997) pointed out that the predominance of theta in the EEG is the best state for "re-scripting" the brain to eliminate destructive emotional patterns that were acquired in childhood.

When people meditate, experience hypnosis, or use any of the brain-training devices previously discussed, they may be producing this amide to create deep relaxation, calm, and emotional stability. By doing so, they can also change their response to charged memories, shifting from agitation and upset to calmness, and as a result may be able to let go of past incidents of emotional wounding.

Deep State Research

One of the earliest deep state researchers, Joe Kamiya (1968), studied Zen meditators and hypothesized that it might be possible for anyone to learn how to control the mind and develop a psychophysiology of consciousness by learning to change states at will. Several investigators have since analyzed the EEG recordings of Zen monks who practiced meditation regularly (Davidson, 2003, 2007). As the monks went into meditation, they passed through four stages. The first stage showed the appearance of alpha waves. The second stage revealed that there was an increase in the amplitudes of the alpha frequency. The third stage showed a decrease in alpha, followed in the fourth stage by an increase in long periods of theta. The further into each session of mediation, the more the theta frequency was produced, although the monks' minds were completely alert. The researchers discovered that compassion is normally found when the mind is quiet (Lutz, Greischer, Rawlings, Ricard, & Davidson, 2004).

Another early investigator into the capacities of the mind was Jose Silva. He became fascinated with the human ability to accomplish most goals through a form of mind training he originally called Dynamic Meditation. Silva described his training as a descent into the deeper realms of consciousness, where information could be gleaned about issues ranging from health to financial success. The Silva Mind Training program began in the 1970s and is still popular around the world. Silva suggested that we come into the world through the delta level and leave at the same level. He believed that with mental rehearsal in an alpha state, we could achieve goals and reprogram the mind for success (Alex Silva, personal communication, July 21, 2003). Figure 7.1 illustrates Silva's formulation

Physical Reality	5 Senses
Mental	**Beta Level** 13-60 cps
Deeper Consciousness	**Alpha Level** 8-12 cps 12 senses Transpersonal
Unconscious Mind	**Theta Level** 4-7 cps
	Delta Level .4-4 cps Intuition, spontaneous decision making, Doorway to the spiritual dimension

Table 7.1. Silva's Formulation of States of Consciousness and Brain Frequencies

of different degrees of awareness, from attending to the neural input from the five senses to increasingly deeper states of consciousness characterized by slower brainwave frequencies.

In researching the theta range at the Menninger Clinic, Elmer and Alyce Green found that this state of deep quiet allowed rich material to come to mind in the form of hypnagogic imagery. The Greens and their colleagues explored the theta state in relation to several processes: creativity, problem solving, and healing mental or physical illness. In the course of their research, they reported that people in their theta training groups experienced many types and levels of improvement, including the following:

- More frequent creative ideas and intuitions
- Increase in the synthesis of ideas
- Improvements in physical healing
- Integrative breakthroughs

- Integrative breakthroughs
- Sustained periods of psychological well-being
- Improved relationships
- Greater tolerance and self-compassion
- Reduced self-criticism

The Greens also found that in the theta state, "information can reach us from levels and by communication channels normally called nonsensory" (Green & Green, 1977, p. 300).

John Lilly and his colleagues explored the deeper states of alpha and theta that often occurred while people were floating in sensory deprivation tanks (Lilly, 1977). They found that with the repeated experience of "restricted environmental stimulation" (REST), many maladies cleared up. Overweight patients lost weight, rheumatoid arthritis pain decreased significantly, depression lifted, anxiety calmed, immune response increased, and people seemed happier overall (Barabasz & Barabasz, 1993). Suedfeld (1993) reported that cognitive processing was slowed in the REST chamber. Turner and Fine (1987) suggested that REST was more than relaxation; it was associated with the release of endogenous opioids, or endocannabinoids. These control many of the body's functions and, in the brain, they modulate neurotransmission and synaptic plasticity; confer neuroprotection; and control metabolism, the generation of neurons and neuritogenesis (the first step of neuronal differentiation), survival, cognitive and motor functions, as well as other higher-order brain functions. Natural cannabinoids perform a number of critical functions in the brain, including registration of novelty, determination of emotional relevance, forgetting of aversive memories, regulation of appetite, regulation of pain threshold, and the regulation of anxiety/fear (Cermak, 2003). People can naturally increase the production of endocannabinoids through the use of deep relaxation strategies such as floating. Budzynski (1990) offered the idea that REST is similar to other consciousness-altering interventions that increase the theta frequency and result in increased creativity, intuition, insight, and calmness.

Peniston and Kulkosky (1989) developed a deep state training protocol to be used with a small group of inpatients being treated for alcoholism. It consisted of temperature biofeedback and autogenic training (in which the person repeats a set of visualizations that induce a state of relaxation) followed by 30-minute sessions of alpha–theta training twice per day for 15 days. Accompanying the deep state training was the use of a visualization where the client rejected the unwanted behavior and imagined the desired outcome. This process was completed several times per day. A follow-up study in 1990 found that a number of personality variables improved in the neurofeedback group relative to a control group. Thirteen months after the original study, 8 of the 10 subjects were still sober. After 10 years, seven still remained abstinent and one had died (Collins, 2009).

The following year, Peniston and Kulkosky (1991) conducted a controlled study in which they used alpha–theta EEG biofeedback with a group of Vietnam veterans who had PTSD. Eighty percent of those receiving the treatment showed significant mitigation of symptoms. Flashbacks, nightmares, and anxiety were greatly diminished after the treatment. In a 2-year follow-up, of the 15 people who received the alpha–theta treatment, only 1 had been rehospitalized, whereas all 14 people who received no treatment were readmitted two or more times. The group receiving treatment also showed great improvement on certain scales of the MMPI, probably the most well-researched and comprehensive personality test available. The researchers demonstrated that with EEG alpha–theta biofeedback training, unmanageable emotional states and behaviors changed dramatically (Peniston & Kulkosky, 1991).

Brain Change Therapy Using Deep States

It is healing to separate from one's normal surroundings and shift into a state of timelessness and silence for a period of time. In that state, in our experience, there tends to be an internal reorganization and a deep connection with what might be called an inner healer. It is within this liminal space that change gently takes place. Here, reclamation, renewal, and a depotentiation of negative life history are all possible. A person can focus on the present and future, free of mental clutter. Awareness expands in this state, and deep reflection leads to an increased joy, creativity, and the emergence of a sense of meaning and life purpose.

Once in the theta state, a deeper level of the mind begins to resolve emotional pain without reference to specific problems. This resolution leads to new perspectives and fewer projections. In this process, clients often find themselves able to extend forgiveness to those whom they perceived had harmed them. Hardt commented that "increased alpha wave activity brings increasing optimism, motivation, and a general state of happiness and well-being" (2007, p. 115). He suggested that the suppression of the slower frequencies due to chronically held negative states results in a person's inability to move fully into forgiveness. Instead, the negative emotional patterns remain in force throughout life. Many traditional therapies are never able to fully resolve these negative states.

Working with deep states can be particularly helpful in dealing with trauma of any kind. When a client discusses past trauma, he or she is often flooded with anxiety, and cognitive processes become impaired. Rather than healing the trauma, a retraumatization may occur. However, anxiety is not experienced in deep states: The two are not simultaneously possible. Thus, time spent in deep states effectively "cools" the limbic system and may allow the client to move into a "witness" state, within which he or she can view what happened in the past from an empathic adult perspective. Of additional benefit, the profoundly calm state is carried over for a period of time after the person returns to normal consciousness. This can lead to a reorganization of understanding and gently "discharge" the emotion from the memory. Because there is amnesia between states of arousal, pain from historical events dissipates so that an upsetting event can be recalled without intense affect.

One client, by then in middle age, still suffered from the memory of a gang rape he had experienced when he was 14. He felt responsible and guilty for the event and, as an adult, he had been unable to sustain an intimate relationship for very long. After helping him develop the ability to feel secure and safe in deep states, we asked him to go back in time slowly and return to that event from his adult perspective. We suggested that perhaps he would notice something he had not previously seen. He was able to review the original event and observe what had really happened. Upon returning from the deep state, he commented, "It really wasn't my fault." After an intense emotional release, for the first time he felt free from the past and able to focus on a more positive future.

We can help the client reach the theta state using either hypnosis or alpha–theta training. Commonly we start with hypnosis; if that is counterindicated or is not showing good results, we move the client to one of the brain-training devices. When the client has reached a deep state, we use a combination of periods of silence and therapeutic techniques to continue deep state work. Designed to create new emotional perspectives, the deep state experience can lead to a restructuring of the consciousness and a repatterning of life habits.

Therapeutic Principles of Deep State Change

Based on our work using deep states for therapeutic change, we have distilled several principles to facilitate therapeutic shifts using the modalities of deep hypnosis and alpha–theta training. Although generally applicable to all types of therapeutic intervention, they have particular relevance to deep state work.

1. *The mind is a significant player in creating "reality" as a person perceives it.* A person who believes that he or she is hungry, even though there are no physical manifestations of hunger, will create the sensations of hunger. A person who imagines an emotion will experience its physical correlates, which will reinforce its seeming truth.

2. *Deep states tend to alter a person's understanding of past events.* More benign explanations seem to generalize into an understanding that judgment without prior inquiry leads to dysfunction.

3. *The liminal space facilitates reorganizing life priorities, rescripting old patterns and themes, tapping creativity, and solving seemingly intractable problems.* In the liminal space, auditory or visual experiences may occur that can inform the client about a past or present dilemma to be solved (Mavromatis, 1987). Alternatively, the client may ask a question of the unconscious mind regarding some personal issue in this deep state. Often, the answer offers a surprisingly different perspective on the matter.

4. *People who are the most self-regulated are the happiest.* Those who can learn how to notice reactions without acting on them have the best management over themselves. Green and Green (1977) suggested that there are three elements to psychophysiological self-regulation: *self-awareness, passive volition,* and *visualization.* For example, a client can learn to become *aware* of the embodied sensations that reflect various emotions. Using *passive volition,* clients can learn to control heart rate and overall body temperature by slowing their rate of

breathing and shifting into the relaxation response (a physical state of deep rest that changes the physical and emotional responses to stress and is the opposite of the fight or flight response). Then they may use *visualization* to practice accomplishing goals. These elements can be used in conjunction with alpha–theta training to process any imagery that comes from the experience, or any insights about a problem.

Those who are heavily armored frequently have difficulty with self-regulation. These people have been overly criticized, controlled, and forced to act in ways that do not suit them. Time spent in deeper states can unhinge armor, neutralize emotional charge, break through old patterns to increase productivity and flow, and open individuals to a better quality of living.

5. *Deep states help clients make distinctions in symptoms and notice slight changes.* We frequently help people notice differences between feeling depressed and fatigued and anxious and hungry (i.e., as a result of low blood sugar). When a client feels bad, categories of distinction become collapsed into one, and everything is negative. Some clients are sufficiently out of touch with their own bodies and their own organismic interface with the world that it is difficult for them to be conscious of positive, yet subtle, differences in focus, concentration, and mood.

6. *Deep states encourage the client's expectation of success.* Some people are so frustrated by the time they come to our practice that they fully expect to fail once again. Every state of consciousness has its own perspective, and such negative states restrict a person from experiencing resources and possibilities. For example, when a person is depressed, the world is perceived through a gray lens, and it is difficult to notice small breakthroughs of color. We might say to a client, "You can notice a change in how you feel in three or four sessions. What will you look for?" Since the client has long viewed the world through a filter of depression and focused only on its symptoms, we may need to help him or her identify and notice change.

7. *Development of co-resonance is particularly critical in deep state work.* Co-resonance is the rapport that occurs through pacing, positive emotional tone, blending (repeating the same behaviors, words, and emotional tone), and leading (suggesting a new behavior or describing future possibilities). It requires making real emotional and energetic contact with a client through empathic and respectful conversation. Writing about resonance, Justice and Justice (2008) note:

Neurobiologically, the brain's limbic system serves as a liminal border across which the physical and psychological, the seen and unseen, the emotional and spiritual interact. Its "door key" is the synapse, which connects cell-to-cell, axons and dendrites for instant intercommunication within and among parts of the brain. The limbic system is so named for crossing the borders of neurons. It is our emotional brain, whose energy can carry outside ourselves.... Having limbic resonance with another person . . . speaks a silent language more moving than words. Such attunement between two worlds—the inner and outer, the unseen and seen, the energy of one person touching another—is not a rare experience. But it is one that neuroscience is giving us more and more technology with which to see into the brain and to picture how the phenomenon works physically. (p. 1)

Stages of the Deep State Process

By whatever means a person accesses the deeper states, there are six discernable stages from normal consciousness (beta state) to profound states and back again: settling, deepening, dissociation, theta crossover stage, deep theta, and reorientation. The clinician should observe the client closely to facilitate the process. It is otherwise possible for a person to access negative theta states and encounter frightening images and upsetting emotions. This may occur if a person remains too long in a state with a dominant brainwave of less than 3 Hz, without appropriate preparation and the ability to lift him- or herself out. We take the same precautions in working with alpha–theta brain training as we do in hypnosis, in which a grounding process precedes the access of any deeper hypnotic states. Grounding may involve having the patient feel the floor with his or her feet, remember in detail a geographical location of real safety, access the sensory qualities of the experience, and memorize the experience. It is never enough just to direct an individual to go to a safe place without making sure that the internal experience is indeed safe and that it involves many senses to which the client can be anchored and which can be remembered for future access. Anchors are sensory references to emotions and states that may come through any of the senses.

The first stage is *settling*, in which the client enters an initial state of relaxation (alpha state). Some individuals become frightened when they first begin to relax, because it feels so foreign. Occasionally, at this point a client will report a sensation of falling. If this occurs, the clinician needs to return to the grounding process and again suggest that the client feel the ground, remember that the chair is upright, and slowly relax with the eyes open before proceeding to close them. Many alpha–theta computer programs have pleasant sounds that accompany the training. Instructing the client to focus on the sound can facilitate the feeling of calm.

The second stage is *deepening.* The client's muscle tension begins to decrease; breathing becomes easier and deeper. Often the person will sigh deeply, an indication that the autonomic nervous system is shifting into parasympathetic functioning. When this occurs, the journey into theta has begun.

Following this stage is a *dissociation* of the conscious from the unconscious mind. The conscious mind quiets or "goes somewhere"; frequently trance phenomena begin to be experienced. Analgesia or anesthesia, trance heaviness or warmth, immobility such as catalepsy, and/ or time distortion, wherein time seems to slow down or stop, may be experienced. Usually the person is completely quiet at this point. As markers of a deeper state, the clinician will observe that the person looks immobile, his or her muscles become flaccid due to relaxation, and often, REM begins.

As the state deepens and the person heads toward sleep, he or she reaches the *theta crossover stage*, where the ratio of theta to alpha waves shifts in favor of theta waves. Without a biofeedback system to monitor this stage, we can discern when a person is in it by the quiet and still state of his or her body. While this crossover is not necessary for a positive response, it does indicate a deep state. At this point the person becomes a conduit for universal images transcending time, culture, and language. Sometimes, voices of loved ones are heard, or an awareness of their presence may be perceived. In this state of reverie, we suggest that the person lightly notice the images rather than try to hold on to them. Being in a receptive state allows the images to flow, whereas if the person attempts to hold on to them, they will disappear. Later in processing the images, we suggest that the client use the images as oracles. We can instruct the client to ask the unconscious for an associated meaning as he or she ponders the message.

The next stage is *deep theta,* wherein the mind may be experienced as quiet or empty. In order for an individual to allow the deepest state to occur, it must be accompanied by a feeling of safety. The clinician may need to do some kind of safety training before this state is achieved. This training might include a discovery process of times the client remembered feeling secure, or the clinician may need to help the client create the feeling by reviewing where in the present time he or she feels safe. It is in this state that movement into healing and regeneration takes place.

In a short explanation before we begin, we often suggest to the client that traveling on the "interstate" of theta creates flexibility, flow, and access to creative solutions because it is possible to receive information from the "dream without distortion" (Kubie, 1943). In this state, the individual moves beyond conditioned beliefs and can perceive ways to achieve that which he or she had thought was impossible.

The sixth stage is a *reorientation* to the client's immediate surroundings. At this point, the clinician suggests that the client slowly begin to reconnect with the body and shift states to one of more activation. This is done slowly to avoid potential headaches or discomfort from reorienting too quickly. We make certain that the client takes enough time to become fully oriented. This is particularly important because the client is likely to be driving a vehicle shortly thereafter and must leave the office competent to do so.

Using Hypnosis to Achieve Deep States

Erickson defined deep hypnosis as "that level of hypnosis that permits the subject to function adequately and directly at an unconscious level of awareness without interference by the conscious mind" (Erickson, 1972, p. 80). The process takes the client into the theta state, where heart rate and oxygen consumption decrease and ego boundaries are loosened. Hobson (2001) suggested that deep trance characteristics are similar to REM sleep dreaming. In both states, there is time distortion, amnesia, visual imagery, and immobility. He noted that "there is clear evidence that memory is state dependent and can be altered" (p. 110). In a Danish study of yoga meditation, Kjaer, Nowak, and Lou (2002) also noticed the similarity of the brain's activation pattern in deep states and in REM. Based on these findings, it may be conjectured that consciousness is restructured in the REM state. REM periods stabilize consciousness and when used intentionally, could potentially speed up therapeutic results.

Further confirming Hobson's work, we frequently observe REM in deep trance and alpha–theta training. Voluntary movement is almost impossible in both REM sleep and in deep trance: the cortex deactivates, the release of certain neurotransmitters is completely suppressed, the independent will goes into neutral, and negative affect is dampened. As a result, motor neurons are not stimulated, a condition known as REM atonia.

To use deep state hypnosis, we begin by helping clients develop a sense of safety and security. When we inquire where clients have felt the safest, they often describe a specific place. We ask them to review this place in detail while in trance and to remember the pleasant feelings and comfort associated with the place. Then we suggest that they move the mind to the deepest place inside, all the way to the edge of sleep. This is a calm, quiet center pervaded by feelings of safety.

We then tell the client that in the following 20 minutes or so, he or she should review the problem and quietly ask the unconscious mind for an answer. What might be reviewed is a life problem to be solved, a disturbing scene from the past, or a confusing circumstance that needs a decision. This is followed by about 20 minutes of complete silence, after which we gently and slowly reorient the person to the present moment.

Amy had a history of abuse and repeatedly found herself in conflict with someone. In working in the deep alpha state, she discovered that her mind took her to a secluded beach in Chile. There she felt a sense of freedom and aliveness, but those feelings were also tinged by sadness. Exploring these feelings further, Amy became aware that she had always identified herself by conflict. Without conflict, she felt empty. We suggested that this was a time of new opening, the beginning of a new life, and that she could redefine herself without struggle and conflict.

Accessing Deep States Through Alpha–Theta Training

As we have previously described, alpha–theta training with neurofeedback involves hooking up the client to a device that records brainwaves and provides positive feedback when he or she is producing the desired frequency. Audio reinforcement of those deep relaxation waves via pleasant sounds of running water and crashing waves helps to create more of the desired state. However, the client must learn to hear the positive feedback sound without becoming too alert, or the brain will shift out of the theta state. Upon reaching the deeper states, the person may begin to access rich unconscious material in the form of striking archetypal images.

We discovered, somewhat by accident, that allowing a client to linger in a deep state could address personal and interpersonal issues far beyond the physiological symptoms of stress or anxiety. At our encouragement, one of our clients, who was having marital stress and was on the verge of divorce, began to do deep state training in alpha–theta using the Cygnet neurofeedback system for stress headaches. To our perplexity, after a few sessions he no longer discussed marital problems. He told us that although there were still disagreements between him and his wife, he realized that he was making too much of the problem. With continued work in deep states, he became calmer and more cheerful, and began making long-term plans with his wife. He developed insight about his own part in the marital problems and began to respond differently to his wife. Most other clients who trained in alpha–theta in our clinic have had similar responses to their daily lives.

Ordinary attention has a "mind" of its own and travels willy-nilly; alpha–theta training teaches the mind how to achieve sustained and focused concentration in deep relaxation. Normal brain functioning drives thoughts, feelings, and images into consciousness based on habitual thinking patterns. These patterns usually involve judgment and reactions to past events, as well as desires for imagined futures. The "movies" that the mind runs absorb energy and maintain a certain level of chronic stress. Over time, these patterns can devolve into automatic thinking that continues beneath the level of conscious awareness. Without some form of deep mind training, longstanding mind habits can overpower a person's resolve, and the mind easily returns to its habitual ways of obsessing or ruminating.

Alpha–theta training begins to deconstruct these toxic processes. Consciousness is transformed; the negative feelings of sadness, worry, anxiety, anger, or fear dissipate, and people begin to feel more compassion for themselves and for others. The result is the integration and elimination of many symptoms that accompany mental health diagnoses. In addition, deep state training can help people access positive inner states at will in order to avoid being overwhelmed by their own negative emotions.

Ella had the most severe case of hives we had ever seen. She had grown up in an atmosphere of heavy criticism and a negation of her very being. Her father frequently told her she was "stupid" and "bad." Children tend to retain these types of early scripting suggestions, and indeed, these pejorative proclamations stayed with her. As an adult, each incident of feeling inconsequential to friends or her husband would set off a prickly sensation in her arms that preceded a breakout of hives. Working in deep alpha–theta states using neurofeedback, Ella began to learn how to turn down the sympathetic system, and she developed a favorite safe place. She visualized walking on Maui's Wailea Beach, crossing an imaginary bridge to a place she called the "eye of the needle," and entering a huge cave where she could hear the soothing sounds of the surf. She began to feel nurtured by "mother earth" and practiced staying in this deep state for long periods of time. This practice led her to manage her state and, consequently, the outbreak of hives.

Combining Hypnosis and Alpha–Theta Training

The combined use of hypnosis and alpha–theta training allows us to determine precisely the brain state a client has reached and to target hypnotic interventions more effectively, based on the readout from an alpha–theta training device. Once the client is in a deep state, hypnotic work is facilitated both by the reward of the sound produced by a neurofeedback system and the client's increased openness to hypnotic suggestion in the theta state.

The treatment of several disordered states is improved through the combined modalities of hypnosis and alpha–theta training. Specifically, anxiety, PTSD, and addictions have been found to respond positively to the combination (Othmer, 2009). In addition, more advanced strategies such as conditioning and "programming" a future goal through visualization in a theta state can be used with the combination of these modalities.

Mary came to us with an unusual problem: She explained that she physically experienced other people's pain. Because she didn't know how to stop it, she was afraid that she was "going crazy." She described growing up in a family where her mother was quite psychic and, as a matter of course, would tell her daughter when a particular person would be phoning. Sure enough, within 5 minutes her mother would be proven right. When Mary took her automobile to be repaired, her mother told her when to call the repair shop because her car would be ready. She was always on target.

For Mary, having similar abilities without knowing how to manage them was very disturbing. She described sitting quietly in church and suddenly experiencing the physical or emotional pain of someone in a nearby pew. As accurately as her mother, she could usually tell which person she was sensing and what was wrong. But Mary could not keep these feelings at bay: They would make her physically and emotionally ill. She felt frightened by her experiences and was reluctant to talk with anyone about them. We suggested she read Judith Orloff's (1997) book, *Second Sight*, to understand that many people have these abilities. We believe that, although usually latent, these abilities could be developed by anyone. However, most people who are not conscious of them do not have an interest in learning to access these nonordinary states of knowing.

In the initial evaluation, Mary spent much of her time in the somewhat dissociated state that many people with paranormal abilities utilize. However, she did not know how to come out of it, how to set internal boundaries or protect herself. The goal of treatment was to help her learn to use her gifts when she chose to do so.

A few sessions of teaching her how to dip into the mental state to pick up information and then move back into a more awake state allowed Mary to feel better. However, she then found that, frequently, she could no longer access her intuitive state. We countered this overlearning with an alpha–theta biofeedback session, and her intuitive capacities began to be available again. During this training, we used hypnotic fractionation (a deepening technique in which the clinician suggests that the client follow numbers down, e.g., 10–1, and when 4 or 5 is reached, the counting starts back up for 2 or 3 numbers and then resumes going back down) to help Mary go into theta and come out again several times, so that she could learn the experience of controlling different states. After a few sessions, Mary felt much more in control of her own mind.

Theta Training Protocol: A Sample Script

Before we begin a theta training session, we instruct the client to call up a sensory experience of safety that has been practiced hypnotically before the theta training. Suggestions about relaxation and developing comfort can be given with eyes closed. We frequently begin with warming the hands to induce relaxation. For example, we might have the person remember a time he or she warmed his or her hands in front of a fireplace or lay on a sun-baked beach. After deep relaxation, we instruct the client to imagine the problem from a distance and notice if there is anything different about visualizing it from a witness perspective. If the client begins to evidence any anxiety or discomfort, we suggest noticing the breath coming in and out of the nostrils until the client returns to a state of comfort. We then explain that the unconscious mind can bring to awareness relevant information that may need processing or relevant people that may need "decharging." Making the trauma or stress interpersonal by discussing it and viewing it from a deeper state can depotentiate emotional reactivity.

The following is a sample script for use with a client who is beginning deep state work. There should be a pause of at least 15–30 seconds between each instruction.

1. "Imagine placing all your anxieties into a container such as a suitcase, a hole in the earth, or a concrete box."
2. "Select an issue or question to focus on. Your deepest mind will know what that might be. Allow it to communicate with you. Wait quietly until something floats into your awareness." (*Pause here longer than 30 seconds. Sustain the pause if the client looks as though something has occurred.*)
3. "Imagine that you can put the issue in a bowl that sits on top of a table. Or imagine that you can offer the person a chair to sit in."
4. "Now take about four steps back, and walk all the way around the table or around the chair."
5. "Look carefully at the item or the person as you walk around. Do you notice that anything has changed?"
6. "Notice any images or sensations that come up."
7. "If an image or sensation arises, ask your deeper knowing, what is the meaning of the image or sensation?"
8. "Listen inside yourself for a response."

Once the session has ended, it is important for the clinician to process the images and sensations that have emerged with the client. Dale Walters (personal communication, August 23, 2002) suggested that the clinician ask, "What is a ___?" concerning the image or sensation and allow the client to give associations to glean a meaning. Continue with the questioning until the client feels satisfied. This protocol can be a useful tool for allowing the client to discover inner resources or identify potential solutions.

Accompanying deep state work, it is important for clients to become aware of any habitual interpretations about life events that are rooted in judgment and fear. These constructs and ways of understanding experience are usually thematic and patterned. They can be discerned by helping the client examine the following statements and filling in the blanks:

1. Life is _____.
2. My partner is _____ .
3. My future is _____.
4. The probability of accomplishing my goal is _____.
5. I am undermining my goals by _____.
6. The extent to which I am aligned with my values is _____.
7. If I looked at my life from an outside perspective, I would see

   _____.
8. Viewing my life from the perspective of my compassionate future self, I want to _____.
9. My personal fears about accomplishing this are _____.
10. My potential future paths are _____.

Techniques and Exercises of Deep State Work

Simply allowing a client to rest in a deep state often has profoundly healing effects. Particularly for clients with issues involving anxiety or stress, the time spent in a theta state may be the most deeply restful period they can remember. A therapeutic silence will also give the client's unconscious the "space" to express its own wisdom—often to the surprise of the client. However, because most clients are not experienced in using silence for self-directed introspective work, they may also benefit from guided exercises. We have developed the following techniques and exercises for use with clients in deep states, accessed either through deep hypnosis or the use of neurofeedback devices.

Deep Dive Inquiry

When clients are at war with their emotions and fight with their own minds, they bring that internal conflict into external relationships and wind up hating the very people they also love. Righteous anger and regret are states of mind that blanket deeper, unexpressed or unresolved emotions and render them invisible. Addictive behaviors may also serve to keep feelings unknown. Neither strategy allows freedom from reaction. Deep inquiry allows the client to gently and calmly express what may have gone unexpressed for years. This process provides an opening to move beyond regret, anger, yearning, and desire into patterns of happiness.

In this case, the client may undertake a "deep dive" into feelings that may have been "stored out of sight" for years. This can be done by guiding the client into a deep state and than having the client ask the following four questions:

1. *"What is blocking me from staying in the target state?"* A focus on the deepest feelings that may have been previously unacknowledged may help shift the client into a profound state of self-understanding and compassion. As a way of understanding these blocks, they can be envisioned as an "unwillingness" to acknowledge yearnings for greater happiness. Delving more deeply into the blocks or defenses can gently break them up.

2. *"What is the purpose and meaning of my life?"* Exploring this question can help a client become clear about what life path he or she wants to follow. By going into an inner silence, a client can connect with a deeper purpose or life direction and what might be called the higher or authentic self. Wisdom traditions throughout history have described this deeper state of being: Buddhism identifies it with the concept of the Buddha nature; Christianity identifies it with the presence of the Holy Spirit; Native Americans with the Great Spirit; and Daoism with the notion of the Source (Scharmer, 2007). Important therapeutic work can be focused in any area in which the person is behaving outside of his or her understood purpose.

3. *"What are the possibilities for my life?"* This question is important to assist clients in moving beyond their own self-created limitations and the fears that hold them in place.

4. *"What is my vision for my life?"* This vision is the specific plan that follows a reflection on possibilities as they become known to the individual. This question may also stimulate the client's interest in developing some type of spiritual practice. Whether it is through meditation, walking in the woods, using silence on a regular basis, or shifting states with any of the brain technologies, an individual can develop a deeper quality of living every day.

Therapeutic Metaphor

The clinician can activate potential resources by retrieving a client's memories of past learning and teaching new skills the person may need by using a story or tale as a therapeutic metaphor. In listening to a story, a client, particularly in the theta state, can make certain associations and understand a different perspective. Personal shifts in feelings and attitudes can happen. Stories have healing power to contain the feelings associated with an experience. Hearing a story about someone else also confirms that the client is not alone in that situation.

Our intention in metaphor construction is to turn on appropriate emotional circuits for therapeutic purposes. Whenever a person hears a story or sees a movie, emotional circuits are stimulated. The interaction of characters with each other or their situations may light up fear circuits, stimulate curiosity and anticipation, or engage care and nurturing circuits. In addition, telling a story about an animal character tends to stimulate some element of age regression.

To construct a therapeutic metaphor, begin by identifying the circuit that needs activation, while taking note of any needs for developmental learning or changes in attitude or behavior. Consider how to end the story to change the client's state, how to make the desired point, and where to place the embedded suggestions. Usually a metaphor involves a protagonist who has an experience, takes a journey, undergoes and resolves a conflict, or just has a conversation. There is a build-up of tension, a crisis, and some type of resolution.

The metaphor can follow a story flow that includes these elements:

1. A person takes a journey into what could be called the Story World.
2. Some means of transportation is used.
3. Certain actions are completed.

4. The experience is quite different from anything experienced in the everyday world.

5. The person is changed by the experience, sometimes in dramatic ways, and returns to the world of origin (Gerrig, 1993; Lankton & Lankton, 1989).

We suggest using therapeutic metaphor while the client is in a relaxed (alpha) state. As deep states are achieved, we suggest that the therapist silently allow the individual to do the deep internal work of integrating the story's points without interruption. Alternatively, the therapeutic metaphor can be offered after the person slightly reorients.

When our daughter Tiffany was 7, she broke an expensive crystal wand that Bill had given Carol. However, she reassembled the broken pieces in the box and said nothing about it. Shortly after that, we accidentally discovered that the wand was broken. At the time, Tiffany had been going through a difficult period and would frequently manufacture stories to avoid taking responsibility for her actions. Bill assumed that the problem was fear- and shamed-based behavior that needed addressing.

Bill spent an afternoon with Tiffany taking a walk, playing, and doing other activities that helped reinforce a strong connection between them. That evening, when he put Tiffany to bed, he asked her if she wanted a bedtime story, and she said yes. Bill told her to lie down, "put your head on the pillow, and let your eyes close so you can imagine what I am saying with your mind's eye."

"Once upon a time there was a squirrel named Benny. He had a beautiful fluffy gray coat with white all the way down from his neck to his tummy. Benny was a very pretty squirrel. One day Benny was busy running up and down his tree to gather acorns for the winter. Benny was responsible and industrious and knew that he needed to prepare for the coming winter, when snows would come and there would be no food to find.

"As Benny was collecting acorns one day, he saw a figure dressed in a purple cloak with yellow moons and stars and with a large purple pointed hat, also with yellow moons and stars, walking down the road. The figure had a long walking stick. Benny became more and more curious about this stranger, so he scampered down the tree and cautiously approached him. As Benny drew closer, he realized that the stranger looked like another squirrel but instead of walking on all fours, he was walking upright. Benny had never seen this before. He asked this squirrel, 'Who and what are you?' The stranger said, 'My name is Merlin and I am a magic squirrel. That is why I can walk on two feet.' Benny's heart began to pound with excitement, and he asked Merlin, 'Do you teach other people magic?' Merlin said, 'Yes. Do you want to learn?' Benny immediately shook his head 'yes.' Merlin told Benny to meet him the next morning at the oak tree in which he lived. Then Merlin went on his way.

"Benny went back to his home and continued gathering nuts. After dinner he went to bed, but Benny could hardly sleep that night. His heart beat quickly; he tossed and turned and could barely close his eyes with the anticipation of this new adventure.

"The next morning, Bennie got up, and following Merlin's directions, he arrived at Merlin's home high in a magnificent oak tree. Benny climbed up and reached the branch that led to the doorway of Merlin's home. Benny knocked on the door. It slowly opened and there stood Merlin, dressed in his wizard's robe and hat. Merlin told Benny to have a seat. Benny asked if he was going to teach him magic. 'Absolutely,' Merlin said. 'To begin, I want you to sit in this chair and concentrate on the magic wand you see on the shelf.' Benny asked, 'Can I pick it up?' Merlin said, 'No, not yet. Just sit patiently and gaze on the wand. I have to run some errands, and I will be back shortly.'

"Benny was beside himself with excitement. The magic wand looked beautifully majestic and the longer he sat there, the more he was tempted to pick up the wand. Eventually Benny could not contain his excitement anymore. He thought to himself, 'It won't hurt if I just pick it up. I won't make any magic with it.' As Benny picked up the wand, an owl flew by and frightened him. He dropped the wand on the floor and it broke in two pieces. Benny was horrified. He couldn't believe what he had done, and the wand was now broken. He thought to himself, 'I am in big trouble now. Merlin will never teach me magic because I disobeyed him.'

"Benny stared at the wand trying to figure out what to do. Fear and sadness gripped Benny, and he stood there frozen. Then, as if a light bulb went off in his head, he said, 'I know what I'll do—I'll put the wand back on the shelf and Merlin will never know I broke it.' And that is what he did. He picked up the wand, put the two pieces together on the shelf, and then left.

"That night Benny once again could not sleep. His heart pounded as if it were going to beat out of his chest, but this time it wasn't because he was excited: It was because he was scared. He tossed and turned and could not sleep a wink. Tears trickled down from Benny's eyes. He was sad because he was not going to learn to do magic. But he was also afraid that Merlin would be very angry. The next morning, when Benny arose, he was still frightened and sad. He paced back and forth in his house. Suddenly he stopped and thought to himself, 'I must tell Merlin the truth. I just can't go on feeling this way.'

"Even though his heart was beating quickly, Benny took a deep breath, held it and let it out, clenched up his little paws, tightened himself up, and then relaxed. He threw back his shoulders, mustering all the courage he could, and went over to Merlin's house.

"When he arrived, he knocked on the door and once again, the big oak door slowly opened and there was Merlin, standing before him. Merlin said, 'Benny, I am surprised to see you. When I came back from doing errands, you were gone.' Benny gulped and asked to come in. Merlin invited him in to have a seat. He asked Benny, 'What brings you here?'

"Benny said, 'I have something I need to tell you. When you were away yesterday and I was sitting looking at the magic wand, I couldn't keep myself from picking it up. I didn't think it would hurt because I just wanted to look at it closer. But I was startled and I dropped it on the floor and it broke. I did not know what to do. I was afraid you would be so angry with me you would never teach me magic, so I picked up the magic wand, placed the two pieces together, put it on the shelf, and ran home.'

"'I see,' said Merlin. 'I am very glad you came back and told me the truth. When I returned from my errands and you were not here, I had a hunch something like that had happened, so I looked at the wand and indeed it was broken.'

"'Merlin, I am so sorry. Will you forgive me?' Benny quietly asked.

"'Of course,' Merlin replied.

"Sorrowfully, Benny said, 'I suppose you won't teach me magic now?'

"Merlin said, 'I am not pleased that you disobeyed me, but you have just passed the first test a magician must take. A magician must have a good heart, and if you are to practice good magic, you must be able to overcome fear and tell the truth. You are not the first student who disobeyed me, but you are one of the few who came back and had the courage to tell the truth. And because you did, I will accept you as my student.' Benny and Merlin hugged and began what was to be a long and productive relationship as teacher and student."

When Bill finished telling Tiffany the story, she opened her eyes and looked at her father, and said, "Would you ask Carol to come upstairs?" So Bill kissed her and went downstairs to get Carol. When Carol came upstairs, Tiffany asked her to sit on the bed. Tiffany told Carol, "Do you know that magic wand Daddy gave you?" Carol said, "Yes, that is a special gift." Tiffany responded, "The other day I picked it up and was playing with it. I know I shouldn't have, but I did. I was pretending to be a magician, and I accidentally banged it into the wall. It broke in two places, and I put it back on the shelf." Carol looked at Tiffany and said, "I really appreciate the courage it took for you to tell me. Why don't we try to glue it together in the morning?"

Tiffany fell asleep and woke up the next day feeling relieved and cheery. The metaphor of Benny the Squirrel had assisted her in changing states from anxious guilt to courage. In hearing its message, she was able to admit to breaking the wand. She discovered that she could handle the consequences of her actions, thereby building a sense of responsibility and self-confidence.

Exercises Based on a New Therapeutic Paradigm of Time

One of the outdated paradigms in psychotherapy is that the past creates the future, and therefore each person is a "victim of the past." Based on that model, a client needed to undertake an archeological dig of the psyche to unearth all of the negative events and then process them in order to free the psyche. This idea still permeates our culture. From a Freudian perspective, analysis of the "root problem" is seen as the means to resolve present dilemmas. And, indeed, the past does influence the present—but the future may have an even greater impact. The new paradigm, informed by quantum physics, suggests that the future creates the present against the background of the past (Wolf, 1990; Pulos, 2003). Every thought or feeling we have about the future becomes a potential future experience. Wolf suggested that every thought we have goes out like an echo wave, and all futures become possibilities. In somewhat simplistic terms, it implies that we have the ability to consider a variety of futures, and that the one on which we focus is the one that often comes to pass. In *Letters to a Young Poet,* Rainer Maria Rilke wrote, "The future enters into us in order to transform itself in us, long before it happens" (1993, pp. 64-65). Emily Dickinson, ahead of her time, wrote, "I dwell in possibility" (1955, poem 657).

Inviting the Future to Create Itself

Deep state work allows a directed access to the wisdom of the unconscious with an ease that few, if any, other techniques can claim. The shift in awareness that occurs in deep states allows a client to open more readily to his or her greatest future possibility and positive destiny.

Rather than living life on the basis of old patterns (the "past that creates the present"), we suggest there is a deeper place from which people can respond. As we explain to clients, it is in this inner space that we can listen to what life calls us to do, by setting judgment aside and opening the heart, mind, and will. It is from that internal space that a coupling with the deepest source of the self can occur (Scharmer, 2007).

The coupling process could be seen as following the pattern of the letter *U*. We move down from life's patterned judgment and reactivity, beneath anxiety and notions of limitations, to deeper aspects of the self. In *Theory U*, Scharmer (2007) suggested that the shift can transform perception, the self, the will, and subsequent action. Whereas he was interested in its application to organizational management and change, we suggest that this is the description of state change whereby the internal movement going down and within transforms the individual.

To receive information from the metaphoric "future," a person must make an internal shift and open to "deeper levels of our emotional perception" in deep reflection (Scharmer, 2007, p. 149). The process begins by shifting states and suspending judgment. As a person moves into deeper states of consciousness, he or she begins to let go of tension and anxiety and enters a place of deep reflection, a calm, quiet center of inner knowing. The movement down the U curve breaks up old attention habits and perceptions and opens the self to deep listening and potentially to an experience of connection with all living things. At the bottom of the U, Scharmer suggested that one can sense the emerging field of the future and use it as a resource. From that experience emerges a wisdom and an understanding of how to proceed and implement some plan of action, if need be.

Meeting One's "Future Self"

Endel Tulving (1993) described "autonoetic consciousness" as a "feeling of remembering" that allows us to distinguish information arising from memory as opposed to information directly from the senses. It is autonoetic consciousness that permits a person to create the experience of the past, present, and future. One process whereby the future and the past "enter into us" is through a kind of mental "time travel." In hypnosis this is called *pseudo-orientation in time*. A common example of pseudo-orientation in time is an adult who, looking at an elderly parent, imagines what he or she will look like at that age. Age progression in deep states can allow the client to imagine him- or herself in the future after a task or goal has been completed and is a method for designing "future memories."

Milton Erickson (1954, 1980) used pseudo-orientation in time for many problems. He would ask the client in an age-progressed state how a problem on which the client was working was resolved. Erickson would then use amnesia for the experience and engage the strategy the client gave him.

Age progression can be accomplished using suggestions, which might include creating an imaginary vehicle for moving into the future, viewing a movie of the future, or reading a special book titled *My Future*. We can use direct suggestion, presuppositions, or the visualization of the older, wiser "Future Self" to help a client move comfortably into an imagined future time when a particular goal has been accomplished. The Future Self then becomes a resource for instruction on how to accomplish the goal and the steps to take in order to do so. In addition, it can become a confidant, counselor, and emotional comforter, one of the client's inner resources to be used on his or her path toward wholeness.

Obviously there will always be events beyond a person's control. Notwithstanding unexpected events, however, we suggest to our clients that they have more power than they believe to direct and control their lives, and to move into the future they most want to experience.

Multiple Future Selves Technique

We suggest that the client take note of him- or herself sitting "here" in a chair and notice the Future Self somewhere in the distance. Then we suggest visualizing a second Future Self that observes both the first Future Self and the client. In doing so, the client has actually created *two* third-person perspectives (similar to the film *Jaws* in which the viewer sees the girl's perspective, the shark's perspective, and the camera's perspective). The two Future Selves can then be invited to share their observations on whatever issue the client is considering. The client may be surprised to find that the second Future Self has observations not yet known to either the ego or the first Future Self.

Quantum Leap to a "Place Beyond Time and Space"

In the Quantum Leap exercise, the client is instructed to develop a deeply relaxed state. The visualization entails having the client "leap" to an imagined "Place Beyond Time and Space." The client can then "retrieve" from the alternate dimension those resources needed for the present time.

The journey to a Place Beyond Time and Space is an imagined experience in which the client moves to a "place" that is unfettered by time and space (or to a "parallel reality" or "alternate dimension"), thereby locating new resources and entering into an empowered state of confidence.

Many cultures have used time projection and the essential experience at the core of the Place Beyond Time and Space exercise in ritualistic ways. Some of these include trance dancing, fire walking, and the Native American vision quest. Meditative practices can also elicit this state. The Australian Aborigines call this state the "dream time." Some expert trackers are reputed to have the ability to follow someone's trail through the Australian outback as much as a year after the fact. They access the information in a trance state and describe being able to walk "beside" the person. From this perspective, they can accurately describe details of the experience.

One friend of ours resided briefly among the people of an indigenous South American culture. While he was there, one family lost their son in a tragic accident. In their grief, the family was terribly upset and distraught. In such a situation, the custom of the tribe was to accompany the family to the woods and dance all night long until the entire tribe experienced a collective vision (or group hallucination). The tribe surrounded the family and sang and danced all night long until all of those present described the same thing: They saw the deceased son, who spoke to them. He said: "I love you, and I am not alone. Our people who have gone ahead are here. I am fine, and it is time for you to go back to your lives." Around daybreak, everyone returned to the village. Our friend witnessed this event and, although he did not personally see the son, he said it was incredible to observe the shift in the family and in the entire tribe. Through the experience, something powerful and meaning-ful had been shifted. This shift brought peace to the family and allowed everyone in the village to return to a state of balance and continue their everyday lives.

Thinking Back in Time

Another exercise that we use with clients in deep state work is to have them think back from the present, in either a professional or per-sonal sense, and examine how events became "organized" to lead to to-day. For example, we might say: "What we are doing now will become the past, and today was once the future, so we are always looking ahead in some fashion. Similarly, the past was once the present, so in another sense, we are always looking back." We encourage the client to notice that what he or she is doing now might be influenced by an unconscious concept of the future.

A playful variant of this exercise is to ask the client to imagine the future 10 or 20 years from now by taking a starship into one possible fu-ture and then thinking back to the present year. We then instruct the client to imagine what he or she wishes he or she had done differently in the present. This exercise can powerfully challenge the organization of priorities.

The Oracle

In therapeutic deep states, clients may receive archetypal information in the form of symbols, hear voices, or sense people being present. The information received is rich in meaning, seems intuitively accurate, and can be used to assist the client's therapy. Elmer Green described receiv-ing these archetypes from the "field of information" and believed that individuals could both create and control synchronicities. To facilitate this ability, Green practiced and taught a process that he called "inter-rogating and programming the collective unconscious" (Green & Green, 1971) to both ask for information regarding a problem and request a certain outcome in a state of autogenic shift, i.e., a state of deep quiet and alertness.

Similarly, Jacob Needleman (1983) described a quality of conscious-ness that is more of a "quality of presence which appears when one is brought in front of the contradictions of one's own life and mind" (p. 174). In deep state work, a client facing such contradictions may more readily recognize them and also discover previously unimagined ways to transcend those contradictions, thereby creating a future that could not have been envisioned earlier.

For many clients, however, the idea of consulting the "unconscious" may be too abstract. In that case, we encourage the client to "take a journey to consult with an oracle." We suggest that the oracle could be a wise person, an animal, or even an ancient tree. In a theta state, the client "journeys" until he or she encounters the oracle figure. At that point, the client visualizes the question or difficulty to be resolved, asks for a comment or answer, and waits for some information to emerge.

Trance Identification

While the client is in a deep state, we may direct him or her to select an individual who has already achieved the client's desired life goal or who possesses certain desired abilities and "merge with" (completely identify with) that person, thereby taking on the desired qualities of that individual. During the day, the client is instructed to maintain the imagined immersion in the other person and to note any changes in his or her perceptions, attitudes, and behaviors.

Case Example: Using Deep State Work to Address Anxiety

Upon her internist's recommendation that she consider "stress management counseling," Deirdre called for an appointment. A woman in her early 70s, Deirdre was still striking, with deep green eyes, pale skin, and white hair that fell in soft waves to her shoulders.

Deirdre related that she had been "plagued" by anxiety for as long as she could remember; she had been taking antianxiety medication for over 25 years. As with many physician-prescribed medications, it was addictive, and, for a second time, the dosage that kept her anxiety at bay was "creeping" significantly. The first time, about 18 years earlier, she had committed herself to a drug rehabilitation program and had managed to stabilize her medication dosage for a number of years. At this point in time, however, her current dose had become largely ineffective and her internist refused to increase the dosage due to possible complications from side effects—particularly a decrease in her balance that, added to severe osteoporosis, meant that any fall might be very serious.

At her first appointment, Deirdre sat in the office with her left hand gripping the arm of the chair so tightly that her knuckles were white, and every tendon across the top of her hand stood out clearly. Coming into co-resonance with the client, Bill could feel his stomach churning. Deirdre made it clear that she had no interest in introspection; she hoped that Bill could "do something" to reduce her anxiety. Listening to her, the image that came to his mind was of a woman dropping off her car for repairs: "Fix it, please. And call me when it's ready."

As Bill progressed with the assessment, he asked Deirdre about her family of origin and she visibly tightened further. She replied that she had no desire to do psychoanalysis; she "guessed her family was like most others." Bill explained that he just wanted to understand how her life may have been impacted by early family experience. Her defensiveness suggested the possibility of early trauma. Attempting to desensitize her anxiety, turn off the fear circuit, and develop rapport, Bill was careful to speak very softly to her.

Over subsequent sessions, Deirdre was able to become increasingly relaxed. Bill used hypnotic empathy and conversational hypnosis to suggest that it was safe for Deirdre to deepen her trust in him, for example, in sentences such as, "Why don't you try this chair? I *trust* you'll find it comfortable."

During her third session, with deep hypnosis to reach a theta state, she related the following hypnogogic vision: She was in an old farmhouse that seemed to be abandoned. She had never been there before. Wandering around, exploring, she saw cobwebs everywhere. There were old papers, musty books, and discarded articles of clothing lying on the floor in different rooms. As she was about to leave, she suddenly heard an infant crying. Startled, she tried to follow the sound of the crying. Going upstairs, she went from room to room. Finally she found another stairway that led to the attic. The crying seemed to be coming from there. When she reached the attic, she realized that part of the roof had fallen in and it was raining into the house. But in one corner, under the eaves, was an old footlocker. It was open, and in it was a naked baby. At first she was afraid to touch the infant. But then the baby turned and looked at her. The baby had dark eyes, and her tiny checks were soaked and red from crying. In the next instant she realized that she was holding the baby. They were both crying, crying together. They were rocking together. She heard herself saying again and again, "It's okay . . . it's going to be okay . . . . it's okay . . . it's going to be okay." As Deirdre related the inner event that she had experienced, her body rocked back and forth and she began to cry. Turning to Bill, she said slowly, "That was me, wasn't it?", and in her tone it was clear that it wasn't really a question.

During a later deep hypnosis session that incorporated an alpha–theta device, Bill suggested that she was now a year older. "Time is different here. It's fluid, like a river. It flows, and you can flow with it. You can flow upstream, or you can flow downstream. Just as your present self could flow into the past and see the baby in what seemed to be an abandoned old farmhouse, you can flow into the future and see yourself as you will be 1 year from now." Bill suggested that her anxiety had largely disappeared and that, on many days, she no longer needed any pills. As Bill spoke, Deirdre smiled slightly. She was open to that future. By the end of the next month, Deirdre had reduced her dependence on the anti-anxiety medication enough that she was able to maintain a comfortable state even with a slightly lower dosage.

In and of itself, the therapeutic experience of alpha–theta states can facilitate profound behavioral changes. While in these deep states, accessed using neurofeedback equipment or deep hypnosis, a client can also be guided to re-envision his or her future or past and return to the present with a greatly expanded sense of what might be possible. In addition to techniques and exercises for deep state work, the chapter offers a sample theta training script.

As we now know, the chronic activation of the fight–flight–freeze response not only leads to dysfunctional behavior, but over time, chronic fear can also inflict significant damage to the frontal and temporal regions of the brain. In the next chapter, we explore ways to resolve fear by using BCT.

CHAPTER 8

Resolving Fear with Brain Change Therapy

The underlying driver of the fight–flight–freeze response is fear, and the chronic activation of that response can express itself in a number of dysfunctional modes. Apart from rage, the primary modes are anxiety, depression, and shame. Since the latter three states are often found as an interwoven set in many clients, this chapter examines the dynamics between them and the therapeutic approaches to resolving them through BCT.

Bruce McEwen, in *The End of Stress as We Know It* (2002), observed that the mind is so powerful that it can set off the stress response just by imagining a frightening situation. A person can literally bring on a complete stress reaction just by conjuring up a worst-case scenario. The chronic activation of the fight–flight–freeze response not only leads to immediately dysfunctional behavior, but over time, can also inflict sufficient damage to the frontal and temporal regions of the brain to precipitate frontotemporal dementia (Bremner, 2005). Frontotemporal damage impairs the ability to control fear as well as the abilities to reason and understand the significance of events (Bremner, 2002), leaving the afflicted person in a generalized state of confusion and anxiety. Fear in its various expressions also increases cortisol in the brain. Cortisol counteracts a brain-nourishing hormone called *brain-derived neurotrophic factor* (BDNF; Bremner, 2002). Loss of BDNF leads to neuronal cell death within the hippocampus, which also impairs memory (Siever, 2009).

The Eeyore Syndrome

Eeyore, a donkey who was so depressed that he found no joy in life and expected everything to go badly, first appeared in *Winnie-the-Pooh* (Milne, 1926). The donkey lived in the Hundred Acre Wood in a place called "Eeyore's Gloomy Place: Rather Boggy and Sad." He held strong judgments about all the other animals and believed them to have no brains—just fluff. A perennial pessimist, Eeyore might have been heard to remark, "The sun is shining. I'll probably get a burn." Whatever it was, Eeyore imagined the worst. He was especially sensitive to events that threatened his sense of internal security. Whether Eeyore had an attachment disorder or suffered some trauma in his early life is unknown.

The "Eeyore syndrome" refers to the tendency in some people to fixate on the darkest element in any situation, no matter how favorable the overall event: the one thoughtless comment made by someone at an otherwise delightful garden party; the one time the driver took a wrong turn and became lost over the course of a 4-day road trip; or the one time the person put quarters into a vending machine and the candy bar got stuck. A person with the Eeyore syndrome might agree with Douglas Adams (1995): "In the beginning the Universe was created. This has made a lot of people very angry and been widely regarded as a bad move" (p. 34). Such people have the unerring ability "to turn even the finest wines to vinegar" and then brood about the situation, grinding a deeper and deeper rut in the neuropathways of pessimism. And some of them become clients.

Anyone can experience an "Eeyore day," particularly during a period of uncertainty. However, clients in whom this tendency is exacerbated are some of the more difficult to treat. These clients are chronically disappointed with life, family, friends, and work, and they frequently have a shame overlay based on their inability to control their state of mind. Depression is often their response to seeing themselves as helpless, as "victims of circumstance." Equally disappointed with the therapeutic experience, they tend to move from therapist to therapist in the hope of solving the chronic sense of feeling bad.

Being continually disappointed and expecting the worst, these clients are apt to discount any positive comment the therapist might make. The clinician can sense that no comment gets past their filters so that it can be experienced as empathic or supportive. No matter the intervention, there is something not quite right about it. Even if the therapist notices that some aspects of the client's life have improved, often the client cannot recognize it.

Robert Sapolsky, a Stanford University neuroscientist, suggested that depression occurs "when your cortex thinks an abstract negative thought and manages to convince the rest of the brain that this is as real as a physical stressor" (2004, p. 354). Sapolsky suggested that stress is anything that knocks a person out of homeostatic balance. The states that usually need to be activated in the Eeyore syndrome are those of curiosity and safety. In addition, using humor will effect a state change. In the process, the therapist will find it helpful to discover what the depression is related to, whether it be early disruption, head injury, or bonding issues that need clinical attention. Frequently, early caregivers of these clients were anxious, fearful, and perfectionistic.

Being unable to shift out of a chronic state is often a matter of brain circuitry and neurological inefficiency rather than some chemical imbalance (Sams, 2006), and using brain-training devices or hypnotic deep state training may be helpful. However, for an individual to be able to move from a sense of hopelessness and helplessness into one of control, the therapist first needs to accept his or her reality and explore the reported areas of the client's life where "nothing is working." By accepting the person's ideas of how things are, the clinician can make the client right about something.

The following is a transcript of how one client was able to move into a more empowering state.

Therapist: You have said you are old and alone. Your house is falling down around you. You have no friends. Your car is in need of repair. There just is nothing working well for you, and even if it did, it wouldn't be long before that too would be in a mess.

Barry: Nothing in my life is going well. I can't remember a time when anything worked well, so I just go to the pub one day a week and numb the feelings by drinking beer.

Therapist: And when you numb the feelings, it is not that you really feel any better; it is just a temporary experience of feeling no pain?

Barry: That's so right. Even though I may like the beer and the band, when I leave the pub, everything is the same.

Therapist: So that experience of everything being the same is a state you return to so much of the time, and it may even be difficult to recognize feeling even a little better. Tell me about the pub and why you go to the same one each week.

Barry: It's familiar; people know me there. Every once in a while, they have a good band.

Therapist: So you see the same people each week and even though you may feel in a rut, there is something familiar. What is *familiar* like?

Barry: Familiar is the same thing over and over again; it can really be boring.

Therapist: Familiarity can be boring and just "more of the same," and sometimes it might be interesting to experience the boringness of familiarity when so many aspects of life are uncertain. [This comment was designed to turn on curiosity about the possibilities of things getting better.]

Barry: I would really like to have a life that wasn't so boring.

Therapist: It is something you yearn for: you wonder what life would be like if you were doing what you really wanted, and you think about how to make that happen. We just went through Hurricane Ike. How was that for you?

Barry: It was scary, and I didn't sleep a wink. The wind was so loud.

Therapist: Were you bored in the middle of it?

Barry: Not really.

Therapist: Someone in our neighborhood put up a sign after the storm that said "Ike, Tina doesn't live here anymore. Go away." (*Client starts to smile.*) And then after a number of days without power, signs started to go up that read, "Will trade favors for power." (*Client continues to smile and adds his own funny stories.*)

For someone who experiences habitually pessimistic feelings, one intervention of stimulating curiosity and humor is a very small event, but it accomplishes two things: It changes the client's state during the interchange, and it helps the client begin to develop the ability to shift states for him- or herself. We followed this shift with more intense work. Gradually, Barry learned how to move into a neutral state by noticing the flowers and plants in his yard and naming them without judgment. In the process, he became aware that he had negative judgments about almost everything. With practice, he became more able to notice elements in his surroundings without immediately assigning them a "good" or—far more often—a "bad" label. In so doing, Barry started to learn to shift his neural patterns, control his mind, and keep it from wandering into Eeyore's Gloomy Bog.

Anxiety

Habituated patterns of anxiety often have their beginnings in early childhood trauma. When caregivers are quick to mete out sudden retribution, particularly for reasons that children may not grasp, the children can develop a nearly permanent state of vigilance, eventually deteriorating into a chronic and unfocused state of anxiety. Additionally, such an individual may have a neurological predisposition toward anxiety.

A wide range of mental health disorders fall under the umbrella of anxiety, including generalized anxiety disorder (GAD), panic disorder, social phobias, obsessive–compulsive disorder (in its intrusive, anxiety-producing ideation or impulses), and PTSD. All anxiety disorders entail a chronic and exaggerated fear of impending doom. Peter Levine, in *Waking the Tiger* (1997), described the core of the anxiety reaction as involving the following characteristics:

- *Hyperarousal*: Increased heart rate, agitation, racing thoughts, or difficulty breathing begins under severe stress; anxiety begins to develop as a short-term solution to undischarged energy.
- *Constriction*: Focus is narrowed, breathing is limited and shallow, and blood vessels constrict, making more blood available to the muscles that are tensed and prepared to take defensive action.
- *Dissociation*: A "split" between mind and body or components of the personality leads to fogginess, feeling spacey, and a heightened pain threshold. This split may occur between various parts of the body and/or psyche; between the experience of self and emotions, thoughts, or sensations; or between a memory and part or all of a previously experienced event.
- *Immobility*: A physical or mental "freezing" accompanied by a feeling of helplessness.

When these characteristics become chronic, they may trigger secondary conditions such as hypervigilance; intrusive imagery; extreme sensitivity to light, sound, or noise of any kind; extreme anxiety; startle reactions or temper outbursts followed by shame or grief responses; disturbed dreams or frequent waking in the night; moodiness; stress vulnerability; and sensitivity to textures and smells.

Even more severe symptoms may ensue: panic attacks; phobias; a fear of dying or having a mental breakdown; the avoidance of other people, including the inability to be involved in social situations; the inability to bond with others; diminished emotional response; and sweating, hot flashes, and trembling. By the time these symptoms develop, the individual no longer has any rational explanation for the reactions. When internal states are discontinuous or inexplicable, people begin to develop ancillary symptoms. In a state of high anxiety, it is impossible to assimilate new information or access other resources, such as one's ability to self-soothe. Attention is narrowly focused, and perception is distorted. Memory declines, and it becomes difficult to hold a thought. Reactions are automatic; thinking becomes concrete. In a full-blown panic attack, lower-order behaviors are accessed, age regression ensues, and primitive thinking, with associations from childhood, can be experienced.

Neurobiology of Anxiety Disorders

Fear, specifically the fear of being unable to prevent the worst possible future from occurring, often underlies the feelings of anxiety. In a study conducted by Richard Davidson (2003), researchers found a positive correlation between the emotions of fear and sadness, increased cortisol levels, and frontal EEG asymmetry. Anxiety and, in its more extreme expression, panic, occur as a result of dysregulated centers in the central nervous system. Fear-producing stimuli are first processed by the amygdala. Aiding the amygdala, the thalamus helps in determining to what extent the stimulus is an actual threat. The hippocampus and cortical regions of the brain also play a part in the evaluation of the information sent from the thalamus. In this process, the interpretation of the stimulus is filtered through past experience and conditioned responses. Messages go out to the peripheral nervous system to increase blood pressure, heart rate, and the fear response of fleeing, fighting, or freezing. Even if an individual "knows" the response is an overreaction, once neurological processing has passed a certain point, it must run the course of excitation, response, and subsequent calming.

Several neurotransmitters are involved in anxiety disorders. Low serotonin levels seem to be a factor, and symptoms tend to improve in many when medication allows more serotonin to be present in the neurons. Compounding matters, individuals with chronic anxiety issues tend to have decreased levels of GABA (gamma-aminobutyric acid) as well as an increase in plasma epinephrine, even when in a resting state. As the levels of serotonin and GABA are reduced in the brain, anxiety and distress increase (Moss, 2003; Berstein, 1995).

Closely related to the experience of anxiety is altered breathing. Anxious people rarely breathe deeply enough. An individual who feels highly anxious may begin to hyperventilate, resulting in decreased carbon dioxide in the blood and decreased cerebral blood flow (Mars, 1998). This reduction results in the stimulation of the sympathetic nervous system, and a variety of symptoms may ensue: fatigue, tension, tremors, stomach pain, difficulty breathing, dizziness, visual distortions, and heart palpitations. As the heart begins to beat faster, the person is apt to become fixated on the physical sensations and is further apt to make negative interpretations of them. What follows is often a closed feedback loop: With increased attention, the symptoms are likely to become more pronounced, which draws even more increased attention.

The individual who is prone to anxiety can eventually become so attuned to bodily sensations that any slight change will be interpreted to mean that death may be imminent. A watchful eye on heart rate, taste, and skin sensations can contribute to the problem. After a time, the anxiety takes on a life of its own, until even a slight stimulus can cause an intense reaction. In fact, the anxious-prone person can set off an anxiety attack merely by thinking it might happen. In essence, the person mentally rehearses it until it occurs.

If the anxiety pattern begins early in life, a person may become so habituated that the discomfort is perceived as normal. This feeling state can become automatic and affect perceptions and thinking. Diaphragmatic breathing and heart rate variability training (e.g., using the em-Wave device) can be useful in changing to calmer states. Teaching clients to discriminate among various body signals, make accurate interpretations of what they feel, and react with appropriate responses is also important. For example, a client may need to learn to distinguish between a normal tensing in the body in relation to feeling excited or surprised and the out-of-control feeling of a panic problem, so that normal tensing does not inevitably lead to panic.

Anxiety disorders tend to run in families, meaning that the likelihood for developing the disorder is higher if someone in the family already has it. In one study, researchers concluded that children whose parents have issues with panic, depression, or both have an increased risk for panic disorder, social anxiety disorder, depression, disruptive behavior disorders, and poor social functioning (Biederman et al., 2001).

For a client with anxiety issues, the voice and the face of the therapist can serve a powerful function as a holding environment and a bridge to new interpretations of experiences. When a client feels genuinely cared for, anxiety can be tolerated more easily and channeled toward change until, eventually, the old feelings and provocations no longer trigger the same negative states of consciousness.

Between-Session Techniques for Clients with Panic Attacks

Panic attacks, or the temporary heightening of anxiety to the point that complete physiological dysfunction may ensue, often drive individuals to seek therapeutic counseling. However, clients seldom have panic attacks in the therapist's office; instead, they occur out in the "real world." For that reason, we recommend "tools" or techniques that they can take with them to address the physiology of a panic attack. In addition to their actual efficacy, the techniques function in part by invoking the placebo effect (the measurable, observable, or felt improvement in health or behavior not attributable to a medication or invasive treatment) and in part as transitional objects (items used to provide psychological comfort, because by association they are connected to a person who represents security). We suggest the following techniques to our clients:

- Use of a *small paper bag*. Instruct the client to breathe into a small paper bag to help regulate breathing until the attack subsides. During a panic attack, a person is likely to hyperventilate, thereby exhaling more carbon dioxide than normal. By breathing in a somewhat enclosed environment (the paper bag), the client inhales air that is slightly more carbon dioxide-rich than usual (slightly less oxygen-rich). By marginally reducing the blood oxygen, the person becomes calmer. Additionally, the entire process gives the client a proscriptive activity and causes him or her to focus on breathing. For clients with panic problems that occur in the car, we emphasize the following: *"Do not attempt to drive during a panic attack. Immediately pull over to the side of the road.* Then use a small paper bag, which can be kept in the car."

- *Use of ReliefBand.* The ReliefBand® is a small device that looks similar to a wristwatch. This device sends a mild electric current into acupuncture points on the wrist, and it can facilitate state change by generating an alpha frequency. Originally developed for motion sickness, the product can be purchased on the Internet under that brand name.

- *Use of meridian stimulation.* Tapping on the acupuncture meridian point between the eyes as well as several other meridian points and breathing from the diaphragm changes the state and can stop anxiety (Wells, Polglase, Andrews, Carrington, & Baker, 2003).

- *Use of the DAVID PAL.* This device can alter an anxious state in a brief period of time.

Case Studies Addressing Panic Attacks

- David was an attorney specializing in contract law who had decided to go back to graduate school. He had always experienced difficulty speaking in front of a group. As a contract attorney, he had not needed to speak in public. However, in graduate school, there was no way to avoid it. Every time he had to make a presentation in class, he experienced an anxiety attack. He would break out in a cold sweat, and by the time he finished speaking, his shirt would be literally soaked. Using hypnosis, we led David to the edge of sleep while maintaining awareness and allowed him to "float" there in a healing theta state for at least 10 minutes. We also suggested he take 500 mg of GABA prior to a presentation to ameliorate the sweating response. Both GABA and 5HTP (5-hydroxytryptophan) have a calming effect on the brain; a severe shortage of these chemicals can actually cause an anxiety disorder. After six sessions, David was able to relax enough to make effective presentations, and he completely stopped perspiring when he spoke in public.

- Mike had a history of emotional and physical abuse by his mother. He was so highly attuned to any bodily sensation that he slid from noticing a slight physiological sensation into experiencing a full-blown panic attack two to three times a day. At the age of 38, Mike was a successful

CPA, but another one of the partners in his firm realized he was near the breaking point and suggested that he look into some therapy. By the time he came to Carol's office, he was experiencing severe insomnia, was in tears more than once a day, and complained of a funny metallic taste in his mouth.

Carol began by working to modify his breathing, which was very shallow. Sitting opposite him, she explained that he needed to breathe more deeply and that they would start by breathing together. Moving her hand up and down to indicate the inbreath and outbreath (like a musical director setting the beat), she began to breathe slowly, and instructed Mike to breathe with her. Twenty minutes later, a smile slowly began to tug at the corners of Mike's face. He reported that, for the first time in many days, he experienced relief.

In subsequent sessions, Mike explained that he had been in therapy with someone who encouraged him to relive the past repeatedly. He had been trying to scream his way to health. We believed that this process was restimulating his childhood trauma and suggested that he stop that process. Carol recommended some other breathing exercises. For example, in one exercise originally developed by Herbert Benson, who pioneered the relaxation response based on Transcendental Meditation, a person visualizes the number *1* on his or her mental screen. As the person exhales, the number moves into the background. With inhalation, the image of *1* returns to the foreground. In addition, alpha–theta training was used to calm his whole system. Before long, Mike had improved enough that he was again working in his office and meeting with his clients rather than having all the work delivered to his home by the office manager.

• Arriving at the office one morning, Carol picked up a telephone message from a man with a strong Middle Eastern accent who said he was calling on behalf of a prince(!) who was in desperate need of treatment. We presumed the message was someone's idea of humor and deleted it. What followed was a complete surprise. Two days later when we were in the office, the gentleman called back. During a half-hour conversation, he asked us to head a treatment team (that would include a psychiatrist) to assist a young man of royalty in the Middle East. We were told that the young man suffered from panic attacks, agoraphobia, and acrophobia. He could not leave his palace either by automobile or by plane without experiencing crippling anxiety. It was close to Thanksgiving, and we were struggling with the decision. A couple of days later, the prince himself called and, in halting English, personally asked us to come to the Middle East to treat him. Not at all certain what we would be getting into, we consented.

First-class airline tickets arrived a day later by Express Mail. Stepping off the plane, we were met by the prince's driver and a couple other security agents, literally waved through customs, and escorted to the hotel. We began to formulate how we might help a young man whose anxiety was so debilitating that he could no longer leave his palace to attend school.

Our initial consultation took place in the palace, a bold modern structure incorporating design elements abstracted from traditional Arabic architecture. We were served a very strong black tea, highly sweetened and flavored with cardamom. Later we learned that the prince drank many glasses of that tea daily and wondered about a possible relationship between a high caffeine intake and his anxiety. Talking to us through an interpreter, he told us that his father and sister also suffered immensely from panic disorder. Thirty minutes into our first meeting, a loud horn sounded. Our host stood up, asked us to wait until prayers had been finished, and excused himself.

As the directors of the therapeutic team, we knew that we would have complete freedom to use any combination of treatments that we felt would be effective and therefore had taken a neurofeedback device with us. By the end of a week of neurofeedback, hypnosis translated by one of his advisors, and an SSRI (that he first gave to one of his attendants to confirm its safety), the prince took us to his mother's palace for dinner. This was the first time he had ventured outside his own compound in 2 years. We encouraged him the entire way and on arrival began to "high-five" his success. Revealing some of the family dynamics and the fact that her son could not do enough to please her, his mother greeted him with evident disdain and scornfully asked why he could not have come the night before. As the dinner progressed, we better understood her curious response. Explaining that the Qur'an allows a man to have up to four wives and that it was the custom for royal men to have four, she complained that she never saw her husband. Generally pessimistic and disappointed with her life, she seemed wrapped in a mantle of permanent defeat. We could only surmise that beneath that defeat lay the rage that she seemed to take out on her son.

On the last day of our visit, the prince personally escorted us to the airport and thanked us for our work. A year later, we heard from him again. He had completed his degree and was busy managing one of his father's businesses.

Shame

Shame is generally an amalgam of inadequacy, frustration, anger, depression, and failure. These emotional states create neural pathways that then often reinforce behavioral patterns of emotional pain, self-neglect, and a sense of victimization. Such self-destructive patterns are warped forms of endurance that are developed early as a means of survival. Clients, of whatever age, may still be under the negative "spell" of someone who was abusive in childhood, when they were conditioned to experience deep embarrassment and anxiety.

There are three key aspects to consider in a shame state reaction: a tendency to experience disproportionate shame, which commonly develops from *excessive early criticism* by someone important in an individual's family of origin; a *fear of someone's judgment* (the individual has been judged and "found guilty"); and, usually, *self-blame* (the individual agrees with the judgment). Collectively, these three factors tend to create a negative trance state in which an individual experiences a negative physiological sensation of "shrinking" accompanied by a flooding of feelings. Not understanding that they can control their states, clients may feel at the mercy of their own ingrained patterns of neural firing and behavior. The therapist must empathically resonate with and attune to a client to help the person move beyond these negative states into areas of possibility and openness, and finally, to states of happiness and thriving.

The Neurophysiology of Shame

The first experience of shame generally occurs around the age of 2, when a child becomes aware of a parent's disapproving tone and negative facial expressions. Schore (2003) pointed out that shame involves the internalized image of a mother's face, whose expression was mismatched to what the child was doing. Shame becomes an imprint of the parent's unhappiness at the child's behavior, to the extent that the child experiences a significant fear of rejection and of the parental bond being broken.

Researchers have discovered that the pain of social rejection is neurologically similar to that of physical pain. Participants in a study played a virtual ball-tossing game, during which they were eventually excluded. During exclusion, their brain scans showed increased activity in the dorsal anterior cingulate cortex and in the anterior insula—the same areas often associated with the distress of physical pain (Eisenberger, Lieberman, & Williams, 2003). Over time, the parent's response results in a "shame signal"—that is, the trigger for the resulting hesitancy and doubt that suppress "bad" behavior and thereby allow the child to avoid the pain of actual rejection.

The experience of shame activates the dorsal medial nucleus of the hypothalamus. This part of the brain produces changes in mood and smooth muscle activity (Schore, 1997). The emotion of shame also activates the parasympathetic nervous system and can immobilize a person in the freeze response. Shore observed that shame rewires the brain and tends to deactivate and prune connections between the limbic and prefrontal systems. The most serious effects, however, are the increased activation of the fight–flight–freeze survival response of the amygdala, the entrenched circuit of FEAR, and the resulting defensive behavior.

In order for the shame-based client to recover, the therapist needs to (1) activate connections to the prefrontal system through empathy and rapport-building and (2) inhibit the shame responses. When intense shame is activated due to poor attachment history, an individual may have difficulty being alone and may even develop manic defenses that cause impulsivity and avoidance of introspection—a reaction that precludes addressing deeper feelings and concerns (Winnicott, 1958). Cozolino (2002, p. 200) suggested that people with manic defenses are frequently misdiagnosed as having attention-deficit disorder.

Differentiating Shame and Guilt

Shame is an emotion in which a person has an overwhelming experience of badness based on an external value system. Derived from presumed external judgments, shame involves a person's self-image in front of others. Shame says, "*They* say I am bad." Shame can be debilitating: The more shameful a person feels, the more likely he or she is to be defensive, deny any wrongdoing, and become anxious or depressed.

Guilt occurs when an individual transgresses an internally held value system, especially in the case of harming another individual. Guilt has to do with a person's self-image in front of him- or herself. Guilt says "*I* did something harmful—something I know was bad."

The therapist will need to distinguish between two types of guilt. One type is an internalized shame carried over from childhood. That guilt adds, "You make me feel so guilty. . . ." The underlying emotion here is resentment, an unacknowledged anger directed at the other. This can be addressed therapeutically within the context of shame.

A different type of guilt arises from adult situations in which, simply put, "bad things happen" that are only partly due to a person's volition. This guilt adds, "I'm terribly sorry." Soldiers who are required to kill other humans often experience major guilt. Automobile accidents in which a pedestrian or bicyclist is killed often leave the driver with profound guilt. Having to consign an aging parent to a nursing home against the parent's wishes, due to the requirements of the parent's care and the larger family circumstances, can cause terrible guilt. The underlying emotions in those cases tend to be sorrow and deep regret. The essence of the work, then, is helping the client to experience forgiveness and particularly to find self-forgiveness, often through some form of reparation or penance.

There is also a middle ground. For example, when a partner needs to feel loved and appreciated in a relationship but does not, this need may be in conflict with the personally held value of commitment to a marriage. If this individual steps outside the relationship to try to meet that need, the breaking of the marital vows may result in either shame or guilt: shame, if the person feels that his or her behavior was largely justified, or guilt, if the person feels it was intrinsically wrong.

Shifting the Experience of Shame

To resolve shameful feelings, we suggest that a client identify the "wave" nature of a feeling. People caught in the web of shame commonly react to situations in which they experienced embarrassment or shame by repetitively reviewing them and engaging in emotional self-flagellation. The rumination can become more painful than the precipitating event. We encourage the client to observe that, if he or she doesn't hold onto it, the feeling comes and goes just as a wave comes into the shore and then retreats. By simply sitting with the physiological sensations he or she associates with shame, a person will notice that, eventually, they dissipate, and a new feeling will arise. The mind chatters incessantly, and if a client can observe the mind's contents without identifying with those contents, he or she can become his or her own mental anthropologist and begin to observe without judgment.

A second, or alternative, antidote for shame is to bring it out into the open. The more an individual can talk about the experience, the more the sensation of shame will abate. Sharing the associated emotions with a clinician who responds empathically can ultimately shift the state from shame to one of less anxiety or depression, and eventually to relief. As long as a sense of disgrace is held in secrecy, its grip on the psyche remains intact.

The final possibility is to have the client embrace the feelings of shame as a way to transmute the energy into insight and awareness. This attempt may interrupt the sensation and allow the person to begin to develop greater self-understanding and forgiveness.

When a client feels shame starting to dissipate through whatever means, confusion about what is occurring may follow. In fact, whenever there is improvement (for example, in the abatement of anxiety), the client will expect and look for the same level of intensity (neural activation) *somewhere*. It is as if the individual's sense of internal homeostasis has become so accustomed to a certain level of activation (whether driven by shame, anxiety, or another habitual pattern) that any alteration feels confusing. We suggest to the client that confusion may be a step toward a change that is getting ready to occur. We encourage clients to allow the "wave" of confusion to pass.

Hypnotic Protocol for Resolving Shame

We have found that hypnosis can assist a client considerably in letting go of shame. This shift is due both to increased relaxation and to increased suggestibility. To use hypnosis in this context, we suggest the following protocol:

1. Ask the client to focus visually on a spot in the room or to focus on his or her breathing.
2. Assist the client in developing a sense of safety by imagining the place where he or she feels most "at home," relaxed, or at peace. This step is particularly critical, because people who have shame reactions

frequently feel insecure. This process begins to shift the internal state to one of comfort. By carefully watching, the clinician will be able to tell from the facial reaction when the person has accomplished this part. Frequently, the client will take a deep breath accompanied by a slight shudder that indicates that a neurological shift has occurred.

3. For emotional grounding, suggest that the client keep his or her feet flat on the floor. We sometimes suggest that the client imagine breathing through the soles of the feet, placing the breath lower in the body in imagination.

4. Assist the client in identifying a figure of comfort, such as an older, wiser individual. When families are working well, parents and/or grandparents validate their children/grandchildren consistently, who thereby learn to trust their own decisions as adults. Parents give compliments, suggest positive futures, and look forward to each child building on the success he or she feels in the moment. Although a client may not have had these experiences in the family or origin, he or she will often have experienced another powerful figure of comfort. If the client has difficulty identifying any figure of comfort, the clinician may develop an imaginary figure who can give a "blessing" to the client. (See the following section for an example of the dialogue used in a hypnotic induction with a figure of comfort.)

5. Find areas of growth on which to compliment the client so that the reinforcement continues in the present. At this point, the therapist becomes the immediate figure of comfort who extends the validation.

6. It may be appropriate to suggest that a client's negative schema or emotional pattern may have come from someone else in the family who felt ashamed. Frequently, children develop a kind of synchrony with a particular parent and end up carrying the negative feelings the parent has not worked through. By suggesting that the shame does not "belong" to the client, it is often easier for the client to let go of it. The goal is to rid the person of the shame reaction and to change the neurophysiological response.

Hypnotic Induction Invoking a Figure of Comfort

One technique for resolving shameful feelings and building self-confidence is to invoke a figure of comfort, such as a mentor, kindly grandparent, a neighbor, or an aunt, who held the client in high-esteem.

Giving a voice to this important figure can enhance the client's self-esteem and underscore the fact that he or she has been loved.

We begin by having the client identify someone in the past or present who acknowledged, perceived accurately, and felt empathy and love for the person. If the client cannot think of anyone, a universal figure can be used: a character from film or television, a grandparent figure, or, if appropriate, a religious or mythological figure.

Particularly when we are working therapeutically with someone who is also a clinician, we may use Milton Erickson as a figure of comfort and tell his life story. Many therapists have imagined Erickson as a consultant for either their professional or personal life. The following is a sample of the hypnotic instructions we might use in this context:

> "Sit comfortably in the chair and take a breath. Close your eyes and shift your attention so you can begin to alter your internal state and shift your brain state. It takes such little effort. Continue the inner process of developing comfort and focus on the pleasant feelings in your body. As you tune into those sensations, all the outside sounds can fade into the background. It is now only you with me, here in this moment. Just the two of us right here and now. Go deeper inside now. There are varieties of experiences along the way that allow the development of such a nice feeling of comfort. You have experienced many by now. I don't know which of those might come to your attention as you think about it, but any would be perfectly all right. As you breathe comfortably, going deeper, deeper, and deeper now. . . .
>
> "Everyone who is able to go to Phoenix, where Milton Erickson used to live, takes some time to climb Squaw Peak, a small mountain nearby. In fact, Erickson used to send people to climb it in order to have a learning experience. With every experience you have, there is learning of some sort. It happened not long ago that we took a trip to Squaw Peak with a friend of ours. We climbed the mountain all the way to the top. The interesting thing was that, as you climb up the mountain, you must lean into the side of the hill to compensate for the steepness and angle. As you go up, up, up, by the time you get almost to the top of the hill, you can see all around the Phoenix area, and it is a spectacular view. When you reach the summit, it is an amazing view. We sat on the top of the mountain and became pensive and quiet, and each of us wondered what learning was occurring.
>
> "We were feeling close to Dr. Erickson, because when he died, his

ashes were spread on this very place. We could imagine his essence being with us. Sitting on the top of the mountain, it was almost as if you could experience Dr. Erickson sitting right there with you. Here was a man who struggled with adversity many times in his life, and yet he had the most positive outlook. He had people throughout his career who made light of him, who were dishonoring, and yet when you looked into his eyes, you could see that twinkle that comes from such a good spirit; that comes from someone who wishes only the best for you. Sitting where we were, we could almost hear Dr. Erickson whisper into your ear: 'You are a good person, and you are making an important contribution to the world. You need to go on with your work. Everyone makes an error somewhere along life's journey, but you can put that behind you and accept your own self-forgiveness. Move on into the future and learn from the experience. Take the learning and put it to good use in the future. My voice will always be with you in the wind and the trees; always with you, supporting you, every step of the way. It is important for you to know: You are not alone. There is always more to learn, and you can be excited about what there is to know. Using that in your particular, special way and implementing it in your unique perspective is your path. As you sit here, you can remember these words. You are here for a reason. Move on with your life and look forward to the future.' As you listen to those words of Dr. Erickson, you can take them inside yourself and really feel full.

"Now, we didn't know how much time had elapsed, but we decided to walk back down the mountain, walking carefully to keep a good footing. As you go back down, you must change your way of stepping carefully, taking one foot at a time and planting it firmly to keep the balance. When we were about three-quarters of the way down, the most unusual thing occurred. We both heard the most interesting music. Our eyes cleared, and we saw who was playing the music. There was a hillbilly band at the bottom of the hill. They were playing jugs, saws, and homemade instruments, and they were making a beautiful sound. Isn't it interesting sometimes when you experience something you would never expect to encounter? A hillbilly band at the bottom of Squaw Peak was an amazing sight. That experience, marked by the music, stimulated our feeling, thinking, and thoughtful meditation.

"You may have someone in your life like Dr. Erickson. Perhaps there was a grandparent you felt close to, or a favorite teacher. And when that person looked at you, you felt really loved. This person believed you would be successful; believed in your positive future and knew you would make a contribution to the world just by being you. Sometimes you don't know how that will occur, but it is nice to know there were people in your life that are now inside of you, and who will stay with you and guide you from an internal perspective forever. It may be now or later that some of that person's words might come back to you. You might remember what that individual said that was so encouraging along the way. Perhaps you might write those words down so as to really remember them and memorize them. You can really appreciate that person's contribution to your life as you go on to make a contribution to someone else's.

"Now, begin to come back gently into the room, taking all the time you would like. Reconnect now with all parts of yourself, slowly and comfortably. Ponder for a while what you have experienced."

Case Example Using a Figure of Comfort

Without any knowledge of the technique, one of our clients used figures of comfort for herself as a child. Her family situation was marked by enormous conflict and chaos; no one felt safe. She knew that her home life was different from that of other kids, and she was too deeply ashamed to invite anyone from school to come over. Watching the *Roy Rogers* television show, she used to imagine herself as belonging to that family and having Roy and Dale Evans as parents. In so doing, she began an internal reparenting process that changed her default state and helped her learn how to feel good about herself.

She told us that one day she decided to write Roy Rogers a letter. She mailed it simply to "Hollywood California" and each day went to the mailbox to see if he had responded. After a while, she forgot about checking. One day, a brown envelope appeared in the mailbox, and her mother told her she had something from California. Her heart beat wildly as she opened the envelope. Inside she found a picture of Roy Rogers autographed to her. She said, in that moment, she knew she was loved. Her recollection of this event continued to comfort her for many years, enhanced her ability to feel good about the person she was becoming, and added to her self-esteem.

Other Hypnotic Tools for Dissolving Shame

We use the following techniques for dissolving shame. As examples, they can also be used as springboards for therapists who wish to create their own techniques.

• Many children who grow up in a healthy family have the experience of sitting between their parents and hearing them both speak warm and empathic words. The therapist can *create a similar inner holding environment* to help a client begin to build a sense of personal security. People who feel secure will recover from an embarrassing incident quickly and are able to refrain from ruminating on the event. Use two imaginary figures of comfort, one sitting on each side of the client. Suggest to the client that they are speaking, one in each ear, at the same time. Through the therapist, the figures express positive ideas and feelings about the client.

• The therapist can *use a transitional object*, which may be any object that represents personal success, power, and competence to the client. Such an object may be either a small gift from the therapist, of symbolic value only, or something that the client already owns. In either case, the therapist's interaction infuses it with an enriched meaning that validates the client. Possessing this object helps the client dissolve early programming that caused the individual to believe that he or she was somehow flawed. If the item is small, the clinician can have the client carry it around in a pocket or purse. For example, the renowned Japanese baseball player Sadaharu Oh (Oh & Faulkner, 1985) always carried a small carved dragon in his pocket. He would touch the talismanic dragon, traditionally symbolizing auspicious power, before he stepped up to bat.

• The therapist can *reparent* through metaphors of early learning. If our evaluation identifies a missing developmental task, we can use a metaphor and construct the learning in a hypnotic trance.

• The *use of hypnotic comforting mechanisms*, such as the sound of the therapist's voice, the sound of running water, or any other soothing, calming tone, will help change the client's internal experience. After discovering what sound is particularly comforting to a client, this can become part of all further hypnotic interventions with him or her.

• The therapist can *retrieve resiliency*. Each person has many resiliency resources based on previous challenges that were conquered or completed. Anyone who has finished school has managed feelings of frustration or even failure and worked through them.

• *Using hypnotic empathy*, the therapist can foster basic trust with the client, as another facet of healing shame. By communicating a sense of caring, warmth, and respect in the way we speak to a person, we can issue a reminder of early nurturing that can build a sense of trust. Once this relationship is established, the potential for growth is unlimited.

From "Less Than" to "Good Enough"

In conversation with a client, we can easily identify the shame-based self-induction (the elements or situations that consistently trigger the sensations and "trance of shame"). Invariably the essence of this negative self-induction focuses on something about the self that is "less than" rather than "good enough." The task is then to shift the focus to the person being "good enough." We might say:

> "You have been discussing how you feel inadequate compared to the people you are around, and it is difficult, when you have that sensation, to remember a time when you felt a bit better. It is difficult, when you are having that experience, even to recognize how that couch you are sitting on gives good-enough support. It is difficult to notice when you receive good-enough responses from people around you. And I wonder what it might entail if you were to really hear a good-enough response from people?"

This response to a litany of shortcomings helps shift the client's expectation that everything will continue to be the same, and it may encourage the client to begin noticing subtle positive responses from others. We further suggest to clients:

> "Perhaps you can begin to notice how you are better on a daily basis. Because the natural state is one of healing, you can find those subtle clues in your environment that help you learn, grow, and develop in ways you really want. It might be that one day when you wake up in the morning and look in the mirror, you can notice something different about yourself that will let you know that an important shift has occurred."

This series of suggestions sows an expectation that the client is improving and will be able to notice *something* that leads toward a better feeling and away from negativity. Since it is possible to practice feelings, the more the client practices feeling well, the less he or she may ruminate on negative feelings. Ultimately, the goal is to move the client to a self-perception of "good enough."

Shame in the Context of Intimate Relationships

Marital partners tend to regulate each other's psychobiological states and can participate in stimulating good feelings or, when upset, create what amounts to shame-based inductions. When couples are getting along, there is a resonance between them, a smooth flow of energy back and forth. Negotiations are easy and the energy exchange is dance-like. Partners have easy access to good feelings, and it is almost impossible for them to remember feeling upset with each other.

But when two people are in conflict, the stress response of fight, flight, or freeze is activated in both. Each person participates in heightening the dysregulation of the other's nervous system and stimulating various high-arousal states. If couples do not have the capacity for self-soothing, they can escalate into name calling, attacking, and demeaning the other person in the most vulnerable and sensitive areas.

John Gottman described diffused physical arousal (DPA), the physiological state of emotional flooding, as a major cause of marital dysfunction. He suggested that the most successful couples do not allow themselves to escalate into this degree of physical arousal. On the whole, these partners have the capacity to keep themselves from being reactive, and they have the ability to soothe the other. The partnership may be considered as an interactive state that, when more stable, contributes to self-regulation from the shared desire to provide healthy responses (Gottman, 1999).

When a person is overaroused, the flooding of emotion activates the sympathetic nervous system. The hypothalamic–pituitary–adrenal axis (HPA) becomes hyperactivated, and heart rates of 15 beats per minute above resting heart rate are reached. Cognitive ability declines, age regression often occurs (wherein partners feel and act younger), frustration tolerance is low, and people respond with defensive behavior. Partners tend to avoid looking at each other directly. When the couple system disintegrates, partners often misjudge intentions and experience the other person as malicious. Gottman (1995) suggests that couples are less likely to be successful in marriage if they incorporate what he calls the "four horsemen of the apocalypse" in their communication styles: criticism, contempt, defensiveness, and stonewalling. Contempt, in particular, is highly destructive and shame-inducing. As Gottman observes, the antidote is to build a culture of appreciation.

Tatkin (2003) wrote that the escalation can involve "the use of primitive defense(s) such as denial, blame, transference, acting-out, splitting, projection, projective identification, avoidance and withdrawal becomes intensified, along with the appearance of core affects such as murderous rage, disgust, helplessness, shame and terror" (p. 76). Panic sets in, and to reestablish control, one partner may attempt to calm down by withdrawing, while the other may attempt to calm down through pursuing interaction. Frequently, these strategies for state change meet with failure. Alternatively, both may move toward complete withdrawal. In this case, both partners experience decreased heart rates, and the emotional pain is often experienced as physical pain (Pelphrey, Singerman, Allison, & McCarthy, 2003).

Shame-based systems may operate in the midst of *retroflection* (a split within the self and subsequent substitution of the self for another, as in doing to the self what one wants to do to someone else, or doing for the self what one wants someone else to do for self). People who imagine that others hold negative judgments about them are often projecting their own sense of personal antipathy and then punishing themselves on the basis of the judgments of "others." The process can be like two mirrors facing each other that reflect a frozen and closed looped state of negativity: No new information can enter, and thus, no corrections can occur.

Because people entrain to the dominant states around them, particularly in the case of partners, we often see couples experiencing this closed loop. In part, this may be a reflection of poor self-boundaries and indicative that a person may not be able to maintain his or her state around someone else. However, it appears that all humans are sensitive, at least unconsciously, to the states of those around them. Tatkin (2003) suggested that how well partners regulate each other's autonomic nervous systems reflects the stability of the couple system. (This is also why we suggest that the clinician, as the primary initiator of state change, should be in the state with which the client needs to align.) In the case of shame, when one person feels embarrassed by a confrontation from his or her partner (i.e., shamed by having been caught), it may trigger a similar feeling in the other partner. In order to break the intolerable feelings of shame, couples may begin to argue. These interactions are painful, unproductive, and often keep partners locked in a continuous loop of negativity.

Negative hypnotic trance states engendered by painful interactions that repeatedly produce shame and anxiety frequently create a pattern of habitual escalation or withdrawal and preclude intimate contact. Couples who are caught up in them have difficulty disentangling themselves enough to work constructively to resolve conflict (Kershaw, 1992). One effective approach to depotentiating the joint negative trance states is the use of conjoint alpha–theta training, a synchrony training wherein the hemispheres of both people entrain to each other in their calmest states. We use the Cygnet software for this training. Each partner is hooked up to a computer (with EEG leads). We have noted, and mention to clients, that in this process of brainwave alignment, they may sense the state of the other as they both become quite calm. When this training is incorporated into marital therapy, partners learn how to shift gears more quickly. If there are shame-based patterns, they can more easily be interrupted and altered. As a couple's physiology calms, frequently, the partners are also able to make more effective use of relationship therapy.

Posttraumatic Stress Disorder

When clients present with intense anxiety, depression, or shame, there are often issues surrounding trauma that may not have been fully processed or even disclosed to the therapist. Issues related to social betrayal and attachment, fear, and memory problems emerge from trauma. Bessel van der Kolk noted the following: "Many traumatized children and adults, confronted with chronically overwhelming emotions, lose their capacity to use emotions as guides for effective action. They often do not recognize what they are feeling and fail to mount an appropriate response. . . . Unable to gauge and modulate their own internal states they habitually collapse in the face of threat, or lash out in response to minor irritations" (2006, p. 1). Because physiological overarousal is at the basis of so many disorders, including posttraumatic states, helping individuals reduce their baseline states of arousal is a key aim in many mental health treatments. Van der Kolk discovered that clients who use neurofeedback as an intervention were generally able to return to full normal functioning. In addition, neurofeedback allows clients to significantly improve their ability to "mentalize"—that is, the ability to observe one's own feelings and those of others without reacting (Fonagy, Gergey, Jurist, & Target, 2005).

In her first meeting with Carol, Patrice reported a remarkable story of emotional abuse in her family of origin and described her former marriage to a man who worked undercover in a U.S. intelligence agency. Her ex-husband had been just as emotionally abusive as her father: He would intimidate her with tactics such as telling her he knew where she was every moment—and then casually add that he could "take her out" any time he felt like it, and no one would ever suspect a thing. Patrice had left him, but she knew that in the year and a half since their divorce, he had broken into her apartment at least half a dozen times and changed small things simply to terrorize her. Her resultant anxiety had become sufficiently chronic and acute that she was experiencing severe insomnia nightly. Her level of daytime anxiety was compromising her ability to perform adequately at her job. Patrice not only felt embarrassed by her situation, feeling that it was "her fault," but she also felt very apprehensive about telling anyone what she was facing. Although she literally feared for her life, she didn't want to "drag anyone else into it" and possibly put that person also at risk. Understandably, Patrice reported feeling depressed. Stating that she was unable to find any respite from hopelessness in anything, she disclosed transient suicidal ideation.

Carol described to her the process of alpha–theta training and its healing potential, and explained that if she could allow her mind to go all the way to the edge of sleep with awareness, she could experience a shift in state to complete relaxation. After 10 weeks of sessions twice a week, Patrice's anxiety was noticeably reduced, and she was sleeping much better. As the shame, anxiety, and depression lifted, Patrice began to feel able to take some concrete actions to improve her situation. Two months later, she moved to an apartment complex with enhanced security features where she felt safer from her ex-husband.

Recognizing that anxiety, depression, and shame are all expressions of fear, this chapter has examined their common underpinning and discussed therapeutic interventions using BCT. The next chapter focuses on the many factors that contribute to weight issues and the BCT approach to assessment and intervention.

CHAPTER 9

A Thinner State of Brain–Mind–Body

Our culture has so accustomed us to using substances—particularly food—to change states that we hardly notice it. American businesses run on coffee. To calm down, people turn to "comfort food": foods with high sugar, high fructose syrup, or simply "high-carb" content, or beverages containing alcohol. Our stress level or our exhaustion dictates our snacks. People also develop conditioned responses to cues in the environment; for example, going out to a movie isn't complete without popcorn and soda. Because a positive, if temporary, feeling follows eating carbohydrates, especially simple carbohydrates, an "addictive response" sets in motion a cycle of desire for carbohydrates, ingestion, temporary satisfaction, and then more craving that can lead to a person losing control over what is consumed. The seeking circuit is highly activated in addictive responses and can lead to a progression from "liking" a food to "wanting" it to "needing" it.

This chapter focuses on weight issues as a result of food addiction. Here we explore the neurochemistry of food, the role of sugar and other simple-carbohydrate craving in obesity; the role of habit, sleep deprivation, genetics, and taste habituation; therapeutic assumptions in addressing weight issues; client assessment for weight management cases; and BCT interventions for weight loss, including case examples.

Overview of the Problem

A serious problem for many, obesity in the United States has become steadily worse. The National Center for Chronic Disease Prevention and

Health Promotion (2010) reports that more than 1/3 of all adults in the United States are obese. Health-care costs attributable to obesity are in excess of $68 million annually. The physical problems that may result include hypertension, type 2 diabetes, coronary–vascular diseases, fatigue, respiratory problems, gall bladder disease, certain types of cancer, sleep apnea, arthritis, depression, anxiety, decreased social interaction, decreased sexual activity, and low self-esteem.

Many variables play a role in weight gain: genetic predisposition, biochemical factors leading to brain dysregulation, the context and social system by which the individual is influenced, the "internal weight manager," susceptibility to external food cues when in a state of anxiety, and learned trance phenomena. These factors work together in an interactive system wherein eating is adjusted in the interests of biological regulation and adaptation to the environment. Some of the factors contributing to obesity can also lead to feelings of helplessness and lack of self-control, which in turn may perpetuate a cycle of dieting and gaining weight. Most dieters have a history of having tried numerous food programs, losing weight, then regaining the lost weight and more. As one of our clients said, "Everyone who has a weight problem is looking for the one program that will finally be the cure-all."

Although this chapter focuses on weight issues as a result of food addiction, the principles discussed here are applicable to many types of addictive behavior. All addictions have several components in common: They attempt to ameliorate emotional or physical distress, generally depression, fear/anxiety, or fatigue. Over time, a loss of control with respect to the substance or behavior occurs. In analyzing drug addiction, Koob (2008) emphasized a two-tier problem consisting of an impulse-control disorder that leads to a compulsive disorder. The impulse-control disorder is triggered by a certain tension or level of arousal that precedes the addictive action; the compulsive disorder is stimulated by stressors or anxiety that the compulsive behavior temporarily relieves. In addiction, behavior progresses from impulsivity to compulsivity in a three-stage cycle: binge/intoxication, withdrawal/negative affect, and preoccupation/anticipation (Koob, 2008, p. 3). Allostasis, which is the process of creating a state of stability by means of change, becomes the driver from substance use to dependence and changes the reward and stress system neurocircuits by flooding the brain with dopamine (National Institute on Drug Abuse, 2008).

The Neurochemistry of Food

Everything a person thinks or experiences—from exercise to visiting some new place—creates new neural connections. Research suggests that there are neural correlates with addictions and, specifically, with eating problems; based on that finding, we need to address the brain in treatment (Grunwald, Schrock, & Kuschinsky, 1991). In studying how the brain prunes or removes certain links (Strauch, 2004), neuroscientists have found that when particular brain circuits are exercised less frequently, the strength of their connection diminishes. Change can occur if certain habits are interrupted and the focus is moved from "my problem" to a viable solution. By shifting the brain–mind state and shifting focus when an urge to eat inappropriately is experienced, over time there is a decrease in the brain activity associated with the problem (Ratey, 2002).

The ventromedial hypothalamus is believed to maintain a satiety center. Stimulation of this area suppresses eating, whereas dysfunction in this part of the hypothalamus may lead to obesity. The lateral hypothalamus also may be responsible for "encouraging" eating behavior. Another part of the brain involved in eating disorders is the cingulate gyrus, located longitudinally through the middle part of the frontal lobes. It allows people to shift attention and change thoughts and behaviors. When an individual is caught in loops of thought or compulsive behaviors, this part of the brain has become overactive. The underlying mechanisms for these regulatory processes involve neurotransmitters and their pathways.

Overeating results in chronic inflammation and can turn on certain immune cells that attack invaders even if they are not present. Researchers discovered that if a certain pathway in the hypothalamus is stimulated, a mouse will consume more food than it needs, and cellular destruction may occur. A few months of overeating can lead to appetite dysregulation and spiraling weight gain (Zhang et al., 2008). Symptoms of Alzheimer's disease can appear with obesity and result in neurodegeneration (Moroz, Tong, Longato, Xu, & de la Monte, 2008).

Food choices can drive many internal states and either advance brain aging or retard it by growing new cells and balancing neural chemistry. Neuroscientist James Joseph (2008) conducted a study on the effect of fruits and vegetables on the brain. With aging, the body's ability to deal with free radicals in the system is gradually reduced. Joseph found that eating a pint of fresh strawberries or a spinach salad every day reduces brain aging. Antioxidants in the diet can forestall oxidative stress, which contributes to neurodegeneration. In fact, "every fruit, vegetable, grain, or source of protein or fat is a precursor to one of the brain chemicals" (Braverman, 2009, p. xv). Four of those key chemicals, or neurotransmitters, are dopamine, acetylcholine, gamma-aminobutyric acid (GABA), and serotonin.

Dopamine

Dopamine is both a neurotransmitter and a neurohormone released by the hypothalamus. Tyrosine, an amino acid found in proteins such as meat, nuts, eggs, dairy products, and beans, is a precursor to dopamine, and dopamine is a precursor of both epinephrine (also known as adrenaline) and another closely related molecule, norepinephrine (or noradrenaline). Epinephrine is implicated in levels of arousal and mental alertness; norepinephrine is released by the sympathetic nervous system to transmit the fight–flight–freeze response. Excessive norepinephrine production contributes to aggressive behavior. Low levels of dopamine lead to an inability to feel satisfied either physically or emotionally and can cause weight gain as an individual tries to consume something that will "fill the gap." Subnormal levels of dopamine also impair the abilities to focus and concentrate. Extremely low levels of dopamine result in lack of energy, sleepiness, depression, and even suicidal thoughts (Robertson, 1996). Moderately elevated levels of dopamine tend to result in sleep disturbances, anxiety, and fear; extremely high levels of dopamine can induce withdrawal, paranoia, or psychosis. Colantuoni et al. (2002) discovered that dopamine is released in the brain not only when we eat but also when we perceive food cues. Sugar tends to deplete dopamine, causing a person to feel fatigued and to search for stimulants.

Acetylcholine

Acetylcholine is an excitatory neurotransmitter in both the central and peripheral nervous systems and is the only neurotransmitter used in the motor division of the somatic nervous system. By influencing the processing of bioelectrical impulses, acetylcholine determines the speed of brain function and is critical for both the storage and recall of memory. A precursor to acetylcholine is choline, a fat-like substance necessary to metabolize fats. It is found in egg yolks, red meat, wheat germ, avocados, and some types of fish and nuts. Memory problems, suspicious thinking, sexual dysfunction, and dry skin and mouth may be manifestations of low levels of acetylcholine. A craving for fatty foods may also be a sign of low acetylcholine.

Gamma-Aminobutyric Acid

GABA is the primary inhibitory neurotransmitter acting to calm and stabilize the brain. GABA is a non-essential amino acid formed from glutamic acid with the help of vitamin B6. Because it cannot penetrate the blood–brain barrier, it must be synthesized in vivo. The GABA precursors are found in complex carbohydrates such as whole grains, tree nuts, lentils, and citrus fruits, as well as fish, meats, and poultry. When GABA levels are deficient, an individual can experience headaches, dizzy spells, short-term memory loss, and anxiety. Low GABA levels can stimulate binge-eating.

Serotonin

The neurotransmitter serotonin is involved in the regulation of such bodily processes as sleep, libido, and body temperature. When serotonin levels are stable, appetite is regulated. Low serotonin levels have been implicated in numerous psychiatric disorders, including depression, OCD, anorexia, bulimia, anxiety, and phobias. Frequently, comorbidities such as depression or OCD accompany eating disorders. (Eating at night can reflect a serotonin deficiency.) Both of these comorbidities involve dysfunction in serotonin levels.

Slightly low serotonin can cause difficulty with concentration and attention; examples are misplacing a purse or wallet, putting strange things in the refrigerator, or going after something in another room only to forget what you needed when you get there. A moderately low serotonin level causes depression and may initiate changes in the bodily functions regulated by serotonin, resulting in sleep disturbance, either significant weight gain or loss, sudden unprovoked tears, and hot flashes. Very low levels of serotonin typically cause the brain to "race" and may be accompanied by OCD, outbursts of rage, "memory torture" (becoming preoccupied with terrible experiences that happened years earlier), and suicidal ideation. When serotonin levels are high, people feel relaxed and reasonably at ease with their lives.

Carbohydrates stimulate the production of serotonin via insulin and the plasma tryptophan ratio, resulting in good feelings. Simple carbohydrates that break down quickly, such as foods made with sugar or white flour, tend to cause a serotonin spike. Complex carbohyrates, such as oatmeal, are digested more slowly and lead to more stable levels of serotonin. Clients with food issues tend to choose simple carbohydrates because of the quicker effect; however, they also find that eating simple carbohydrates increases their cravings and may lead to a self-reinforcing cycle that perpetuates overeating. Consuming foods high in sugar or other simple carbohydrates also causes blood sugar levels to rise and fall dramatically, which can lead not only to carbohydrate craving but, on a longer-term basis, to diabetes.

An increase in the ratio of the amino acid tryptophan to the amino acids phenylalanine and leucine will also increase serotonin levels. Tryptophan is present to different degrees in all protein, but particularly in turkey. Fruits with a good ratio include dates, sour cherries, papaya, and banana. Other foods that increase serotonin levels are asparagus, avocado, pecans, pineapple, eggplant, spinach, walnuts, and oats. Foods with a lower ratio, including whole wheat and rye bread, inhibit the production of serotonin.

Cocoa has also been found to increase serotonin levels in the brain, but since most chocolate is high in sugar, it causes blood sugar levels to spike. When the blood sugar level drops, the serotonin level also plummets. For this reason, chocolate with a cocoa content of 70% or higher is recommended for clients who find themselves compelled to reach for candy bars to "lift their spirits."

Although it appears counterintuitive, research also suggests that eating a diet rich in whole-grain carbohydrates and relatively lower in protein will increase serotonin by causing the secretion of insulin, which helps in amino acid competition. This is because insulin lowers the blood levels of most amino acids, with the exception of tryptophan. Consequently, once insulin has cleared the competing amino acids from the blood, tryptophan is free to enter the brain. A diet with a 40:30:30 ratio of daily calories obtained from carbohydrates, proteins, and fats, respectively (popularized as the "Zone" diet by nutritional biochemist Barry Sears), balances two main metabolic hormones: insulin, a precursor of serotonin that promotes the storing of excess calories as fat; and glucagon, a hormone secreted by the pancreas that raises blood glucose levels and promotes the burning of fat.

Factors That Contribute to Weight Issues

Weight gain is a complex phenomenon with many contributing factors, ranging from deep biological processes to habit patterns and taste thresholds. Here we consider five categories of factors that impact the consumption and metabolism of food: genetics, sugar and other simple-carbohydrate cravings, habit, sleep deprivation, and taste habituation.

Genetics

A new area in the study of genetic signaling, known as *epigenetics*, examines changes in gene activity that do not involve an alteration of the genetic code, per se, but that are nonetheless passed down to at least one successive generation. These patterns of gene expression are governed by the cellular material—the *epigenome*—that sits on top of the genome, just outside it (the prefix *epi-* means "above"). Epigenetic "marks" tell genes to switch on or off, to speak loudly or whisper. It is through epigenetic marks that environmental factors such as diet, stress, and prenatal nutrition can make an imprint on genes that are passed from one generation to the next. Studies in epigenetics have shown that lifestyle may alter gene expression over generations (Pembrey et al., 2006). An ancestor's habits of overeating, heavy drinking, and minimal exercising can contribute to the expression of "fat" genes.

Research has not yet fully demonstrated the ability to manipulate a broad spectrum of epigenetic factors, but there are at least two studies suggesting that possibility. It takes only the addition of a methyl group (one carbon atom attached to three hydrogen atoms) to change an epigenome. When a methyl group attaches to a specific spot on a gene—a process called *DNA methylation*—it can change the gene's expression, turning it off or on, dampening it or making it "louder." At Duke University, Robert Waterland and Randy Jirtle devised an experiment using mice with an "agouti" gene (i.e., a type of gene that affects coloration) that gives them yellow coats and a propensity for obesity and diabetes when the gene is expressed continuously. One group of pregnant agouti mice was fed a diet rich in B vitamins. Another group of genetically identical mice did not receive the B vitamin supplement. The B vitamins caused methyl groups to attach more frequently to the agouti gene in utero, thereby altering its expression. Simply by providing increased B vitamins—without altering the genomic structure of mouse DNA—Waterland and Jirtle induced agouti mothers to produce healthy brown pups that were of normal weight and not prone to diabetes. The control group of mice produced regular agouti offspring (Waterland & Jirtle, 2003).

A second study concerning gene expression was conducted by Dean Ornish. In a pilot study of 30 men with prostate cancer, Ornish found that changes in their diets for 3 months (mostly fruits, vegetables, and whole grains) led to 453 genes being turned off. The PSA level (prostate-specific antigen, a blood marker for prostate growth) of the men in the study dropped by an average of 4%, whereas it increased by an average of 6% in the control group. Ornish, Weiner and Fair (2005) suggested that the implications of this study go far beyond the ability of the body to heal itself under favorable conditions. Also implied may be an ability to change gene expression, such that heredity may not be a given (Hitt, 2003).

Jeffrey Friedman discovered a gene that activates the hormone leptin. Normally, leptin acts on receptors in the hypothalamus where it inhibits appetite; people who completely lack leptin eat copious amounts and are morbidly obese. For these individuals, treatment with synthetic leptin leads to dramatic weight loss. Leptin is manufactured primarily in adipose (fat) tissue, and the level of leptin is proportional to a person's total body fat. For this reason, when most people diet, their leptin levels decrease—which is one reason that keeping the weight off is difficult (Friedman, 2001). However, as Friedman (2001) pointed out, we are the guardians of our genes, not victims of them. Jirtle, Waterland, and Ornish would agree with him.

Sugar and Other Simple-Carbohydrate Cravings

Lenoir (2007) at the University of Bordeaux in France did a study in which she found that rats that had been given cocaine preferred sugar water to cocaine. Excessive sugar in the diet can overstimulate the sweet receptors in the brain and lead to addiction and loss of control. Another researcher experimented with two groups of mice to determine the differences in response to walking over a hot plate with and without ingesting sugar. The group that ate a sugar solution prior to the experiment took twice as long to lift their feet from the hot surface (Cleary, 1996). In a third experiment, researchers measured isolation distress in baby mice. The researchers noted that when the baby mice were taken away from the mother, they cried over 300 times in a 6-minute period. However, eight baby mice given sugar water cried only 75 times in the same period. When the second group was given the drug naloxone before the sugar water, the chemical blocked the effect of the sugar. Then the second group of baby mice cried as frequently as the first group (Blass, 1986; Blass & Watt, 1999).

Sugar not only slowed the response time to a painful stimulus of the hot plate, it also seemed to depress a painful reaction to being isolated from the mother. From these studies, the researchers concluded that sugar blocked emotional as well as physical pain. Other researchers suggest that human beings may have a similar response to sugar, as the lead element in the sugar–insulin–tryptophan–serotonin cycle. To increase serotonin levels and change states, cravings for carbohydrates, alcohol, or sweets may arise. When an individual gives into the craving over multiple times, an addictive cycle may be set up (Colantuoni, 1992). Once the problem cycle is in place, any environmental stressor that is "medicated" with food becomes self-reinforcing, slows metabolism, and places the brain in a state of dysregulation. Over time, the addictive cycle is difficult to break (Yudkin, Kang, & Bruckdorfer, 1980; Fields, 1983; Ceriello, 2000). In addition, sugar consumption can increase the slower brain frequencies, which can slow thinking processes and learning (Molteni, 2002; Christensen, 1991).

The sugar–insulin–tryptophan–serotonin cycle provides a clear rationale for the fact that taste is affected by serotonin levels: The lower the serotonin level, the more sugar is required for a person to detect its taste—inducing a person to consume more sugar under low serotonin conditions. As mood stabilizes, the desire for sugar decreases (Heath, Melichar, Nutt, & Donaldson, 2006).

Habit

Shifts in energy levels during the day are associated with the biological rhythms of state change, and people may be especially prone to overeat during these periods of biorhythm shift. Ultradian cycles are expressed in patterns, and we see them in what are called *endogenous biological rhythms* (Thayer, 2001). Driven by these biologically-based rhythms, individuals tend to develop habit patterns; the coffee break and the cocktail hour are culturally institutionalized examples of this biological propensity.

Habit is one of the most commonly overlooked factors in obesity. As we mention to our clients, "No one becomes significantly overweight in a day. The pointer on the bathroom scale creeps up over time as the effects of eating habits accrue." Entrenched eating habits may become practically unconscious. Particularly under stress, people often activate automatic and trance-like eating behavior. Frequently, clients report no memory of feeling hungry or the subsequent act of eating. Trance phenomena such as amnesia (loss of ability to recall) and analgesia (loss of ability to register physical sensation) keep anxiety low and awareness of overeating from the conscious mind. We commonly find that a client's patterns of feeling, thinking, and behaving, once set in motion, continue almost unconsciously.

Professor Ben Fletcher of the University of Hertfordshire in the United Kingdom has demonstrated that if a person can break the habit that made him or her overweight in the first place, he or she can lose weight without focusing on it. Fletcher (2007) conducted a psychological experiment in which people had to select and follow a behavior pattern that was different from their usual habit/style, chosen from a pair of contrasting behaviors each day. Samples of paired behaviors were lively/quiet, reactive/proactive, introvert/extrovert, passive/assertive, generous/stingy, shy/flirty, etc. For example, introverts would act in a specifically extroverted manner. Twice weekly, they would have to try something outside their comfort zone, such as eating something they had never tried before, turning off their cell phone for a day, or going dancing. The participants were not on a diet; they were simply taking part in a psychological study. Losing weight turned out to be a byproduct of the experiment. The striking result was that after 4 four months the subjects had lost an average of 11 pounds simply by selecting activities that did not conform to their previous habit patterns. Six months later, almost all had kept the weight off, and some continued to lose more.

Sleep Deprivation

Many Americans have a stoic idea about how much sleep a person should need. Often we hear people boasting that they can get along on 4 or 5 hours per night, with the implication that sleeping is largely a waste of time. However, enough sleep is crucial for psychological and physiological health. Dr. Emmanuel Mignot researching sleep disorders, noted: "In Western societies, where chronic sleep restriction is common and food is widely available, changes in appetite regulatory hormones with sleep curtailment may contribute to obesity" (Mignot, 2004, Conclusion section., para. 1).

Research has found that sleep loss impacts several hormones related to appetite and food intake. Two hormones, in particular—ghrelin and leptin—are thought to play a role in the interaction between short sleep duration and high body mass index (BMI). Ghrelin, primarily produced by the stomach, triggers appetite: The higher the ghrelin level, the higher a desire to eat. Leptin (derived from the Greek word *leptos*, meaning "thin") is a hormone produced by fat cells. Leptin controls eating and expenditure of energy and actually can rewire the brain to facilitate the process of slimming. Low leptin levels promote appetite and are a signal of metabolic starvation. The study data showed a 14.9% increase in ghrelin and a 15.5% decrease in leptin in people who consistently slept for 5 hours compared with those who slept for 8. For people who slept less than 8 hours per night (74.4% of the sample), their increased BMI was proportional to decreased sleep. Increasing sleep duration therefore may prove to be an important way to treat inappropriate weight gain (Taheri, Lin, Austin, Young & Mignot, 2004).

A shortage of sleep reduces the capacity of the body to perform basic metabolic functions such as processing and storing carbohydrates. The changes induced by sleep deprivation in one study included profound alterations in glucose metabolism, in some situations resembling patients with Type 2 diabetes. "We found that the metabolic and endocrine changes resulting from a significant sleep debt mimic many of the hallmarks of aging," said Eve Van Cauter, director of a study examining sleep deprivation in healthy young adults. "We suspect that chronic sleep loss may not only hasten the onset but could also increase the severity of age-related ailments such as diabetes, hypertension, obesity and memory loss" (Spiegel, Leproult & Van Cauter, 1999, p. 1437). People deprived of sleep for 4 nights exhibited signs of pre-diabetes and, because of a drop in leptin, showed a tendency to a high carbohydrate load (Peykar, 2008).

Even while sleeping, the brain can sense the smallest amount of light, and this can contribute to poor quality sleep. The hormone melatonin is secreted by the pineal gland; its level rises with dusk and subsides with sunrise, thereby regulating periods of sleep and wakefulness. Without a sufficient period of darkness, melatonin production may be impaired. In a French study, researchers demonstrated that melatonin prevented the development of obesity in animals fed a typical Western high-fat diet (Prunet-Marcassas, et al., 2003).

A lack of sleep may contribute to weight problems even in very young children. A study done by Harvard Medical School showed that 14% of preschool children ages 1–3 years old who slept less than 11 hours were overweight, compared to children who received at least 13 hours per night (Taveras, 2008).

Taste Habituation

The brain is wired to seek novelty in the case of taste, as in other experiences. For each different type of taste, the tongue has a detection threshold (or recognition threshold), meaning the point at which a person can first detect a particular taste. For example, sweetness is detectable at roughly 1 part in 200 of sucrose in solution. Bitterness (often indicative that a certain plant is toxic to eat) has a much lower detection threshold, at about 1 part in 2 million for quinine in solution. Taste sensors reach their maximum intensity after approximately 1 minute of stimulation; at that point habituation occurs and the perception is that the tastes "fades." If a person takes a bite of one food followed by a bite of a second food, there is more novelty and the tastes of both seem more intense. When the same food is presented to taste buds repetitively, adaptation will result in the discernment of fewer individual flavors and a decreased overall flavor intensity. After the third or fourth spoonful of ice cream, the rest of the carton—if consumed in one sitting—does not taste as interesting. Because of this fading effect, an unconscious drive to regain a previously experienced intensity of taste may be a contributing factor in some overeating.

Therapeutic Assumptions in Addressing Weight Issues

A weight problem may be symptomatic of many different issues. Often, there are issues of early abuse, and weight keeps a person from being sexual. Until the abuse is resolved, successful weight loss will be impossible. Another issue is that in a family where all the members are overweight, family loyalty may be defined by weight. One client who came from a family in which the women were quite overweight found that they all chastised her for wanting to lose weight. For others, the issue may have to do with the stability of the marital relationship. We have had clients who were concerned that if they lost weight, they might want to leave their equally overweight spouse. In that situation, to engage support for the new pattern, we normally suggest that the partner also come for joint sessions. However, in all cases, certain therapeutic assumptions form the foundation of our work with overweight clients. These are outlined below:

• *People have the ability to manage their weight* (or other addictive behavior). In most cases, the person was not always overweight. We suggest that the client has the capacity to change states and deal with cravings and anxiety-driven eating. Cravings are emotionally driven and/or physiologically driven obsessive thoughts or sensations that a person does not know how to manage.

• *Addictive behavior functions to mask or medicate unresolved issues.* When a person is unsuccessful with many weight loss attempts, there are frequently deep emotional conflicts that must be addressed therapeutically. Once the veil of illusion regarding an addiction is lifted, the feelings that were hidden from awareness by overeating can be revealed, and the quest for self-understanding and mastery becomes possible.

• *The motivational circuit of determination must be activated.* Determination may be located in non-food-related arenas (Panksepp, 1998). People already know how to motivate themselves toward goal attainment. Those resources can be redirected for food management. Although weight loss based on either incentive or threat is usually short-lived, it may be enough to bridge a person into the target state. However, an individual must develop other motivation in order to stay there. Ultimately a person must learn to change the neurological patterns driving brain–mind states and the behavior that led to being overweight in order to maintain of lower weight.

Milton Erickson was a master in utilizing the problem and eliciting resourceful states from people. In treating an obese young woman, Erickson utilized her intense pain about her weight by asking her to stand in front of a full-length mirror and really notice how much she disliked all the fat. He continued: "If you think hard enough and look through that layer of blubber that you've got wrapped around you, you will see a very pretty feminine figure, but it is buried rather deeply. And what do you think you ought to do to get that figure excavated?" Erickson reported that she "excavated" 5 pounds a week (Erickson, Rossi, Ryan, & Sharp, 1983, pp. 267–268). With his intervention, Erickson elicited positive motivating anxiety by using the client's own pain and redirecting it toward action. He helped this woman find the real body she had long been unable to see.

• *A client's weight issues are frequently embedded in a relationship and must be addressed within that context.* The system in which an individual operates may serve to keep a problem active. Usually clients with weight issues are aware of many conflicts surrounding food and have good insights, but they may be less aware of the ways in which the present system is reinforcing negative behaviors and attitudes. In one case, the client's wife unintentionally played a role in the reinforcement of symptom behavior. She was so worried about him dying from his overweight condition that she would watch him at night. When he would sneak into the pantry and begin eating, she would jump out and tell him, "I caught you." He would then become angry and have more urge to binge. To interrupt the marital dynamics around this issue, we asked the wife to purchase a Sherlock Holmes hat and wear it at night. Her husband was to purposefully sneak into the pantry. She was to then jump out with a flare and announce, "I caught you." After doing this twice, they were both able to laugh about this "game" and then stop it.

• *Most clients with weight issues visualize themselves gaining back any lost weight.* Often they use the negative practice of envisioning the worst possible future, although this visual practice is usually outside awareness until the therapist begins to ask about the idea of future success in keeping the weight off. Since we generally tend to achieve the goals we visualize, it is important to be certain that the client's future is seen as a thinner one. In fact, we suggest that clients imagine themselves thinner up to the end of life.

• *Clients may be using trance phenomena in a negative manner to shield themselves from awareness of their own behavior.* Many clients with weight problems are skilled in using dissociation from body sensations such that they cannot distinguish anxiety from hunger or recognize feeling full. Often they employ amnesia for bingeing episodes and only later, if prodded, may recall a recent specific event. In trance, the client can be directed to attend to his or her bodily sensations and become more conscious of bingeing behavior and exactly what was eaten during the bingeing. By learning to listen to the body, the client can become aware of its ability to provide immediate, meaningful feedback, bring him- or herself out of a dissociated state, and access more conscious choices in terms of food selection.

• *Client education may be necessary.* As needed, client education may include techniques of state change, basics of nutrition, how to recognize hunger and distinguish it from other sensations, and how to recognize the feeling of being full. In some cases, we may even teach simple facts about neurochemistry (e.g., the carbohydrate–insulin–tryptophan–serotonin cycle) so that the client has an understanding of the neurological basis for certain cravings.

• *Teach clients about* kaizen. The Japanese have a word for continuous improvement through small changes; the word has spread from the business community into common usage: *kaizen* (Imai, 1986). We suggest that even one small change can be the tipping point for greater change. Success does not have to be an "all or nothing, right now or never" affair. It can be achieved through *kaizen*—a succession of countless small changes in habit and behavior patterns. These can shift a person's diet from one high in simple carbohydrates or in fats to one that is primarily fruits, vegetables, and lean protein with lots of variety for novel eating. After a period of time, the desire for sugar, starches and fat fades. However, if food management begins to wane, adaptation to previously well- known lethargy, sensations of bloating, inflammation, etc., will recur and weight will begin to climb (O'Mahoney, 2007).

Client Assessment for Weight Management Cases

When applying BCT to clients who come with weight as the presenting issue, the first step, as with all clients, is taking a detailed history while establishing rapport. In this case, the clinician will want to focus specifically on the client's "food history," which should include answers to the following questions:

1. Ask for a history of the weight problem, including the age of the client when it began.

2. Ask the client to describe any particular cravings or tendencies toward binges and the circumstances under which these occur.

3. Inquire about family-of-origin messages regarding food. Examples are: Food equals love; food equals "good times"; "You should eat because children in name-of-remote-place are starving." For the now-aging Baby Boomer generation, there may have been a carryover from Depression-era circumstances, during which their parents were taught to clean their plates at every meal. Frequently, clients report anxiety around mealtimes when growing up.

4. If the client is married, ask about the "contract" made regarding food and how slim each partner would remain over the years. Sometimes weight gain becomes an arena for power struggles.

5. Listen for the "food language" that a client may use unconsciously. For example, "I could really taste that success"; "That idea is something you can really get your teeth into"; "This is food for thought." This language can then be used by the therapist in conversational hypnosis to focus attention on the impending change to a slimmer individual.

6. Discover the client's "motivating anxiety" and consider how it might be engaged. A person needs to feel determination and positive anticipation in order to move toward goal attainment. If the client's affect is flat,

it is useful to mildly activate the anxiety circuit by helping the client identify some truly motivating positive reason to lose weight. The weight loss client usually enters therapy because he or she "failed" at dieting on his or her own, so there is already an intrinsic motivation. However, "I can't do it alone"—which brought the person into therapy—is not enough motivation to succeed. Together, the client and the therapist must discover some compelling, emotionally based reason to lose weight *from the perspective of the client* (not from the doctor's perspective or the spouse's perspective or even the client's own intellectually based perspective).

7. Most people have an "internal weight manager" that tells them how much weight gain is too much. This may be found by asking how the client maintains the present weight. Frequently, people use a scale or notice how their clothes fit as their internal weight manager.

8. Ascertain whether or not the client knows when he or she feels full.

9. Find out how the client related to food when he or she weighed less. For example, the therapist might ask, "How did you maintain your weight then? Were you more interested in other things? How did you comfort yourself then?"

10. Identify the trance phenomena the client may be using to keep the problem going. Inquiries might include: "Do you remember when you overeat (amnesia)?"; "Do you pay attention to feeling full? (dissociation)"; "Do you notice your hand floating to your face when you eat?" (Hand levitation is an unconscious movement of the hand, and most anxiety eating includes this behavior.)

11. Ask about expectations regarding treatment.

BCT Interventions Applied to Weight Loss Clients

Many of the BCT tools stimulate a renewed ability for self-regulation, particularly for the self-regulation of weight, so that an individual has more control, peace of mind, and self-discipline for personal success. We use the following protocol as our guide in working with patients whose focus is weight loss.

1. *Assist the client in becoming consciously aware of and, specifically, able to articulate to him- or herself what emotions or feelings*

he or she is experiencing in stressful situations. Help the client develop descriptive labels of his or her feelings using the client's own
words. For example:

- "I feel caged."
- "I get the 'elevator feeling'—too many people all pressing in
  around me."
- "I feel like a pack of fierce wild dogs is coming after me and I can't
  run fast enough to escape."

For easy reference, these can then be shortened to "caged," "the elevator feeling," "can't run fast enough." Instruct the client to watch for the
feeling and make a mental note of the circumstance in which it arises.
Encourage the client to become honestly curious (turns on the seeking
circuit) about whether he or she is hungry or is, in fact, anxious. If the
answer is "anxious," suggest that the client deepen his or her breathing
for 2 minutes as a refocus of attention. This focused breathing can even
be formalized by watching the minute hand on a watch.

2. *Utilize and reframe the problem to expand the number of solutions and turn on the seeking circuit.* Resistance to losing weight can
be framed as the person choosing to be fully in control of his or her behavior and deciding when and how he or she will lose weight. This is
particularly appropriate for clients who feel "helpless," a "victim of their
circumstances," or "out of control" when in fact none of those is the
case. The pivot point is when the client can see that he or she is *already
making controlled choices.* The seeking circuit is activated any time
the client self-inquires, "What is really going on here?"

3. *Retrieve resources to assist in a resolution of the problem.* Clients with weight issues need to experience a sense of renewed determination to succeed. By remembering several incidents where a person
strongly experienced determination, he or she can transfer the strong
affect associated with the original success to resolve the weight problem.
For one client, the deep determination to stay involved in the lives of his
adult children and wanting their approval was associated with demonstrating success in the area of food management.

4. *Help the client learn to differentiate states and manage state
change.* More often than not, the physical sensations of hunger and anxiety are poorly differentiated by clients with weight issues. Because the

act of eating and the digestion of food may change a stressful state to a relaxed one, food becomes associated with relaxation. When a person can learn to turn on the relaxation response and practice it, there is much less urge to use food to alleviate anxiety. We have found that clients who use regular relaxation techniques or devices such as the DAVID PAL can interrupt their desire to overeat. Clients also need to learn how to turn on the circuit for nurture, care, and comfort without using food— for example, by curling up with the family cat.

5. *Use deep state training to bring down the set point of arousal.* The set point of arousal is the point at which stressors begin to set off a stress response. Frequently, individuals do not have a body sensation or memory of what it feels like to be completely relaxed without a substance or food. Deep state training reteaches an individual how to reconnect to a state of total relaxation.

6. *Use deep state training to dislodge negative and limiting core beliefs, so that an individual can believe the process of losing weight can be successful.* We note that in the deepest state of profound calmness and openness, the client may be in the most receptive state of mind. A desire to be in control dominates the thinking of many clients with weight issues. While a person may experience him- or herself as out of control, we frequently find that the individual is demonstrating a remarkable ability to eat in a way that closely maintains the weight over a number of years.

7. *Use deep states to make direct suggestions about control of self, management of food, and feeling full on less food.* If the clinician is using hypnosis to achieve deep states, it may be useful to conduct the hypnosis while the client is connected to a biofeedback system to access more precise information about the person's brainwave states.

8. *Use future orientation in time to help the client to envision a time at which the problem has been resolved.* Ask the client to bring in a photograph of him- or herself at the target weight and to remember how he or she felt when at that weight. This image can be used in a trance induction involving future orientation in time. In hypnosis, various scenarios of being thinner and enjoying looking as he or she did in the photograph can be employed. Self-regulation can also be encouraged by having the client visualize his or her ideal future body on a regular basis—for example, as he or she exercises.

Case Example: Imagining a Life of Her Own

Nearly in tears of frustration, Kimberly told Carol, "I just have no control over my eating when I am upset, lonely, or bored." This belief controlled her behavior and had been strongly reinforced by attending a self-help group that underscored the belief that she was uncontrollably addicted to food. In the process of gathering a history of Kim's overeating, Carol learned that her mother had tried to control her by being intrusive about what and when she could eat. Kim recounted that the refrigerator had been "practically a lockbox." About her mother, Kim said, "It was like she always had a mental inventory of the fridge and could tell by looking if anything had been moved—or removed" [history of eating disorder]. Introducing the family to someone new, her parents would refer to her with embarrassment as "our little chub" [food message]. Early on, Kimberly said, she had became enraged by her mother's attitude toward her and decided that *she* would be in charge. In later years, any attempt on her part to limit her food intake was met forcefully by her own resistance and resentment, just as it had been elicited originally in the context of the family dynamics.

Listening to her, Carol pointed out that *she truly was in charge* of whether she gained or lost weight—just as she had been as a child [therapeutic assumption that people have the ability to manage their weight]. It was totally her decision, and Carol would support her ability to decide. This therapeutic position took Kim out of the victim role, placed her in charge of herself, and eliminated the basis for blaming anyone else for her decision. Perhaps for the first time, Kim consciously grasped the reality of her own empowerment.

Carol suggested that if she decided to lose weight, it would not be a matter of willpower, of constantly trying to "just say no" to food, as Kim put it, but one of focusing her mind on the goal and allowing any other thoughts or feelings to just come and go, like shooting stars. This verbalization gave her a *positive focus* rather than a negative one. Carol also used alpha–theta biofeedback in conjunction with guided visualization to reinforce the fact that it was entirely Kim's decision to choose "bad" foods or not. The visualization continued to place her in charge and, ultimately, she chose to skip the high-fat, high-calorie foods most of the time while keeping the option to have them on occasion.

Determination or persistence is a resource that all people have in different contexts. During one session, Kim mentioned that when she was 9 and her two older brothers were both riding their bicycles "hands free," she became absolutely determined to be able to do it too. Practicing in secret, it took her a couple months and quite a few falls, but she managed it. Having located the previously developed resource of *strong persistence* as an internal state [motivational circuit], Carol used conversational hypnosis to help Kim review the feeling and overlay it onto the goal of managing her weight.

Kim also became fascinated [internal circuit of curiosity] with how slimmer people keep their weight under control. In the process of studying other people's behaviors and strategies for mood regulation, she also learned a little about the neurochemistry of nutrition and became more educated in managing her own mind states [client education, in this case self-directed].

After 4 months of therapy, Kimberly had lost 23 pounds; she had also become aware of the ways in which she had structured much of her life as an unconscious means of "just saying no" to her mother. And for the first time, she was ready to actively address the question, "Who would I be—and what would my life look like—if I started to 'just say yes' *to me?*"

Additional Specific Interventions

In addition to the general guidelines provided in the protocol described above, we recommend the following specific interventions for consideration when working with clients who have weight issues:

• *Help the client develop a self-hypnotic feeling of fullness by remembering a time when he or she was really full and then attempting to feel the sensation again in the stomach.* If the client reports difficulty identifying this sensation, we normally suggest drinking a glass of water in the session. After the memory is stimulated (or the sensation created during the session by drinking a glass of water), the client can memorize the feeling and recall the sensation.

• *Advise the client to return to a food plan and an exercise routine with which the client has had success (at least, temporarily) in the past.* If the client does not have either of those, assist the client in creating them. For example, the client may need encouragement to engage a personal trainer at a gym for a period of time in order to fashion an appropriate exercise regimen. Particularly for clients with diabetes, high blood pressure, or other medical complications, make certain that they are also coordinating with their internist or cardiologist.

• *Teach the client to interrupt the agitation of wanting something not on the food plan with an internal sound or song.* This could be the word *click*, the song line "I want to be in that number . . . " (from "When the Saints Come Marching In"), or a sound like "yeeeeeeeeee". Almost anything, however brief, can be enough to shift a person's attention. The intent is to replace the object of desire by interrupting the focus of concentration long enough for a different thought to enter.

• *Help the client identify ways to reward progress with something other than food.*

• *Encourage the client to develop the habit of consistently practicing the relaxation response by focusing attention on the breath and allowing any thought or sensation to pass by without judgment.*

Case Example: Weighting for the Light

Aaron, a physician whose specialty was oncology, knew the dangers of obesity with clinical exactitude. Nonetheless, he was 100 pounds overweight and had struggled with eating problems all his life. Coming from a family in which anxiety was calmed by food, both his parents and brother were obese. His father had died from a heart attack, and his brother had been hospitalized recently with heart trouble. Aaron reported that his overweight mother used to act like the "food police" and tell him what he should and should not eat. Not surprisingly, he responded with rebellion, anger, and resentment.

Aaron had already worked with a number of therapists, consulted nutritionists, and tried many weight loss programs. He had spent years in analysis and had substantial insight into the issues underlying his weight, but he still could not stop bingeing. His excess pounds were a constant source of frustration, grief, embarrassment, and self-loathing. He said he was waiting for "the light to come on"—for the one insight that would be illuminating enough to propel him to success.

He had binged for years by stopping at four or five restaurants on his way home from his office at the end of the day. Whenever he was surprised by having to be on call with little notice, a resurgence of the old anger and resentment toward authority triggered further bingeing episodes. He felt victimized when his answering service called him after-hours for an emergency, even though being on call was an unavoidable part of his medical practice.

A key to making change is being able to access internal resources for problem resolution and solution maintenance. In the first hypnosis session, we suggested, "You can go back in time and discover two or three experiences when you were completely determined to succeed." Immediately, he described his "full" focus in medical school [food language] and ability to complete the work. Another resourceful memory was the unwavering determination to spend time with his children after his divorce, even though his ex-wife attempted to keep the children from him. We suggested: "You can fully remember these feelings—first one event and then the other. Really savor the flavor of your determination [food language] to succeed. Then, remember what you looked like, how your body felt, and how people responded to you when you were 100 pounds lighter." These resourceful memories "jumpstarted" the loss of weight. [Access internal resources for motivation.]

Aaron returned to a food program with which he had previously had some success, but the bingeing continued. After each frustrating day, he would stop at three or four restaurants and feel a growing level of shame as he progressed from one to the next. Curiously, his report of these events lacked much emotion. When we asked him where the missing feelings were, he became aware that there was little positive motivating anxiety driving him to resolve the problem. But the pattern clearly had to be interrupted for him to succeed.

We realized that Aaron needed to find a way to manage his attitude regarding his work and a way to change his brain state in order to interrupt the bingeing episodes. He reported that he always felt exhausted before he binged.

He agreed to use the DAVID PAL device, which shifts the brain into a state of relaxation and calms the whole body (Seiver, 2003), before leaving work each evening. By this means, he achieved a more positive state of mind, managed to let go of the day's tension, and rediscovered the ability to drive straight home. He was successful until he had a particularly upsetting and stressful workday, at which time he binged again. Obviously, more drastic measures were needed. [Facilitate state change.]

At the next session, we asked him what he would be able to do if he had the motivation to take charge and manage his weight differently. He replied that he could easily lose 1 pound a week without any struggle or feeling of deprivation and could keep himself from bingeing.

We then asked Aaron to name the person or persons whom he most hated. After much thought, he said that it had to be the American Nazi Party. We asked him to take out his checkbook, write a check for $1,000 to the American Nazi Party, and to leave it in the office. He was told that if he could not maintain his commitment to lose a pound a week and cease bingeing, the check would be mailed. *Cautionary Note*: An intervention of this sort should not be used with any client who has a previous history of abuse or trauma. Such a client might well feel that he was being asked to "collude in his own emotional blackmail," or it might feel "punishing" and the effect could be highly counterproductive. [Access hidden determination.]

He suddenly imagined being placed on the group's mailing list and receiving their literature for the rest of his life. What would his letter carrier think? Would word of this reach his rabbi? Of course he could blame it on his therapist, but would anyone really believe him? What would his Jewish neighbors think, to say nothing of his friends and family? All of the color drained from his face, but he wrote out the check. "Aaron, you've been waiting for the light to come on," we said. "Perhaps you could imagine the swastika rotating and a beam of light coming from its center each time you see an unhealthy food or a fast-food restaurant. Can you see the light?" [Increase motivating anxiety.]

Because we did not know the address of the American Nazi Party, we asked Aaron to look it up on the Internet. He had the address at the next session and confided that he had searched the Internet late at night so that no one in the family would know. Positive motivating anxiety was now activated, and he lost 3 pounds the first week. For the first time since he had started bingeing, he was successful in controlling his state and behavior.

Thus, for a short time Aaron's motivation was his fear of an external threat—that we would mail the check. In essence, as therapists we were temporarily carrying his motivation for him. However, as soon as Aaron could demonstrate a measure of success—most importantly, to himself—we needed to reinvest him with an internally driven sense of motivation. We asked him to bring in a picture of himself at a time when he was at his target weight. The photograph that he showed us was of a lean and tanned younger man, confidently smiling at the helm of catamaran. That photograph became an icon of the man he wanted to reclaim and connected him to the motivation that eventually took him to his target weight.

Aaron began eating five times per day, including a protein and a complex carbohydrate each time he ate. We encouraged him to eat fibrous vegetables with protein in the evening and avoid white carbohydrates after 5:00 P.M. Exercising with light weights three times a week and at least 20–30 minutes of aerobics were suggested. Whenever Aaron had lost weight previously, he realized, he had visualized himself as heavy again. This time, we instructed him to practice two visualizations while he exercised each time. One was to visualize himself as thin and enjoying others admiring his physique. The other was to develop an image of himself as healthy and old.

We included alpha–theta training to teach Aaron methods of self-soothing. We also used deep hypnosis to allow Aaron to practice various scenarios in which he could make healthy food choices. Suggestions for the proper balance of protein, complex carbohydrates, and vegetables were paired with feelings of comfort, delight, fullness, and enjoyment of a lighter sensation (Blum & Tractenberg, 1990). Over time, he responded by feeling less stress daily, being in a more positive mood, and continuing to losing weight.

By the time Aaron terminated therapy, he had lost 100 pounds. With his consent, we kept the $1,000 check in our office fireproof file cabinet so he could remember that this assistance would always be in our office. At follow-up 8 years later, he reported that he had not binged again.

This chapter discussed the neurochemistry of food, including simple carbohydrate craving and the four key neurotransmitters, dopamine, acetylcholine, gamma-aminobutyric acid (GABA), and serotonin. It explored the roles of genetics, sleep deprivation, habit and taste habituation in weight issues; therapeutic assumptions in working with clients having weight issues; client assessment for weight management cases; and BCT interventions weight loss.

In the next chapter we describe the use of three combined treatment modalities—hypnosis and meditation used to harness the power of the unconscious mind, alpha–theta training to augment the healing ability of the CNS, and group relational support—in treating life-threatening or chronic illnesses. Working with a small group of participants to explore all three possibilities, we developed applicable mind-training techniques, qualitative themes, a collaborative process for the creation of individual healing journeys, and group metaphors for healing.

CHAPTER 10

Interventions in Life-Threatening and Chronic Illnesses

Psychotherapy, or "healing the psyche," comes from Greek. For the ancient Greek physicians, the word *psyche* was a rich and complex term that included the concepts we now name separately as *soul, mind, consciousness*, and *self*. In essence, it was the invisible component of a living being; it was everything that was not the *soma*, the body. Psyche was the animating principle, the mysterious element that disappeared at death. In life, its preeminence to—and its influence upon—the body were assumed. Comments made by the fictional character Doctor Zhivago (Pasternak, 1957) offer a more contemporary articulation of the same perspective: "Your health is bound to be affected if day after day you say the opposite of what you feel; if you grovel before what you dislike and rejoice at what brings you nothing but misfortune. Our nervous system isn't just a fiction. It's part of our physical body, and our soul exists in space and is inside us like the teeth in our mouth. It can't be forever violated with impunity" (p. 483).

For good or ill, there is a reciprocal relationship between the *psyche* and the *soma*. Chronic stress, persistent negative thoughts, attitudes, the destructive emotions of anger and anxiety, personal coping styles, and family dynamics can influence the development of health or illness (Schwartz, 2003). Over time, chronic stress lowers the immune system which can lead to the onset or exacerbation of illness. In families, chronic conflict upsets the natural psychobiological rhythms of all the family members.

However, the same dynamic interaction between *psyche* and *soma* permits the healing of physical illness to be facilitated by the brain–mind, particularly through the use of hypnotic psychotherapy and deep state training. These may be targeted anywhere from the level of gene (Rossi, 1993) to the level of social dynamics where habituated dysfunctional transactions result in responses that include elevated blood pressure, interrupted breathing, negative patterned trance behaviors and marked incongruence between what is experienced and what is expressed. Often spawned from this incongruency, chronic anxiety can cause the occurrence or exacerbation of physical disequilibrium and the ability of a person to manage the symptoms.

As our work in developing the BCT approach progressed, we became acutely aware of the potential healing power of combining treatment modalities: specifically, hypnosis to harness the power of the unconscious mind, alpha–theta training to augment the healing ability of the CNS, and a group format to provide relational and social support. We reasoned that the deeper states tend to stimulate the healing response, and the specific use of these states might provide a significant adjunctive treatment format for individuals with life-threatening or chronic illness. The relational group, we hypothesized, could utilize deep interpersonal connections, shared hypnotic experiences, therapeutic metaphors, deep state training experience, and the group connection for healing the body–mind.

Overview of the Psyche–Soma Interface

In 1975 a study by Ader and Cohen (1975) launched the field of psychoneuroimmunology, which seeks focused on gathering empirical evidence of the role of belief, expectation, and emotion in impacting the mind-body. Ader and Cohen's research demonstrated that the immune response responds in particular ways in relation to conscious expectations. The researchers first suppressed the immune system of rats by feeding them water mixed with saccharine and cytoxan (a drug that causes nausea and lowers the immune response). The rats learned to associate the sweet water with nausea. When cytoxan was no longer added, the rats still responded to the sweet water by developing nausea and dying of infection. The rats had been conditioned to suppress their immune systems and were unable to make a distinction between poison and nonpoison (Ader & Cohen, 1975).

Candace Pert, a leading psychoneuroimmunologist who discovered endorphins, the body's natural opiates, suggested that emotions exist in two realms: the mind and living matter. Neuropeptides mediate between emotions and thoughts and seem to be a key to the body's healing response (Pert, 1999). "Thus, we might refer to the whole system as a psychosomatic information network, linking 'psyche,' which comprises all that is of an ostensibly nonmaterial nature, such as mind, emotion and soul, to 'soma,' which is the material world of molecules, cells and organs. Mind and body, psyche and soma" (Pert, 1999, p. 2).

Illness is influenced by many factors, including genetic predisposition, lifestyle, exposure to pathogens, perceived stress, and immune system competence. But unless interrupted, the body's natural drive is toward healing. Various studies suggest that a combination of hypnosis, brain change technologies, and interpersonal support can positively affect health and, in some cases, retard or reverse illness (Dillon, Minchoff, & Baker, 1985; Spiegel, 1991; Siever, 2004). In a hypnotic state, people have been able to raise blisters on skin without heat, interrupt the inflammatory process of potentially severe burns (Ewin, 1994), successfully manage asthmatic attacks (Kershaw, 1987), stop chronic pain (Barber & Adrian, 1982), reduce the need for insulin by people with diabetes (Achterberg & Lawlis, 1980; Kershaw, 1979), and effect a variety of other mind–body repairs. In addition, some of the brain technologies that include neurofeedback and audiovisual stimulation have been shown to reduce pain and inflammation, lower blood pressure, increase blood flow, and train the CNS toward more flexibility (Othmer, 2009).

Other state change approaches such as meditation can have profound effects on the body. Meditation has long been shown to lower blood pressure. Additionally, in a study of 60 people who had atherosclerosis, all of them showed decreased thickness in the arterial walls after practicing meditation for 9 months (Johnson, 1996). State-changing techniques used on a regular basis can eliminate addictions to alcohol, tobacco, and drugs (Alexander, 1997).

Stress is a central issue in many chronic illnesses. Personal core beliefs that have led an individual to perceive the world in certain ways may lock in restrictive behaviors, attitudes, and emotions. Tracy realized that she had "invited" her breast cancer; from the time she had been a small child, she had known death would come from cancer in her 30s. Her family had constantly encouraged her to think of herself as ill, weak, and fragile. The narrative constructed by Tracy's family members painted a future without any possibilities than early death. Agreeing with them, she had become locked in their belief system. Ultimately, she realized that a powerful core belief she had carried for years was exactly that: a belief—but not necessarily a fact. At that point, Tracy was able to reject that self-image and create a new one as a survivor—which she certainly was, on many different levels.

Beliefs, such as an expectation of illness or early death, can lead to dysfunctional mind–body communication in the form of heightened states of arousal. The inner dialogue in which all of us engage has psychobiological consequences. That dialogue generates emotions that become psychobiological events and may lead to anxiety, shallow breathing, elevation of blood pressure, increased pulse rate, and a release of various hormones and chemical messengers that drive the body into the "biological stress syndrome" (Selye, 1978) characterized by: "(1) the initial complex adaptive [stressor] response of alarm and arousal and (2) the eventual maladaptive consequences of the prolonged stress response when arousal becomes chronic, leading to mind–body problems" (Rossi, 1993, pp. 70–71). The consequences can be lowered immune surveillance, hyperactive immune response, and increased risk of disease.

All the cells in the body are in uninterrupted communication and constantly influence each other. Under certain conditions, a genetic predisposition toward a system breakdown can be stimulated during prolonged stress responses. We know that emotional states correlate with changes in the immune system (Davidson, Scherer, & Goldsmith, 2002) and, frequently, illness follows stressful life events. Collectively, studies strongly support the view that people have the capacity to negatively influence their physical health simply through long-held beliefs and expectations; equally, people have the capacity to maintain self-regulation, self-healing, and long periods of wellness until death. This capacity can be enhanced by mind0training methods as well as by positive social interaction.

Mind Training Applied to Life-Threatening or Chronic Illnesses

When a person becomes ill, in addition to treating the body through a traditional medical approach, adjunctive treatments can improve mood and increase the sense of hopefulness, personal control, and relaxation.

The application of mind training in the context of life-threatening or chronic illness can employ any or all of three basic strategies: stress reduction through state change, physical wellness enhancement via improved immune functioning, and an emphasis on improving the quality of life, for example, by increasing the patient's sense of self-mastery and hopefulness.

Working with a small group of participants to explore all three possibilities, we designed a treatment plan combining hypnosis and meditation, alpha–theta state training, and group therapy. We were interested in noting the impact, if any, on the course of the participants' physical illnesses. We also wished to explore the participants' phenomenological worlds by examining their experiences in depth and learning how each constructed and understood his or her life. Additionally, we noted each participant's level of overall stress, a subjective measure of quality of life, and any descriptive data from client medical tests that addressed change in immune function before, during, and after the 52 weekly sessions.

A group program was created to provide 20 minutes of alpha–theta state training, 25 minutes of group support, and 20 minutes of group hypnosis that included imagery, metaphor, and suggestion to enhance immune functioning as well as overall well-being. As part of the group hypnosis, we constructed metaphors for healing in the context of a group process. (Two of these healing metaphor scripts are included later in this chapter.) We focused on (1) using trance phenomena in a group setting for stimulating healing resources, (2) addressing the relationship dynamics between the participant and family and physician, and (3) exploring aspects of the inner life that needed attention. Additionally, the group members utilized a daily self-report scale that evaluated behaviors indicative of stress as well as positive events. Trance phenomena, such as hypnotic analgesia, dissociation, and time distortion, were taught to group members to enhance suggestions of their brain–mind–body's ability to improve their health and well-being and to deal with discomfort. Therapeutic metaphors evolved from the group process each week. Self-hypnotic techniques and meditation training were offered to group members for additional work at home between sessions.

Murakami (2006) suggested that the mind can turn off genes that trigger cancer and turn on genes that provide healing to the body. Hayashi et al. (2006) found that blood glucose levels were lowered after Type 2 diabetes patients listened to comedy acts. They found that 23

genes designed to promote immune system response and signal trans-
duction can be mentally activated. Based on this data, we suggested that
group members add regular comedy to their routines.

The seven participants, three adult men and four adult women, were
referred by other therapists and the M.D. Anderson Cancer Hospital in
Houston. The group consisted of:

- An HIV-positive man who had been symptom free for 11 years
  and who had chosen to manage the disease with nontraditional
  methods, including special diet, exercise, and hypnotic methods,
  such as future orientation in time with an image of himself as an
  active, vibrant, old man.
- A man who had passed the 4-year marker since his chemotherapy treatments for a malignant melanoma. He had selected a combination of traditional and nontraditional treatment. At the age of
  58, he continued to participate in strenuous physical exercise,
  such as triathlons to enhance his confidence in his physical ability. He also learned a variety of meditative and hypnotic methods.
- A third man was currently in chemotherapy treatment for a malignant tumor and had come into the group somewhat skeptical
  that any alternative approach could be beneficial. He believed
  that he would die within the next year.
- One woman was undergoing chemotherapy for metastasized
  breast cancer. Her remarkable and contagious "fighting spirit"
  and interest in mobilizing her inner mind to enhance immune
  functioning impacted all of us.
- A second woman was fighting uterine cancer and had recovered
  from a heart attack and brain aneurysm. She used both traditional and nontraditional methods for healing. Having little difficulty
  in asking for what she needed, she was described by the group as
  courageous and spirited.
- The third woman suffered paralyzing arthritis and needed braces
  to walk. She was depressed but curious about what she could
  learn in the brain–mind–body group experience.
- The fourth woman was 3 years past her diagnosis of breast cancer
  and came into the group believing that her psychological makeup
  and past behavior had "caused" the cancer. She had steeped herself in "New Age" thinking that she was completely responsible
  for her physical condition and carried much pain and guilt.

Through conversation during group meetings, members explored in-depth personal health-related ideas, feelings, and behaviors. All group members perceived serious illness as a life marker event, which stimulated great change in other areas of life. Becoming aware of and naming chronic somatic and emotional complaints was one of the first areas considered. Many members found some physical correlation between a chronic emotional complaint and a body tension or connected issue such as insomnia. Most thought that there was an emotional component to their illnesses but not that the emotional had, in itself, caused the illness. Because there can be so many different triggers for illness, we pointed out that these emotional complaints may not have had anything to do with becoming ill.

Individual Self-Assessments

The group participants were asked to keep a log of daily stress on a scale from 1 to 10 (with 10 being extremely stressed), based on a self-evaluation. The stress measurements were averaged weekly. Each member was also asked to evaluate any emotional states such as anxiety, depression, etc. By monitoring their stress levels, some members realized that they were experiencing more stress than they had been consciously aware of before the self-check.

Each member summarized his or her family-of-origin health–illness history and family messages about being well and maintaining health. Physical and nutritional information was documented, including weight, eating habits, and amount of exercise. General health information was gathered, such as the frequency and number of colds per year as well as any other illnesses. Particular attention was paid to patterns of developing illnesses over the years. Overall physical and emotional functioning as self-reported was discussed throughout the year-long process. Additionally, beliefs and expectations about an individual's ability to impact health and illness were discussed.

Another focus of examination was each member's primary defensive or coping style. Among these were humor, denial, distraction, optimism, and pessimism. The particular characterological style of each member was noted in understanding attachment style as reflected in the unique resistance or openness to making contact with other group members. For example, the man who believed that he would die soon kept to himself in the group. When he did comment, his remarks were cryptic and cynical.

One of the most important aspects of the personal assessments was that people discovered inner resources of which they had been unaware, such as overlooked social, emotional, and physical abilities upon which they could build new responses.

Qualitative Themes

A number of themes emerged from the year-long group process:

- The illnesses had acted as a "wakeup call" to the group members to reorient life priorities so that time spent with family and friends came first. Their illnesses had also been a stimulus to resolve relationship conflicts and to focus on enhancing experiences with others.

- The participants believed that their group experience led to a greater quality of life; self-reported feelings of general well-being improved.

- Some members believed that they had been living out certain hypnotically suggested stories or "life scripts." For example, early suggestions from the family of origin of several members included ideas that they could only live in a particular area of the country or that they must get married or, conversely, must stay single. In each case, the members' illnesses led them to question these assumptions.

- A resource for each member was a personal "fighting spirit": Members discovered a personal resilience that surprised each of them.

- Due to their illnesses, members had dropped certain psychological defenses and placed personal honesty with others and themselves as a high priority.

- Members focused on psychological and spiritual development, and talked about developing extreme clarity for their goals.

- Members reviewed their lives with an emphasis on examining unmet goals, life experiences they had longed for, and taking care of "unfinished business."

- How a person envisions the future influences the perception of the present; developing an image of being old empowered members. Bringing in representations of wise old men and women symbolized life on many dimensions.

- Patterns that led to a poor quality of life were identified (e.g., feeling driven by time; the desire to accumulate material wealth, status, and power; feeling driven to achieve or maintain relationships that did not serve them well). These were replaced by new patterns that seemed better oriented to physical and emotional health.
- The ordinariness of life became more appreciated as a "special magic."
- Death could be talked about as a developmental stage and transition; it could be grieved and accepted.

Results of the Group Work

All group members reported a positive change in their perceived ability to influence their bodies toward health. With the exception of the woman with ovarian cancer, at the end of the 52 weeks, group members had better medical reports than when they began the program. Each member also experienced an increase in the perceived quality of life. Although it is difficult to determine what degree of healing the group experience provided, it was clearly meaningful to all members.

The results of this exploration are not sufficient to support the conclusion of a causal effect from the hypnosis, alpha–theta training, and group interaction in improving the overall health for most of the members. However, they do seem to support Spiegel's (1991) observation that group therapy combined with hypnosis may offer a viable treatment model for people with chronic or life-threatening illnesses. Kiecolt-Glaser, Marucha, Atkinson, and Glaser (2001) reported that using hypnosis was like hitting a reset button that tended to raise the immune response. Hopefully, further studies will statistically examine the immune system response to hypnosis, deep state training, and group work to quantify the efficacy of this approach in the adjunctive treatment of chronic illness. Our own clinical observations working with other cancer patients and those with chronic illnesses have indicated that deep state training can reduce or eliminate many treatment symptoms (e.g., nausea) and improve immune function.

Developing Healing Journeys

As a leading clinician who works with people who are chronically ill or have life-threatening illnesses, Dr. Rachel Naomi Remen has suggested that "healing happens between people. The wound in me evokes the healer in you, and the wound in you evokes the healer in me, and then the two healers collaborate" (as cited in Markova, 1994, p. 56). This collaboration process is the basis for the following protocol that Carol developed for utilizing the group connection for healing psychodynamic issues and stimulating individual psychobiological healing:

1. Listen for the theme and tone of the group discussion. Group members will often develop a common subject for discussion and will relate to each other around the topic. Themes can range from how supportive pets are to the process of dying. On any particular topic, the conversational tone can range from serious to quite humorous.

2. The therapist or group facilitator should allow the theme and dynamic of the group to stimulate an idea, image, phrase, or complete storyline that can be expanded into a therapeutic metaphor to be used in the hypnosis session, while maintaining an externally oriented trance (therapist's primary focus is on the group interactions, outside the self). After the therapist develops the goal for the hypnosis portion, based on the group's theme, evoked images or storylines can be organized by deciding how the metaphor will end. Working backward from the goal keeps the focus clear and allows the unfolding metaphor to stay within a particular structure.

3. Focus group members on their inner awareness of mind–body experiences in shifting states. For example, the therapist can ask, "What are you aware of now inside of your mind–body? . . . and now? . . . and now?"

4. After a formal trance induction, the therapist should mentally step into the image or storyline and begin to enlarge upon the metaphor or tell the story using sensory descriptions of the experience to involve the clients at a deeper level.

5. Notice and incorporate ideomotor behaviors (any unconscious movement) from the group members. Attention to certain involuntary movements from the members caused by suggesting various motoric be-

haviors can assist in the development of a trance state. We might say, "As you breathe more deeply, your immune response is resetting itself to provide healing and regeneration."

6. Incorporate direct suggestions of adaptation, healing, and regeneration of the mind–body . Suggest that the mind–body is already in a state of healing. Cells are constantly being replaced, tissue is regenerated, and all systems are responding and adapting to the environment, to internal thought processes, and to the intake of nutrition.

7. Members of the group may evoke various archetypal images from or in each other. Weave these images into the metaphor or story and give them back to the group. Examples of universal images representing different aspects of a person's process include the "warrior," the "earth mother," and the "trickster."

8. The hypnotic work should last around 20 minutes and then should include a silent period in which each person's unconscious awareness may sense the positive healing intent of the others in the room.

9. Suggest that participants can do inner work to resolve personal issues connected to the ones discussed in the group. Allow enough time to pass for the ideomotor or nonverbal responses to indicate that some shift has occurred. This may be observed in people taking deeper breaths and "settling in" more deeply.

10. Outside of the formal hypnotic session, group members may often find themselves in a negative trance state as they focus on aspects of their illnesses. Therefore, before delivering specific suggestions, the conscious mindset of the group should be disrupted. This can be accomplished with a change in breathing or body posture, by telling an anecdote, using humor, etc. Then an unconscious search for state- dependent resources can be initiated. Clients have had experiences being well before the onset of illness. It is useful to engage in a search for the mind–body memories of feeling and being well. Also, a focus on retrieving the resources of safety, courage to carry on, persistence, facing fears, and making a commitment to a goal can encourage a client during the management of chronic illness. (See sample metaphor scripts later in this chapter.)

11. Discuss any insights the group members developed during the trance work. Participants often develop insights during the silent interaction phase of the hypnosis session, and they can suggest ways to implement those insights.

Within the structure of the healing metaphor, various hypnotic suggestions can be emphasized to stimulate healing, promote hope, and reinforce the fact that the mind can influence the body. Suggestions such as the following can be interspersed or delivered in a direct fashion within the context of the metaphor. The redundancy below is intentional; repeating the same communication in slightly different words helps the mind to hold it.

- The mind–body can heal itself.
- The body is in a constant state of adaptation, healing, and regeneration.
- All of the mind–body systems can work together to resolve psychobiological problems.
- If there is any emotional issue connected to the physical problem, the unconscious can communicate this to the conscious mind via a symbol or picture or word or some other way.
- The mind–body is one and works together for healing and well-being.
- The mind–body can develop a healing image for the healing process.
- The mind–body can release the right biochemicals for ridding the body of confused diseased cells and creating a balance between the old cells being normally eliminated and new healthy cells replacing them.
- The mind–body can work together with medical treatment for health and well-being.
- The mind–body knows how to heal itself and develop "chronic health."
- The mind–body can begin to communicate with the part of the self beyond the symptom.
- The mind–body can develop a deep rapport with the self.

We felt privileged to work with these clients, and one of the effects was to ask ourselves the same questions they were constantly asking: "Is this what I want to be doing with my time?" "Is this the quality of life I want to have?" Being a part of each person's struggle to live touched us deeply, for they were not only each others' mirrors, but ours as well. They cried together, sang together, shared dreams, and when each went for the next medical report, they held their breath together in hopes of good news.

One of the members carved a small statue. On it, he placed *milagros*, symbols of each person's particular body part that was impaired, and led the group through a healing ceremony in which the carving was passed around, held, and given a personal blessing. The carving sat on our desk during the group experience to watch over the sacred space created by the participants' coming together.

Toward the end of the year, the woman with uterine cancer became so ill that she was transferred to a hospice. The group gathered in her hospice room and began to sing a Jewish song that she recognized from childhood. They held hands and gently touched her to say goodbye for the last time. She died several hours later.

Many times over those previous months, as we all contemplated our own mortality, but especially as we sat together in the hospice room, I (Carol) was reminded of my own grandmother. She had been a model for me of how a woman can successfully run her own business and develop the artist within. Grandmother had also been married three times in an era when divorce was not at all socially acceptable—something I hoped not to emulate. She loved to paint the Texas countryside with its familiar bluebonnets and, as an artist, went on many trips to capture the sweeping Texas landscape on canvas.

I remembered my grandmother's funeral and the smaller group who came out to honor my grandmother's life at the graveside. While the preacher droned on, a huge black bird flew up and began to make loud calls to interrupt the sermon. My grandmother, who was half Cherokee Indian, would have loved this. She was always making jokes; I felt it was her spirit that came to share a last chuckle.

After the internment, an elderly woman dressed in a long purple robe-like dress with a huge floppy hat and knurled wooden cane came up to me and said, "You must be the doctor! Your grandmother spoke so highly of you and was ever so proud. We painted together, and she spoke of you often." I had been the only member of my family to graduate from college, thanks to the support of my parents, to say nothing of earning a doctoral degree. Her words were stunning and touched me so deeply that I stood there and wept. What a lovely gift she had given me with her memories.

As we all gathered at the woman's bedside in the hospice, I knew that she too had given each of us a treasured gift. In her dying was a peaceful letting go and, in that, she helped the rest of us relax into the idea that our own dying would be all right. Time flows swiftly. We all knew that she had preceded us only by a little.

Group Metaphors for Healing

The following are two group metaphors we constructed following a discussion time that focused on fear of the future in terms of illness, healing emotions as well as the body, and desires for certain life experiences. The metaphors were designed to shift the group's state from fear to curiosity and to underscore the fact that the body is always in a state of healing.

Discovering Keys

"Close your eyes . . . and begin to turn your attention to your breathing . . . just allow your mind to settle, kind of like a feather might drift down and land gently on the ground . . . landing very gently and seeming to be quite comfortable. I would like you to just notice your breathing and notice that as you shift your awareness to attending to a deeper place inside, you can enter that pleasant state of deeper comfort.

"We are looking forward to the day this week when the temperature is predicted to change, cooling off things . . . always a marker of a beginning shift in the seasons. You can look forward to feeling cooler . . . Most people, when they begin to feel a little cooler, feel a little more energetic . . . a little more enthusiasm . . . remembering how pleasant it is to have a break in the hot weather . . . and the leaves begin to turn and if you listen carefully, even the birds' songs changes . . . and already signs of a coolness in the environment. In some places you can watch the seasons change rather dramatically but here, you have to notice the subtleties.

"As I have been talking to you, perhaps your own temperature has shifted, and I don't know whether your body begins to feel heavy . . . maybe a comfortable heaviness . . . breathing more deeply and allowing your mind and your body to go even deeper into your experience of this moment . . . extending into a longer moment . . . where time can go by, but it can seem as if it has completely stopped for now. Every season that changes brings with it an anticipation of a gift. . . .

"Now, in a moment I'm going to count down from 10 to 0 and just allow yourself to be more comfortable as each number becomes smaller. Beginning to count now . . . 10 . . . 9 . . . going deeper . . . 8 . . . 7 . . . 6 . . . drifting down . . . 5 . . . 4 . . . 3 . . . 2 . . . 1 . . . and 0. In a moment, I will count down from 3 to 0 and imagine each of these numbers count 10. Your inner mind won't mind how comfortable you can become now and in the future . . . 3 . . . 2 . . . 1 . . . 0.

"Not long ago a man was walking in the country and enjoying watching the sunlight as it filtered down among the pine trees, enjoying the crisp air, taking a morning walk to begin a lovely day. As he walked down the path, he found that the tress became so dense that it was difficult to see the path on which he was walking. But the birds were singing and the clouds were gently moving overhead. He came to a place where the trunk of an old tree had fallen over, and he sat down on it to take a nice deep breath and look around. His eyes caught the reflection of the sun bouncing off something on the forest floor.

"He was curious so he walked over and, almost buried beneath one of the large pine trees, was a set of three old keys. He sat back down on the trunk and, brushing off the encrusted dirt, he examined the keys one by one. He couldn't help but wonder what they opened . . . was it a treasure of some sort? . . . or perhaps, they were keys to an old farm house. Each of the keys looked different. On one of the key handles was what looked like a word, but on closer examination, he saw that it was an arrow. He thought this was odd that someone would have inscribed an arrow on a key. He took the keys back where he'd found them and set them up again in the same way he'd found them. He noticed where the arrow pointed. It pointed to the next tree and to the right of it was a large boulder. He wondered if this were some code or map, or if maybe he'd been watching too many movies.

"He went to the boulder and began to dig around it. Finally, he heard the clang of a large piece of metal. In fact, there was something there, so he kept digging. Finally, he discovered an old metal chest with a huge lock. He looked at the keys and wondered if any of them would open the lock. He took the first key and tried it. It wouldn't even fit in the lock. The second key fit in the lock, but it wouldn't turn. He fiddled with it gently but the lock would not budge. He took the third key with the engraved arrow and placed it in the lock. Immediately the lock opened— and his heart began to pound. He wondered what he would find when the chest opened.

"Perhaps he would find a great treasure . . . and perhaps it belonged to someone a long time ago and he really shouldn't disturb it, but his curiosity drove him to open the chest. He opened the chest slowly and as he peered inside, he discovered seven more keys . . . and each key had inscribed on it a different symbol. Underneath the keys was a map with seven locations matching the symbol inscribed on each key. The map indicated seven treasure chests, one in each location.

"When you are walking down a path and you discover something that is a surprise, you certainly have a variety of choices . . . about what to do . . . about whether in fact to take the adventure that might be presented or to keep that potential experience in the back of your mind . . . or to use your keys to open a lock to an inner discovery that might lead to a whole other adventure in itself. . . . As he sat there looking at the map, he already knew what he would do.

"Now as you let yourself enjoy this nice inner state of mind and body . . . allowing yourself to open to that inner healer . . . that can be triggered by changing states of mind, breathing more slowly, and enjoying your own inner state of sanctuary. In fact, your inner healer has many capacities to stimulate the natural state of healing. The adventures that you want to have . . . you can determine to accomplish in the near future . . . and in this state . . . perhaps discover something important about yourself that you didn't know before. And sitting here with this group and all of the support that you feel from each other, you can take this healing energy with you through the week and know you are connected to each other through your own caring and good energy for a better tomorrow. In a moment, you can begin to come back here and bring back this comfortable state with you. That's right. . . ."

Finding a Special Place of Regeneration

"Take a nice deep breath and allow your breathing to be a bridge from one state of consciousness to another . . . almost like you would begin to walk across a bridge from one shore to another . . . and as you breathe in and out, just allow yourself to become a little more settled and centered. The mind can become quiet as the body becomes still. This is the entry into the healing internal space . . . into your own internal medicine being received here by being together in this group. The Eastern ideas of healing suggest that we all have energy points called chakras that are in alignment from the base of the torso right up to top of the head. I would like you to imagine that each of these points is beginning to spin like a ball, starting with the crown of the head, spinning in a clockwise direction from your point of view. All seven points begin to spin, and allow you to feel more comfortable.

"Allow your breathing to become slower and whatever sensations begin to develop, just allow them to occur . . . knowing that it is only your unconscious mind beginning to speak . . . and consciously and unconsciously I would like you to develop good intentions for each person here. Take a few moments to hold each person in your mind and bathe that person with positive feeling. And now hold the same feeling for yourself.

"Every living thing is constantly in a process of regeneration. Your body . . . is always in a state of regeneration. So appreciate how this process automatically occurs without your awareness.

"And think about this: One woman found her spirit tending her own garden. As she grew strawberries, tomatoes, and herbs, she relaxed into what she called her special place inside where nothing could bother her state of ease. For her, her garden became her special place. As she nurtured the plants, caring for each one as it needed, her whole garden nurtured her. Every person has a special place. Maybe it is a place outside and also a place inside you. Maybe it is only a place inside you. Take a few minutes to let your awareness roam over all of the places that have touched you deeply. Feel each of the places and find the one that is your special place. Maybe you know immediately where it is. If you do not discover it now, allow yourself later to return to the question and the answer will come to you.

"Connected to your special place is a feeling, a state. It is a state of freedom, of relaxed openness. As you experience that state inside of you just now, fully enjoy your ability to create it within yourself and around others. In a moment, I will ask you to come gently back here and bring this feeling with you, knowing that you can take it with you as you return home."

Case Example: Managing High Blood Pressure

Marjorie was an investment advisor in her mid-50s. Given the vicissitudes of the stock market, she frequently had clients calling her in a state of anxiety—some of which she admittedly picked up. She was not overweight, but she did have a family history of stroke. Other than a fairly high-torque career, her life appeared stable. She reported being comfortably settled in her marriage of 23 years.

Marjorie entered therapy because she had extremely high blood pressure, and the beta-blocker medication her physician had prescribed made her feel sluggish both physically and mentally. She wanted to see if she could change her diet and stress level enough to control her blood pressure without the drugs and requested help with that.

We used a combination of alpha–theta training and hypnosis, and her blood pressure began to come down. At one point in a deep state, she commented that she felt her deceased mother in the room with her; the mother told Marjorie that she was happy and fine and not to worry so about her. Marjorie began to weep with relief. She said that at that moment she felt an enormous release of internal pressure and guilt that she had not been or done enough for her mother.

Although she had said in the initial evaluation that her blood pressure had become critically high about a year and a half earlier, she had not mentioned that it had happened about the same time that her mother had become unable to live independently and the family had decided that she must move to an assisted living situation. In fact, until then Marjorie had not consciously connected the two events. As she explained near the end of that hour, her mother had been very unhappy in the assisted living facility and had died 6 months later.

That session was the turning point in Marjorie's efforts to control her high blood pressure. Under her physician's supervision, she began to lower her blood pressure medicine until she was off of it. She continued to attend to diet and exercise and monitored her blood pressure twice daily. Her physician asked her to come in monthly to be certain she was functioning well. During a follow-up phone call a year later, we learned that she was still maintaining a blood pressure low enough that she did not need to take medication to manage it.

In this chapter, we have explored the ways in which BCT, by combining the treatment modalities of hypnosis, alpha–theta training and a group support format, can engage or augment the healing ability of the mind–body in the context of life-threatening or chronic illness.

In the next chapter we embark on a journey toward peak performances and optimal life experiences. Enhanced performance—in every arena—is achieved through training the mind by training the brain. We explore the factors involved in optimal performance, ways of accessing the zone or state of flow, client assessment issues, and how to design a personalized brain change training program, among other related topics.

CHAPTER 11

Enhancing Performance in Professional Arenas

From NASA astronauts to executives, from actors and athletes to countless individuals who simply want to function in an optimal state, there is increased interest in enhancing human performance. Whether it is in professional sports, the performing arts, or behind the executive desk, people need to respond to situations with speed, accurate analysis, consistency, expert focus, and stamina (Sams, 2006).

All performers must attend to three areas of concern. First, they rely on the body's ability to deal with the physical demands of an activity. Whether playing a sport, an instrument, or singing, the performer's body is either part of the instrument or the entire instrument and must be exercised both adequately and correctly to allow it to work properly. Second, performance carries high psychological demands. In fact, a high incidence of psychiatric disorders (e.g., panic, performance anxiety, other mood and anxiety issues, insomnia, and eating disorders) can be found among musicians and performing artists (Nagel, 1998). Third, and bridging between the first two, emotional stress can generate body tension leading to physical injuries (Zinn & Zinn, 2003).

Enhanced performance in every arena is achieved through training the mind by training the brain. A critical element in performance is matching the responses of the sympathetic nervous system to the demands of the performance activity (Moss, 2003). Controlling attention, quieting the mind, and becoming unattached to thoughts and outcomes are the keys both to performing well and to living more fully. As in most pursuits, the brain needs to be able to make state shifts easily and quickly. Superb performers eventually pick up these skills, but success needn't be so hard won. The basic techniques of BCT facilitate their intentional acquisition.

Performance Factors

Several categories of factors typically affect performance: environmental, situational, nutritional, skill level, and mental state. The environment is the golf course, the weather, the performance hall, the office, or anything about the setting that may aid or deter performance. Situational factors involve whether the performance will be judged or how much is "riding on" it, such as a musician playing an audition for a symphony chair, or an athlete competing in the Olympics. Generally, the more important the event, the more difficult it is to maintain concentration. When crowds are screaming, weather conditions are less than ideal, and there is little margin for error, it is normal to become tense, worry about the result, and lose mental focus and concentration. This level of arousal is similar to the fight–flight–freeze response. Athletes and performers "at the top of their game" have learned to override the natural response, refocus their attention, alter their level of arousal to an optimal level, and give themselves the best chance for peak performance.

Performance states need to shift quickly and with flexibility. Good nutrition is crucial to activating the brain. To achieve peak performance in different athletic activities, diets with varying emphases will be advised by coaches, but in all cases attention needs to be paid not only to nutrition that supports strength and endurance but that enhances the speed of neural processing. Neural circuits activate and show precise coordination with brain centers that modulate energy homeostasis and cognitive function with food consumption, and foods specifically affect brain function. For example, the omega-3 fatty acid, which is mostly obtained from eating fish, can affect synaptic function and cognitive abilities by providing plasma membrane fluidity at synaptic regions (Gómez-Pinilla, 2008).

Naturally, skill levels affect performance in important ways. The performer must "overtrain" using correct style and form. Mistakes not corrected in practice will become like a virus that spreads into the performance. Once the activity has been practiced to the point that it has become an automatic movement directed by the unconscious, the athlete or artist can let go of the idea of performing.

Mental factors involve the ability to notice small errors with little or no affect and return to a focused mind. However, becoming "caught" by any thought will take the mind out of the moment and disrupt the state of flow. Beliefs also act as a lens that either expands or limits the performer's personal reality and sense of what is possible. As an example, beliefs based on past performance often determine what goals a performer will try to reach. For these reasons, the ability to maintain a conducive emotional state and a supportive set of beliefs must be developed and practiced just as assiduously as physical skills.

By building on abilities honed through practice in each of these areas, the tools of biofeedback, hypnosis, and visualization can give a performer a critical edge. Chartier, Collins, and Koons (1997) confirmed the usefulness of these approaches. In a study using neurofeedback training and mind–body skill integration practice sessions with golfers, 14 out of 15 subjects showed significant improvements as measured by pre and post scores; furthermore, 10 out of 12 who took the Profile of Mood States (POMS) assessment earned the "iceberg profile," a mindset usually seen in elite athletes where no situation caused them to lose focus. The iceberg profile is a low score on the POMS in all six categories (except for vigor): tension/anxiety, depression/dejection, anger/hostility, vigor/activity, fatigue/inertia, and confusion/bewilderment. Improvements were also noted in the obsessive-compulsive scale on the Symptom Checklist–90.

State Flexibility: Open and Closed Focus in Performance

Complicated situations often require immediate assessment and decision making followed by complex actions. All of these necessitate numerous rapid and sensitive changes in brainwave states. State flexibility, the cornerstone of BCT, allows rapid transitions between passive and active engagement; from looking and listening to analysis; from the visualization of possible outcomes to decisions and from there to action.

"Open focus," according to its originator Dr. Les Fehmi, the director of the Princeton Biofeedback Center, is the effortless orientation to any waking activity (Fehmi & Robbins, 2007). He suggested that one's attention can be equally spread among body sensation, thoughts, feelings, sounds, and other input while doing any task. Fehmi characterized attention as simultaneously falling somewhere along two continua: objective–immersed and narrow–diffuse. *Objective attention* is distances the person from the object of attention. In contrast, *immersed attention* is one in which there is little or no separation between the person attending and that to which attention is directed. *Narrow attention* restricts itself to one or a few things, whereas *diffuse attention* is inclusive and three-dimensional, awarding equal attention to all internal and external stimuli simultaneously. Diffuse and immersed forms of attention result in an open focus and are organized by the right hemisphere of the brain, exhibiting a high degree of alpha waves. Most people's habitual orientation falls into a narrow–objective mode of attending organized by the left hemisphere and focused on whatever is stressful. In that mode, mental flexibility is lost. Open focus is demonstrated when a quarterback can read the defense, peruse the field, locate open receivers, and remain aware of and dodge onrushing linemen. A closed focus is useful when the player needs to lock in on a receiver and deliver a pass, often between two defenders. The goal is to develop the ability to flexibly shift between these states.

The ease with which an individual can shift back and forth between an open and closed focus exemplifies the power of mind. For example, in team sports or in a dance company, the peak state will predominantly require an open immersed focus of attention with quick shifts to closed focus, as needed, and then a return to open focus. For soloists, a narrow immersed focus may be primary with quick shifts to open diffuse focus. To the extent that a brief shifting to thoughts or feelings does not include internal criticism, the more the performer has control. Optimally, the performer's concentration is completely focused in the moment; the past and the future disappear. Such concentration cannot be forced, but it can be developed (Nideffer, 1993, 2001). As illustrated in the next case example, BCT can assist a performer in learning to shift more easily between open and closed focus.

Case Example: Falling into the Music

Even finest athletes make minor errors. The same holds true for excellent musicians. No musician goes through a complex piece of music without making extremely small errors and, because a good musician's hearing will always exceed his or her capacity to play, every one of those errors is *heard* by the performer. Preferably, a musician will hear a small error, make a mental note, drop back into the music and again become absorbed in the sound.

However, a performer also needs to make contact with the audience. That contact communicates the musicality to audience members and enriches their experience of the concert. One needs only to attend a concert with Itzhak Perlman as soloist to understand how enjoyable a performance can be, not only for the quality of the music but for also the intimate contact Perlman makes with people. Knowing that there are music critics in the audience, the artist "forgets" the critics and connects with the *people* (including the critics). This process becomes more complex for a soloist leading an orchestra. Not only must the soloist be focused on playing and connect with the audience, but he or she must also maintain contact with the conductor and, through him or her, be aware of the rest of the orchestra. Managing this level of complexity requires frequent shifting between closed and open focus and demands a relaxed concentration.

Sarah, a promising violinist, came to Bill for assistance in developing a secure state when she performed. She had an amazing work ethic and would practice for hours. However, her left hand was developing carpel tunnel syndrome due to incorrect technique compounded by all the practicing. Adding to the problem, she had a slight familial hand tremor. As a result, she was also experiencing a level of anxiety that was further eroding the quality of her performance. Sarah's violin teacher worked with her on technique and Bill taught her to go into trance and "fall into the music" (right brain, open focus) while performing. In trance, the anxiety disappeared and, in shifting the state, the signals sent from the brain to the hand were altered, which completely stopped the tremor. When Sarah would make a small error, she learned to make a quick note of it for future reference and move on. Later, she learned how to drop into the music, shift out to connect with the audience, and then move back into the music.

Case Example: Topping a Personal Best

Howard was a pole-vaulter whose personal best was 3 years behind him at the time he came in to work with Bill. Over the intervening years, many of Howard's friends, whom he had previously beaten, had caught up and surpassed him. He was frustrated because he had been unable to meet his own best again and was on the verge of giving up. After a few sessions using hypnosis, he learned to develop a very narrow focus of attention and to block out external stimuli. In trance, he remembered that his muscles knew what to do in competition, and he focused his attention and let go of all concern about the height of the bar. Taking that learning into the field, the tension he had experienced previously evaporated. He altered his level of arousal by remembering feeling of tense, tight, and nervous and then consciously shifting his state to one that was relaxed and calm. Very shortly, he not only matched his personal best, but finished second in a conference championship. From there, he went to the regional competition, where he had the best jump of his career, giving him "All American" status.

Peak Performance: Accessing the Zone or State of Flow

A state of consciousness that makes optimal performance feel practically effortless has been variously described as being in the "zone" or in a state of "flow." Both extraordinary performers and ordinary people describe the experience of being in the zone as a transcendent state or a psychological space in which consciousness of the self disappears. In the zone, time seems to slow; athletic movement becomes transformed into near-ballet; and performers report an amazingly crisp clarity and focus of attention.

In that state, a relaxed concentration and an experience of being one with the activity is easily maintained. The mind state of "at-oneness" has usually been experienced at least once in a person's life. This dissolution of the boundary between self and other allows a performer to drop any critical thinking or judgment, which inevitably precludes a state of flow by separating the mind from the activity. For a condition of flow, the internal critic—often one of the most difficult factors to manage—must become silent.

The study of the state of flow has ancient roots. Patanjali, an Indian philosopher-sage who lived some time around 250 B.C.E., is best known as the author or collector of the *Yoga Sutras*, one of the most revered classical Sanskrit texts. Structured as terse aphorisms, the *Yoga Sutras* deal with training the mind to achieve oneness or pure liberation. To this end, they describe four levels of attention involved in developing the state of flow:

1. *Pratyahara* is a narrowing of focus wherein all external distractions are eliminated with a tunnel or laser vision.

2. *Dharana* is the focusing or concentration on an object or state of consciousness. In the realm of performance, the athlete or artist can completely focus on a ball or music or a novel to be written.

3. *Dhyana* is the undisturbed or uninterrupted attention on the object of contemplation, such that the flow of attention to the object is constant. This might be the equivalent of the performance "trance" where time seems to "stand still."

4. *Samadhi* may be said to occur when a person experiences total clarity and the sense of being one with the object of concentration. No longer is there a sense of differentiation between the individual focusing and the object of the focus.

Contemporary Research

Numerous contemporary studies have also researched ways to maintain the state of flow under pressure (Csikszentmihalyi, 1990; Jackson, 1996). However, despite more than 2,000 intervening years, contemporary descriptions of levels of attention accessed by peak performers are remarkably similar to Patanjali's stages. Further, the *Yoga Sutras* perceptively note that "suffering" comes from identification with either the contents in the mind or the outcomes of events. Peak performers have experienced this principle firsthand: Attachment erodes performance. The challenge, then, is in learning how to detach from the results of a performance, whether great or mediocre (Prabhavananda & Isherwood, 1953).

Dan Landers and colleagues at Arizona State University in 1991 examined peak states in successful archers. They discovered that in the peak state, the archers' minds were producing alpha rhythm, indicative of a relaxed but concentrated focus. Landers suggested that the elite athlete must allow the right hemisphere to take over when performing a skill. The researchers noted: "The archers who increased alpha activity in their right hemispheres improved their performances, while those who increased left-hemisphere activity saw their accuracy decline. That may be because the right hemisphere is involved with simultaneous processing and spatial relations, while the left handles sequential thinking and language" (Landers, 1991, p. 222).

In another study, Paul Mahoney and Peter Terry worked with Malaysian trapshooters (as cited in Dingfelder, 2008). They found that different trapshooters evidenced different patterns of brain activity: Some athletes showed alpha activity just before a successful shot, whereas others displayed even slower brainwaves. Mahoney and Terry hypothesized that those who excelled showing the alpha wave activity may have needed to be more alert, relatively speaking, whereas the athletes who performed well with slower brainwaves may have benefited from a more meditative state. As a result, Mahoney and Terry trained each athlete to reproduce the exact brain frequencies that occurred when he had his best shots. The participants all improved their accuracy and reported increased concentration.

Japan's Babe Ruth

Sadaharu Oh, born in 1940 and active in professional baseball through 2008, was considered to be Japan's "Babe Ruth." He hit 868 home runs, more than any other professional baseball player in history. Oh was a first baseman for the Tokyo Giants and retired after 22 seasons. In addition to consistent practice, he developed a philosophy that kept him in a peak state. He believed that when he stepped into the batter's box, he entered into a special relationship with the pitcher. He and the pitcher were one; in fact, he, the ball, and the pitcher were one. There was no separation, no adversary. He could not bat without the pitcher, and the pitcher could not pitch without the batter. The notion of harmonizing with a player on the "opponent's" team allowed him to develop a focused concentration that led to a superb batting average (Oh & Faulkner, 1985).

Oh said he learned that mastery of any kind takes time, commitment, patience, and keeping the mind in shape. Attention to hand position, weight transfer, waiting, focusing, and anticipating require a great deal of effort before the process appears effortless. Oh added that one must also learn to wait. One must wait for the right pitch, the right swing, the right attitude, and the right focus. Ultimately, however, even technique and practice are not enough: It is the Zen Buddhist ideal of a state of no thought that produces the ideal swing and extraordinary performance. The Zen Buddhist philosophy states that all that exists is this moment; everything else—past and future—are illusions. In fact, every situation (e.g., every pitch) is unique and requires a unique response rather than one that has been memorized. For this reason, the mind needs to concentrate, remain flexible, and adjust to situations almost instantly. Body and mind must then act as one, a process that can be enhanced by learning to breathe rhythmically. However, the Zen Buddhist approach to martial arts suggests something very important: that while the mind must always be attentive to the opponent, *there is never an enemy*. This is equally true on the playing field, in the concert hall, at the boardroom table, and in combat: There is no enemy—not the opponent, not the self, and not the circumstances.

Client Assessment

Before embarking on any interventions, the clinician should fully understand what kind of difficulties the performer is experiencing. An assessment must identify and analyze what is bothering the performer both from an internal and an external perspective. The following questions provide a useful outline for a diagnostic inquiry:

1. What is the general nature of the problem?

2. What part of the problem stems from what the performer is doing? What is the performer's level of reactivity to the situation? Is something happening internally that causes the problem?

3. What part of the problem stems from what others are doing?

4. Does the performer become too nervous, too aware of outcome, of a bad score from a judge, or of losing the game?

5. Does the performer become too focused on small mistakes and unable to take in the information, make the correction, and move forward?

6. Has the performer fallen into a negative trance, no longer trusting in his or her innate skill level and expecting to fail at some point in the performance?

7. Does the performer hold any core beliefs that are at odds with the idea of winning or being successful?

8. Is the performer experiencing any problem in shifting states—for example, in being able to be absorbed and in love with the music and then shift to make an emotional contact with the audience?

9. As a crucial element in building rapport, throughout the assessment, the clinician will want to keep in mind one additional question: What can realistically be done to make at least a small improvement in the situation?

Case Example: A Shift in Attitude

Jason was the best discus thrower in the state; his coach referred him to Bill. The problem was that after doing very well one time, anxiety would cause him to tank the next two throws [Assessment questions 1 and 2]. The means of improvement was to change Jason's attitude and performance on the first throw [2 and 4]. As a metaphor, Bill used the Houston Rockets who won a title by coming from behind in every game in the playoffs. Bill focused on the theme of having confidence even though doing poorly the first time and then surging from behind and enjoying the process [3, 4, and 5]. When Jason went to the state meet, he had the worst throw of his career. But instead of tanking the next two throws, the second throw was a state meet and personal record. So dramatic was the change, other coaches were all but conceding defeat. That throw was the second best throw of the entire state meet, and Jason first place easily. The small change had to do with shifting to an attitude that he could come from behind and succeed [8 and 9].

Designing a Personalized Brain Change Training Program

The design of a brain change training program, whether for an athlete, a performing artist, or an executive, is similar. We work with the client to determine what consciously applied strategies may help and, if needed, what states and resources might be accessed at the unconscious level. Then we develop a plan for change that usually includes the following components:

- Training in self-regulation
- Strengthening of emotional state and retrieval of seemingly unrelated inner resources (see also "Resource Activation," Chapter 4)
- Accessing the zone or state of flow
- Engaging in visual imagery for success, including identifying a successful role model to emulate in a process of trance identification
- Conducting mental rehearsal, usually done in very light, self-induced trance
- Imagining the activity or seeking creative business ideas in deep trance
- Aligning core beliefs

Frequently a second part of the assessment process follows the development of the personalized training program and is accomplished using a neurofeedback instrument. Through a series of hypnotic suggestions, we ask the person to remember a time when the state of flow was achieved. If the person is able to return to that memory while hooked up to the computer, his or her brainwaves will create a peak performance map. For example, Joel Lubar (Personal Communication, July 18, 1999) hooks up golfers to an EEG machine, has them take their stance with the golf club, and then has them remember the peak state. In that moment, he captures a reading of the person's unique peak performance state on the EEG. Through neurofeedback training, the performer then trains to recreate that specific state. If the client is not able to recapture the sense of flow, we can still assist the person in learning to "step into" the state; we simply don't have the unique neural "signature" with which to work.

Interventions for Optimizing Performance

When people attempt to force a new behavior, things frequently get worse. Willpower may be successful for a short period but usually cannot sustain a change in behavior. Therefore, we encourage the performer to learn how to develop a different state of consciousness that *allows* a new behavior. To enhance performance, he or she may need to correct attitudes, improve the ability to shift focus, or reduce performance anxiety. These can all be accomplished with deep state training.

Typically we use hypnosis rather than brain-training devices with performers because we need to assist them in acquiring new skills that are more complex than just learning how to hold particular brainwave configurations. Performers need to learn how to (1) relax sufficiently to access a variety of states of arousal; (2) link to emotional resources such as the pleasure of performing; (3) practice mental rehearsal so that muscles can further refine the skill; (4) shift core beliefs and dysfunctional programming; and (5) develop the capacity to problem-solve rapidly both when a problem arises in the actual activity and, as training for that, in the hypnotic trance. A reorganization of the conception of a problem, accompanied by new associations accessed from a different state of consciousness, can transform an apparently limited situation into one with more possibilities.

Logan was 11, doing poorly in school, and had significant anger issues when his parents asked Bill to try to help him. He was also a committed baseball player on a team that had been rated one of the top 20 teams in his age group in the country. However, Logan's anger was spilling out there and affecting his performance on the team. At bat, he would sometimes act out when he hit a foul ball or struck out.

Using conversational hypnosis, Bill recounted some baseball anecdotes, structuring them as metaphors for state change underlying behavioral change. One story was based on an incident that occurred in 1956 when the Washington Senators' pitcher Pedro Ramos was pitching to New York Yankee slugger, Mickey Mantle. Ramos threw a ball that hit him and knocked him down. In the next game that Mickey faced Ramos, the Yankees were behind 1-0. With Mickey at bat, Ramos threw a fastball and Mantle connected with it perfectly. The ball sailed off in a high drive toward right-field and looked like it was on its way to becoming the first ball to go completely out of Yankee Stadium. It got caught by a stiff breeze and missed clearing the roof by only about 18 inches. But it was that close.

"That's what focus can do for you. When something goes wrong, you just stay focused," Bill explained. He suggested that with every pitch, Logan's focus would become more narrow in a pleasurable way [link to emotional resources]. Other metaphors focused on not holding onto mistakes in a way that allowed them to become distractions. He also suggested that Logan could become more relaxed right before he stepped to the plate by shifting his focus from the upcoming performance demand to a mental check list of the details of a good swing [relax to access appropriate state of arousal and practice mental rehearsal].

Logan, as an 11-year-old, was not particularly motivated to address his academic performance or his outbursts of anger, but by reorienting the therapy, Bill helped him to learn to alter his habitual response patterns [shift core beliefs and dysfunctional programming]. Logan came to see that his issues were not so much "getting mad and getting bad grades" as they were losing focus because he let himself be distracted by an error or an emotional response [reorganization of the conception of a problem, accompanied by new associations accessed from a different state of consciousness, in this case, initiated by the therapist rather than the client]. As Logan developed new ways to sidestep tension and anger in the context of baseball, without even thinking about it, he also began to apply those same skills in his home and school life.

This process is equally appropriate for performance artists, athletes, executives, and anyone involved in a complex endeavor. If the performer has a problem with concentration or there are brain issues such as a brain frequency in which the amplitude is too high (i.e., too slow), we also use the brain-training technologies.

In the next sections we describe various interventions we use to address particular problem areas toward the goal of optimizing performance in the client's chosen arena.

Sidestepping Mental Interference

Fear of failure and overthinking a situation interfere with performance and block access to creativity. If an individual begins to ruminate over all the possible things that might go wrong, anxiety is raised, and the ability to access the zone is compromised. Greene (1998) suggested a three-step mental exercise to do just before a performance, which our clients have found helpful:

1. Close the eyes, take a breath, and focus on the air flowing into the nostrils. On exhalation, relax all the muscles in the body.
2. Take another breath, exhale, and place the attention on the body's center, two inches below the navel.
3. On the third inbreath bring to mind a cue word or phrase associ-

ated with your best performance, such as in focused and relaxed, or effortless playing. With the third exhalation, open your eyes, focus on a specific place outside, and say a positive phrase such as "Be here."

Self-Regulation Training

Neural focus and state change can be used to turn on appropriate emotional circuits and to accomplish goals. We begin by teaching individuals how to change sensations in their arms and hands by just focusing and going into a light trance state. Clients practicing with self-hypnosis can develop heaviness, lightness, numbness, or tingling in the arms and hands as signs of calm. To improve the ability to focus calmly and maintain concentration, the performer can practice using an inexpensive GSR or electrodermal device to notice when anxiety gets in the way of focus. An anxious thought usually results in activation of the sympathetic nervous system and increased electrical conductivity of the skin. A return to the object of concentration will reactivate the parasympathetic nervous system.

Script for Strengthening the Emotional State

State strengthening, or the conditioning of more productive states, may be necessary for the enhancement of self-confidence and expectation of success. This may involve retrieving experiences from the past where resources were experienced and recorded at the unconscious level. Confidence, feelings of safety, positive risk taking, curiosity, motivation, the ability to say both "yes" and "no," being in the zone, an internal knowing that others believe in one's ability to accomplish goals, and the perseverance to finish the game or the activity—all can be accessed in a hypnotic state. When a client reviews positive past experiences in terms of their sensory elements, the success state can then be accessed and practiced for an upcoming event. We encourage the client to take the feeling and attitude of success, review it, and keep it in the body before the athletic or artistic event. Following is a script for emotional state strengthening:

"Take three nice and easy breaths and allow yourself to relax. When you relax, you have access to many abilities you have developed over the years. Allow yourself to go deeper into that feeling of comfort, and feel all the tension evaporate just like the mist rising from a lake early in the morning. Sweep your mind through your whole body, and sweep out any unnecessary muscle tightness. The more you relax now, the more you can relax later.

"Everyone has been a little baby who first learned how to crawl. One day, you picked yourself up and stood up for the first time. The world looked very different, and you began to experiment by putting one foot in front of another. Perhaps you fell down, but you got up again, and it really wasn't so difficult. You gave falling down little thought. You continued day after day, balancing, swinging the arms, moving forward. One very important day, something happened that changed you forever. You walked across a room all by yourself, completely unassisted. Now, a whole new world opened up.

"But, what did you learn when you learned to walk? Certainly you learned a very complex skill in coordinating all of those motor movements in the body. However, you also learned important emotional building blocks that you would use the rest of your life. You learned how to have courage; one must have courage to try something difficult and challenging. You learned how to take a risk. You also learned that if you fall, you can get up again, and you learned how to face your fears and walk through them. You learned that every new endeavor has a learning curve, and the more you persist, the easier the task becomes. You also learned how to make a commitment to a goal. All of these learnings went into your unconscious mind for your use in future endeavors.

"When you went to school for the first time, you called upon the courage, confidence, and ability to face the unknown. When you learned the A-B-C's for the first time, you called upon the persistence you learned. First you learned how to recognize the letters, how to keep the lowercase letters separated from the uppercase ones. You learned that some of the lowercase letters have flags, like a d, a p, and a q. All of this went into your unconscious mind, just like learning to tie a shoe or a button a shirt. Isn't it nice to know that you have so many resources to call upon now?"

Script for Accessing the Zone or State of Flow Directly

Once the client has learned how to move into the zone with deep state training, we can teach the technique of retrieving the state in any situation. This is the formation and practice of the "performance-ready" state.

In the script below, the performer is instructed to create a signal or cue to retrieve the state. This cue can be further developed while the client is working in a deep state and then practiced in a light self-induced hypnotic state. This script for hypnotic induction can be used to assist a client in accessing the zone or state of flow:

"Sit with your feet on the floor. Take a few easy and gentle breaths and turn your attention inwardly. Allow a natural settling to occur and then go deeper into that quiet center inside you. If you have any concerns, let them drift away. Focus on your breath or, if you like, keep your eyes open and focus on an object outside until your vision begins to distort a little. Feel a natural heaviness develop and enjoy the comfort that is beneath conscious attention. This comfort is always available. Sometimes you are aware of it; sometimes it is resting just beneath your awareness. This comfort is focused in the present moment. It is focused in your breath.

"Let your memory slip back in time, back to a time when you were really in the flow. Perhaps it was an athletic event or performance of some kind, or it may have just been a time when you felt completely centered. Anything you tried, you accomplished. Everything was effortless. You didn't have to do anything. It just happened and you were part of it happening. It all came together. And it was just . . . exactly . . . right.

"When you are in the zone, there is no separation. When you create music, there is no separation between you and the music. No separation between you and the instrument. [For other types of performers, vary the script appropriately.] You are all one, working together in an attentive but relaxed state. You are the creation and the creation is you, and it is a lovely feeling. Imagine that now; no separation, just being one in a comfortable, relaxed state of mind and body. You are the music and the instrument. You are the one who is playing and the one who is played. You are you and you are the audience. And everything comes together. This is the synchrony state of mind. You can memorize this state and call it back whenever you wish by giving yourself some personal signal. Create the signal now; it might be putting the first finger and thumb together. It might be calling up the feeling as you take a nice deep breath. (Pause for 15–30 seconds.)

"Now, when you really need to focus in a relaxed state of mind, you can narrow your concentration and become still, ready, and alert. This

state of mind can enhance your ability to develop solutions to problems, to plan certain movements, to study ideas or allow something
you may not have noticed before to come into your awareness. Like
peering through a lens that magnifies whatever is behind it, that particular target becomes large and easy to see. You may shift from this
narrow focus to a broader view and find the shifting process easy. Seeing the broader perspective is as important as seeing the narrow one.

"If you mind catches an error, just allow it to go by. Errors are only
information for later correction. You can be so in the flow that the focused experience is one of bliss.

"In a moment, begin to allow yourself to come back and know that
you may call up the state of relaxed or focused attention any time you
need it."

Script for Accessing the Zone State through Deep Identification

Some clients may have difficulty accessing the zone state directly
through recall of their previous experiences of it. Another technique is
to access it indirectly, by introjecting the persona and known (or presumed) zone experience of a meaningful role model. To identify with a
successful role model by imagining actually being that person, via full
sensory engagement, silences the critical mind and allows the athlete to
perform without self-imposed limitations. We therefore suggest that the
performer identify an individual from the past who was outstanding in
his or her field. The athlete should study this individual: his or her life
story, motivation, mental attitude, strategies for success, and methods
for entering the zone. Then, whether accessed through hypnosis or
through alpha–theta training equipment, deep trance identification as a
mental practice is effective in facilitating entry into the zone state. The
following script can be used (adapted) by the clinician:

> "As you find just the right comfortable space inside, and you feel your-
> self floating and relaxed, imagine _____ [successful uber-figure]
> sitting across the room. Notice the relaxed smile, confident attitude,
> and pleasant demeanor. This is your friend and confidant who will
> show you everything about the zone. As I count down from 10 to 0, you
> and this special person begin to merge. By the count of 0, you and he
> [or she] are one. (Count down.) Now, you can see the athletic field
> with his eyes, hear with his ears, feel the easy and confident attitude.
> Feel the power in your arms, hands, and legs. [Vary the script appro-
> priately for other endeavors.] You can feel his swing. As you connect

with the ball, your body and his body are moving as one body. Through his eyes, you watch the ball arc out across the field. In this merging your body can learn what he knows intuitively. Instinctively, it knows exactly what to do."

Script for Sensory Alteration

The following is a sample script to elicit trance phenomena of sensory alteration. This script is designed to encourage the client to realize that if he or she can change physical sensations, he or she can also change and even direct state of arousal (or calm) and constancy of focus on the object of attention:

> "Sit comfortably with your back and shoulders supported by the chair and focus your attention on the back of one of your hands. As you continue to observe your hand, you may notice how the hand's sensations change. You may or may not become aware of a variety of the following feelings. Perhaps you might notice a developing heaviness in that hand. You may be aware of developing warmth in the palm of your hand. You may be aware of a slight tingling in the fingers. Please keep your focus on the back of your hand and gently tell me which sensations you notice."

After the client reports which sensations are experienced, the clinician may want to suggest that the client can expand those sensations into even greater ones:

> "Now that you have noticed a feeling of heaviness, I would like you to allow that sensation to continue to develop. Everyone has picked up a heavy suitcase and felt the weight of that suitcase in the arm. Just allow the heaviness to continue to whatever depth you would like."
> *Or*:

> "Notice how that warm feeling in the palm of your hand can spread. Perhaps it will move over the hand and up the arm so that you now have a heavy, warm feeling." *Or*:

> "The tingling sensation can increase, if you like, and begin to allow the fingers and hand to feel a little numb. Isn't it interesting how you can develop a different sensation just by focusing on your hand. And there are so many other abilities you have that you may not know yet you have."

Researchers Erik Peper and Andrea Shapiro found that when athletes worked in pairs by taking turns having one concentrate and the other attempt to distract the person, they developed much better concentration in actual performance situations (as cited in Schmid, 1998). Practice with focusing attention in the peak state allows the performer to call up the state when needed.

Visual Imagery for Success

We recommend that performers visualize their success from two different perspectives: their own and that of someone else important in their lives. In visualizing success from their own perspective, we suggest that they have the experience of seeing themselves achieving the much-desired goal as though they are viewing an event that seems to be in the past from a point in the future—in other words, as though it has already happened. Visualizing the success as happening at some future time may appear to leave it more open to chance; the past, as most people consider it, is "already set in stone." When performers visualize themselves through the eyes of someone who believes in them, the likelihood of fulfilling that image increases. It is easier to believe in oneself when others, particularly significant others, validate that belief. In essence, someone else's expectation of their success translates into actual success.

Mental Rehearsal

Mental rehearsal is a powerful technique for learning new skills and for refining skills that are already well developed. Karl Pribram (1982) described the process by which the brain develops an image for a successful outcome. He later noted:

> What the data suggest is that there exists in the cortex, a multidimensional holographic-like process serving as an attractor or set point toward which muscular contractions operate to achieve a specified environmental result. The specification has to be based on prior experience (of the species or the individual) and stored in holographic-like form. Activation of the store involves patterns of muscular contractions (guided by basal ganglia, cerebellar, brain stem and spinal cord) whose sequential operations need only to satisfy the "target'" encoded in the image of achievement much as the patterns of sequential opera-

tions of heating and cooling must meet the setpoint of the thermostat. (Pribram, 1997, conclusion, para. 1).

In essence, Pribram is saying that the mental image precedes—and drives—the muscular achievement.

We suggest that the performer or athlete can develop a detailed sensory image that allows him or her to practice and, ultimately, to perform in a relaxed state of mind. In effect, this visualization is done in a light, self-induced trance. A visual image enriched by multisensory components activates minute muscle groups at an unconscious level. This process functions to teaching the body the right moves even though no discernable motion is involved. Clients can extend the learning to times outside of the practice environment. They can also extend the image beyond the simple physical motions to a larger image of their field of endeavor. For professional performers who often practice for hours every day, mental rehearsal carries the added benefit of not further taxing the physical body, which may already be practicing at the limit of its ability to maintain and restore itself.

When Carol was 8 years old, her parents enrolled her in a swimming class. In order to graduate from the class, each child needed to swim across the pool. Every time it was Carol's turn, she would swim out to the center of the pool and make a sharp right turn. The class was coming to an end and Carol was worried about being the only one not to graduate. So she began to visualize herself getting in the pool and swimming correctly across the pool until she felt it in her body. Her mental rehearsal paid off on the final day: She successfully swam across the pool and avoided the embarrassment of failing. This memory also became a resource for her for the many times in her life when she needed to feel self-confident.

Imagining the Activity or Seeking Creative Business Ideas in Deep Trance

This practice differs from visual imagery and mental rehearsal in that there is a greater depth of trance and intensity of focus. While in deep trance, the client mentally practices the activity or examines the business situation. During this time, the clinician should watch for ideomotor cues; for example, a pole-vaulter might move his or her feet slightly or a violinist's fingers might move slightly as if he or she were playing. Also, rapid eye movements occur often when the person is practicing. The clinician should be very attentive to ideomotor clues or rapid eye movements as a means of determining when the client is completely involved in the process. An absence of such clues generally indicates that the trance should be deepened.

Aligning Core Beliefs

Whether through visualization or trance identification, we suggest that the performer focus on feeling positive, empowered, and focused. However, it is critical that the individual be clear that no unconscious beliefs or attitudes are in conflict with achieving the desired goals. For example, in the case of the athlete who overtrains to the detriment of his body, the unconscious belief may be "I should not have to rest or take days off" or "No pain, no gain." Such beliefs may set up a person for injury. Frequently, the unconscious belief is revealed in the language used, through incongruent behavior, and by not following the instructions of the coach or trainer. Often, the fear of failure generates resistance to success. This may take the form of establishing an unrealistic standard with the accompanying expectation that this standard will be impossible to achieve. The person ends up not enjoying the activity, which again sets up failure. If the person is focused on only external rewards, there will never be success.

If there is conflict between unconscious beliefs or attitudes and achieving the desired goals, the clinician will need to help the client clear or resolve the conflict before he or she will be able to move forward. Resolution can be achieved in a hypnotic state through mental dialogue with the conflicted part and via emotional stabilization with the neurofeedback, enabling the brain to achieve the right level of arousal for each specific task. Another way to help the client move beyond the conflict is by encouraging him or her to improve by very small increments—for example, by suggesting doing better by just 1 inch or (whatever fits the athletic event) . . . then 1 inch more . . . then another. This is an example of fractionation. Eventually this practice will produce a significant change.

Case Example: Beating a Bum Rap

Carrying the weight of old emotional baggage puts any performer at a disadvantage. Debra, a triathlete, had suffered for many years from her father's referring to her as a "bum." Viewing herself through her father's eyes, she felt unworthy, unintelligent, and invisible. In her first session, she talked about how painful it was to be referred to in that way. Several months into therapy, we asked her to think about the word and find associations. She immediately replied, "It sounds like *numb*" In fact, she felt that she had been numb for many years. We asked her to scramble the letters in *bum* and notice what the word would be backward; we asked if it could it be an acronym. *MUB* could stand for "Magnificent, Unsurpassed Beauty" or "Measures Up Best." *MBU* could stand for "Matchless Body Undaunted." *UBM* could stand for "Ultra Blazin' Mamma." That *bum* that her father referred to could be "Bravo, Unstoppable Marvel!." This neutralizing intervention caused her to change her state into feeling proud, more relaxed, and open. Debra also recognized that her emotional reactions before an athletic event could both stimulate hives and cause them to disappear. It was only exposure to deep state training with the alpha–theta program that Debra realized, for the first time, what it was to experience a sense of deep comfort. As these interventions built on each other, she was able to shave minutes off her time.

Corporate Executives

Like elite athletes and performing artists, some corporate executives are driven to "go for the gold." Also like them, the executives generally enter therapy because they have recognized an issue that requires resolution and they are looking for creative direction. However, in the process of addressing the issue at hand, they realize that "more is possible." Highly motivated to learn to function at a peak level or maintain the state for longer periods of time, they are interested in maximizing their performance in terms of accurately analyzing situations; developing creative ideas, strategies, and solutions; and implementing them in ways that are effective and efficient.

In working with executives, most of our assessment is conducted in conversational exchange. However, our standard assessment also includes several psychological tests; among them are Cattell's 16 Personality Factor Questionnaire and, occasionally, the MMPI. In essence, we are looking for indications of underlying issues, emotions, or unconscious programs that may be blocking someone from functioning effectively in terms of leadership style or from achieving his or her goals. We also use the Test of Variables of Attention to gauge focus and concentration, since these may need improvement as adjuncts to techniques of creative problem solving.

We ask specifically what the person's goals are for the therapeutic interaction and then discuss how achievable these are in light of the individual's available time and resources. Issues that we commonly address include major career decision points, achieving an improved balance between personal/family life and career, effective communication, better methods of reinforcing motivation, and better stress management tools during crises.

Executive Interventions

Often, executives who have already worked with us in a personal context come back when they need assistance with executive decision making. If a client has been working diligently on a problem and cannot come up with a solution, we may suggest that he or she put it aside mentally while simultaneously asking the unconscious to take note of anything going by in the outside environment that might be useful. Then often a song on the radio or something from television may spark a completely new train of thought. Suddenly, cascades of interesting ideas emerge into consciousness, and the person just knows what to do. We also use the following version of the deep state protocol for accessing possible business solutions:

1. Go into the future to a time when the present problem may need to be solved again.
2. Envision the ultimate solution or ideal system such that the present solution is just one step in the right direction.
3. Recognize that the problem exists within a framework of interactions and interlocking systems. The best solution now will eventually become a transitional step to a better solution. Every solution can be viewed with the knowledge that it will not only lead to change but will probably be changed.
4. Allow the information to come in from the deepest state.
5. Process the images and associations after the experience.

Another envisioning exercise is going into a "futuring" laboratory where a client can develop many futures. To assist in this, we may say:

"Write down all of the futures that you would like to experience and remember that change may not be linear. Notice that even discontinuous change can start a chain reaction." The person practices visualizing the future and, with our coaching, begins to create a concrete plan of action. The individual also begins to identify elements that may block success, such as a hidden belief that it is not okay to be successful. A tremendous release of energy and sense of freedom occur when a person can identify unconscious beliefs.

Case Example: Heeding the Wisdom of the Unconscious

Frank knew that he wanted to create a future in which he had become a consultant to others in the oil business. He had years of experience and excellent contacts but could not find the courage to go out on his own and start a company. Upon trying to visualize this future, his unconscious mind pictured a future in which he lost money, lost his valuable network, and lost credibility in the industry. We suggested that he needed to heed that message, that it meant that he did not yet have a business plan that he intuitively knew would succeed. Frank began to work on this and developed an innovative idea that no one else had produced. Six months later, with a well-developed business plan that included his business model, a marketing plan, and realistic financial projections, he started his company. Two years later, he was doing so well that he was expanding into related areas and was approached by a private equity firm potentially interested in buying him out.

Case Example: Improving a Leadership Style with Deep State Work

Allen came in to work with Carol in order to deal with his lack of confidence and depression. As the president of a steel mini-mill that specialized in making pipe, he was highly successful but was unable to hold a positive regard for anything very long. Because he felt anxious and on trial whenever anyone questioned his opinion, his leadership style was abrupt, authoritarian, and often demeaning. The turnover rate among his management team was high, and he knew that he had repeatedly lost good people due to "clashes in personality." Eventually he recognized that the only managers who stayed very long were all "yes men" who

presented him with a bland mask of deference but who brought no vision, no energy, and no creativity to the firm.

In talking about his family of origin, Allen revealed that his father had
been extremely critical and demeaning as well as physically abusive. Alpha–theta training was used to take him to extremely deep states so that
more positive self views could be conditioned. He also worked on his
feelings about his father and was able to come to a point of feeling forgiveness toward him. As Allen came to understand that he treated himself in the same way that his father had treated him, he began to treat
himself with more kindness.

Realizing that all that his employees would show him were their
masks, Allen also requested that the "veil" be lifted so he could see and
hear others and better understand them. Suggestions were given that he
could understand others and the pain that often dictated their behaviors—because he could understand the pain that had dictated his own
choices in response to his father's behavior. As he slowly learned to listen without feeling threatened, his staff members learned that it was
safe to share their ideas, their hopes for the business and, ultimately,
more of themselves.

Recognizing that of all the elements involved in optimizing performance, mental state is the most crucial, this chapter has examined different BCT techniques by which a performer can achieve a chosen
mental state, direct his or her focus, align unconscious beliefs with conscious goals, address performance anxiety, solve problems, and deal
with distractions.

In addition to healing the psyche and stewarding the body toward optimal performance and well-being, BCT can be applied to foster emergent states of consciousness, including states of thriving and happiness
and beyond, to "supramental" and "unity" states—the subject of Chapter 12.

Thriving and Beyond

Humans have extraordinary abilities that are largely undeveloped. Among those are the capacities to love, to create, and to learn (Leonard & Murphy, 2005)—capacities whose outer reaches are far beyond where most people venture. People innately possess the abilities necessary not only to thrive but to explore and, ultimately, shift into deeper levels of living. BCT rests on the understanding that a person's brain–mind states are major determinants of both illness and health. Becoming aware of these states and learning how to work with them is crucial to healing the psyche and stewarding the body. The development of these skills is even more critical if one is to experience life in ways that are richly satisfying. Going even beyond that, they can enable a person to access and explore emergent states of consciousness.

Thriving

Thriving is an emotional state of mind encompassing certain perspectives and behaviors that contribute to high functioning. In a state of thriving, a person maintains high levels of emotional, psychological, and social stability and well-being characterized by positive feelings and functioning (Keyes & Haidt, 2002). Keyes identified 13 "symptoms" of what he termed "flourishing":

1. Regularly cheerful, in good spirits, happy, calm and peaceful, satisfied, and full of life (positive affect)

2. Feels happy or satisfied with life overall or domains of life (avowed happiness or avowed life satisfaction)

3. Holds positive attitudes toward oneself and past life and concedes and accepts varied aspects of self (self-acceptance)

4. Has positive attitude toward others while acknowledging and accepting people's differences and complexity (social acceptance)

5. Shows insight into own potential, sense of development, and open to new and challenging experiences (personal growth)

6. Believes that people, social groups, and society have potential and can evolve or grow positively (social actualization)

7. Holds goals and beliefs that affirm sense of direction in life and feels that life has a purpose and meaning (purpose in life)

8. Feels that one's life is useful to society and that the output of his or her own activities are valued by or valuable to others (social contribution)

9. Exhibits capability to manage complex environment and can choose or manage and mold environments to suit needs (environmental mastery)

10. Interested in society or social life; feels society and culture are intelligible, somewhat logical, predictable, and meaningful (social coherence)

11. Exhibits self-direction that is often guided by his or her own socially accepted and conventional internal standards and resists unsavory social pressures (autonomy)

12. Has warm, satisfying, trusting personal relationships and is capable of empathy and intimacy (positive relations with others)

13. Has a sense of belonging to a community and derives comfort and support from community (social integration)

Keyes and Haidt argued that both positive feelings and positive functioning are crucial to mental health and should serve as its definition. On the other hand, they noted that most adults fall into a category they called "languishing"—a state characterized by decreased psychosocial, and even physical, vitality, although lacking any specific mental illness. These individuals are twice as likely to experience a depressive episode compared with generally mentally healthy adults (Keyes & Haidt, 2002).

As clinicians, we need to exemplify thriving and promote this state to our clients rather than helping them only solve problems. To stay in a state of thriving requires mental training; one must learn how to regulate the mind and overcome the inevitable challenges and setbacks of daily life. His Holiness the Dalai Lama noted that "suffering and pain are understood to be a function of an untamed and undisciplined mind, while happiness and joy are understood to be a function of a tamed and disciplined mind" (as cited in Parvin, 2008, p. 1).

Habits of thought become habits of life. Thich Nhat Hanh, a Vietnamese Zen Buddhist monk, spoke to this notion when he said the following:

> Traditional writings describe consciousness as a field, a piece of land, on which all kinds of seeds are sown—seeds for suffering, happiness, joy, sorrow, fear, annoyance and hope. And tradition describes the memory of feeling as a storehouse that is filled with all our seeds. As soon as a seed is manifested in our consciousness, it will always return to the storehouse stronger than before. . . . Every single moment during which we perceive something peaceful and beautiful waters the seed for peace and beauty within us. . . . And during that same time, other seeds like fear and pain remain unwatered. (as cited in Klein, 2006, pp. 118–119)

Eastern psychology and religion suggest that the seeds for happiness and well-being lie deep within each person. We would simply call this state "thriving" and suggest that both clients and clinicians can learn to spend more time in that state.

Lassoing Happiness

Matthieu Ricard (2008), a molecular biologist who became a Buddhist monk and is considered by some to be the "happiest man alive," noted that it is really the *state of mind* that determines states of well-being or misery. He defined happiness as a deep state of well-being and wisdom that is present in every moment and may extend to an experience of states of clear, thoughtless concentration. Research shows that people can increase their happiness by making a conscious effort to "count their blessings," reframe situations in a positive light, or perform kind acts (Lyubomirsky, 2008). In *The Art of Happiness* (Dalai Lama & Cutler, 1998), Howard Cutler, in a conversation with His Holiness the Dalai Lama, noted: "The systematic training of the mind—the cultivation of happiness, the genuine inner transformation by deliberately selecting and focusing on positive mental states and challenging negative mental states—is possible because of the very structure and function of the brain" (p. 306). Because pleasant experiences are not usually as intense as negative ones, they tend to be more difficult to remember. To be better retained, states of well-being need to be practiced. Pleasant rituals performed regularly assist in reinforcing states of well-being (Newberg, 2006).

Berns (2006) discovered that experiences that contain both moderate novelty and challenge produce a neural response that leads to feelings of satisfaction. Novel experiences stimulate the production of dopamine, the chemical of anticipated satisfaction, which reinforces the development of commitment and motivation, two important elements for achieving life success.

A person cannot be directly aware of the central nervous system's functioning. What can be noticed and regulated, however, are emotional states of mind, body sensations, and the content of consciousness. Another way to assist clients in achieving enhanced well-being is by teaching them to distinguish states of mind that can be defined by levels of arousal and notice the ones that enhance, uplift, enchant, heal, or open awareness to wisdom. A clinical goal therefore is to learn how to shift into these states when an individual so chooses. Learning to harness negative thinking is the first step toward achieving the ability to *choose* to be happy.

Harnessing Negativity

Most people engage in habitual negative thinking. The mind, a brilliant but conflicted tool, keeps churning on and, in the process, further develops the art of using negative language (Mipham, 2005). Expressing anger repeatedly, for example, only serves to reinforce the feeling. If, instead of gripping the anger, a person can allow the ideation of it to move through the mind and the emotion of it to move through the body, the anger will naturally diminish. The same is true for any nagging thought, whether it is to eat something unhealthy or to engage in self-criticism. The nurturance of constructive states of mind entails practicing self-respect, integrity, compassion, generosity, love, and relationship

(Goleman, 2003, p. 68). From an Eastern point of view, it is an indulgence to allow the mind to stay in a state of upset.

We suggest to clients that negativity can be harnessed and used as an advisor. For example, we might explain:

"When there is negativity, most likely some life pattern has been stimulated. A disturbing sensation or feeling can indicate an opening either into some new aspect of the self or an old and disowned one. It is important to identify and acknowledge those aspects of the self that may be unconsciously expressed in a relationship through withholding or passive anger. Allow the thought to come into awareness, being curious about it, and then let it go. This is important in cultivating the happiness skill."

Engaging a natural curiosity can help a client identify the source of negative feeling. Knowing where it came from may provide an element of closure that makes it easier to let it go. Understanding what emotional circuit may have been triggered can also be useful in developing mental control. Once clients realize how they contribute to their own discontent, it becomes possible for them to see that it is a matter of active choice either to let a negative thought pattern play out to the end or to bring the mind back to a neutral space, shift mental gears, and change emotional states. At that point, negativity can be further harnessed. Not only can it alert a client to the activation of a negative life pattern; it can be thought of as a small bell ringing, simply reminding a person to bring the mind back to a neutral space.

The Awareness Wheel

The Awareness Wheel was developed by Sherod and Phyllis Miller as part of their Core Communication program, which teaches communication skills (Miller & Miller, 1997). It is based on the observation that, whether an individual is consciously aware of them or not, there are five key types of information or sources of relevant data in any situation. They are:

1. *Sensory data*, both external and internal: all the information picked up by the five senses as well as bodily sensations (e.g., a

suddenly clenched stomach, a headache, or a sudden surge of adrenaline).

2. *Thoughts:* the meanings assembled from the sensory data as informed by a person's ideas, beliefs, assumptions, judgments, interpretations, meanings, and expectations.

3. *Feelings:* the embodied response to thoughts (interpretations) of the sensory data. These include the physiological expression of what the Millers identify as the six basic emotions: happiness, sadness, anger, fear, disgust, and surprise.

4. *Wants:* the desires, hopes, aspirations, dreams, and yearnings that someone has for him- or herself and for others.

5. *Actions:* a person's actual behaviors on a current basis, in the past or in the future.

As a client is beginning to examine his or her life in light of intermittent experiences of thriving and with the intent to increase the degree of thriving, the Awareness Wheel can be presented as an introspective tool for examining situations or experiences, making decision, resolving conflicts, and cultivating a deeper understanding of the self and other. For simplicity, the Awareness Wheel can be compressed into five questions:

1. What do I see/hear?
2. What meaning do I make of it?
3. How do I feel about it?
4. What do I want from it or in terms of it?
5. What am I willing to do to, for, or about it?

We use the Awareness Wheel as an adjunct to BCT to assist a client in shifting his or her state to one in which a broader range of possibilities can be envisioned. Joseph often felt so caught in responsibility toward his elderly, divorced mother that before entering therapy, he would often give up his weekend plans to drive over to her house and work his way through her detailed list of chores. Increasingly exhausted, he finally acknowledged that his life was no longer his own.

We used the awareness wheel to help him move out of the bind he experienced. He asked himself: "What do I see/hear? My mother crying to me for help. What meaning do I make of it? I must rescue her from her pain. How do I feel about it? Guilty, if I don't respond as she wishes; angry and resentful when I do. What do I want from this situation? I want to be free from having to do things for her on her schedule and free from guilt. What am I willing to do about it? I can give myself permission to put myself first when I need and want to. I can talk to her about hiring a handyman and help her find the right person. I can decide what gift of my time I will give her."

The Awareness Wheel allowed Joseph to articulate the double bind that he was in and see that he needed to release himself from the burden of over-responsibility. He became conscious of the fact that it was not in his power either to keep her alive or happy. What he could do was decide what "portion" of himself he could give her freely and thereby remain in charge of his own mental states.

Neuroconditioning Processes

Negative emotional life patterns are often activated just outside of conscious awareness and result in a feeling of generalized anxiety. This anxiety, in turn, dictates nearly unconscious behavior designed to relieve it—like rain relieving the pressure of colliding weather systems. Over time, the relieving behavior becomes a habituated response. However, because two different mental states cannot be held simultaneously, practicing an alpha state of mind and focusing on compassion or a loved one can lower anxiety or other states of arousal over time and thereby break this pattern.

The goal of each of the following exercises is to decouple or decharge counterproductive neural pathways that have been conditioned over time and activate optimal pathways. In addition, the exercises attempt to inhibit anxiety. As Grawe (2007) recognized, "it becomes clear that the creation of an anxiety-inhibiting brain state will be a core aim of all therapeutic activity" (Grawe, 2007, p. 404). Furthermore, positive states lead to improved performance in any setting (Ashby, Isen, & Turken, 1999). As we introduce these exercises to a client, we try to make certain that the client understands that we are not suggesting that he or she should not have feelings about other people's behaviors and the situations that arise. What we are suggesting is that, from the perspective of a calm state, a person can remember that we are all interconnected and, probably based on some similar experience in life, can intuit why someone else may have done something disturbing. This may help the person view those behaviors through a more compassionate lens.

We suggest that a client start with the first exercise, practicing for 5–10 minutes daily for at least 2 weeks. At that point (or sooner), we ask the client about his or her experience with the exercise. When the client feels comfortably proficient with the first exercise, we introduce the second one. After the client has become proficient at the second exercise, we suggest that he or she can choose when to use each one, as it may be appropriate to the current circumstances. However, some clients are particularly "left brained": logical and perhaps not entirely comfortable with visualizations, conceivably feeling them to be nothing more than a matter of "imagining things." For those clients, we recommend starting with the third exercise and later adding the second exercise.

Neuroconditioning Exercise 1

1. Take a breath and exhale.
2. Find the calm center inside by taking a few long inbreaths and exhaling twice as long as the inhalation.
3. Pair the feeling of the calm center with an imagined calm and relaxed location. Continue the breathing pattern noted above and bring to mind the place (e.g., a secluded spot by a waterfall on Maui).
4. Relax the tongue from the back to the front. Let it "float" up to the roof of your mouth. (A relaxed tongue will naturally rise until it rests up against the hard palate.)
5. Bring to mind someone (or a pet, a plant, or even a treasured object) that you love and focus on the feeling of loving that person/pet/plant/object.
6. Breathe slowly in and out and just notice your thoughts coming in and going out again.

Neuroconditioning Exercise 2

We encourage the development of a balanced state of arousal because it is the foundation of a balanced and flexible emotional state. Neurologically, this state includes enough alpha brainwaves for self-comfort. A person's self-perception of this state might be described as feeling "A-okay" or "at peace with myself and the world." For most people, alpha wave activity is decreased by everyday stresses. Hardt (2007) noted that, as examples, the following mindsets hinder alpha wave activity: doubt, drowsiness, distractibility/worry, aversion/ill will, and boredom. Conquering an emotion such as fear, he said, can be done by imagining the worst-case scenario and then "flooding the brain with alpha waves" via positive emotions.

It turns out that music/song can be used to elicit a more balanced state of arousal. In a study at the University of Texas, Baker (2000) found that music stimulates several different brain areas. Because music and language structures are similar, it was suspected that by stimulating the right side of the brain with music, the left side would begin to (re) make connections as well. Based on this research, melodic intonation therapy (MIT) was developed for stroke patients. Even when patients cannot speak words, often they can sing music. For this reason, patients are encouraged to sing words rather than speak them in conversational tones in the early phases of MIT. Studies using positron emission tomography (PET) scans have shown Broca's area (a region in the left frontal brain controlling speech and language comprehension) to be reactivated through repetition of sung words (Blood & Zatorre, 2001).

If a client needs to be in an active and alert but calm state, consider the following neuroconditioning exercise, which is more energizing and can result in balanced arousal:

1. Sit erect in a chair and take a deep breath.
2. Remember an activating song and mentally rehearse it from the beginning to the end. It might be a song from your childhood, a patriotic song, a favorite hymn, or maybe a ballad. We had one client who would mentally sing Louis Armstrong's "What a Wonderful World." Let your breathing match the phrasing of the music, just as though you were singing out loud.
3. Notice the alert and comfortable feeling at the end of the exercise.

Neuroconditioning Exercise 3

In order to interrupt emotional reactions, we can focus our attention on different phases in the reaction process:

1. Identify the emotional state as it is perceived in the mind, for example, "discouraged," "exasperated," "grim," or "resentful."

2. Attempt to identify the triggered schema (negative life pattern). Ask yourself, "Where do I remember this emotion from earlier in life?"

3. Observe the body's expression of the reactive emotion. How does the emotion feel at a somatic level?

4. Mentally step away from the feeling. For example, imagine floating up in a hot air balloon or just shift the mind away and focus somewhere else.

5. Breathe deeply and change states.

The Monk and the Rock

The purpose of each of the exercises above is to depotentiate long-used but dysfunctional neural pathways and activate optimal ones. The following story describes the same outcome achieved in a different manner:

When Bill was on his first extended Zen meditation retreat, the purpose of which was to become mindful and focused in the here-and-now, he meditated 6–8 hours a day with a group of other students. Meditation sessions ran for 50 minutes, followed by a short break and then another 50 minutes. There were also periods of mindful work around the center and meals. The retreat was conducted in "noble silence," which meant that the students could not speak unless absolutely necessary, and then it was to be in hushed tones. They could not read anything, text anyone, use their cell phones, or listen to any podcasts or music. The only conversation they had was each day was during a brief meeting with the monk who led the retreat. He would ask "How is your meditation proceeding?"

After Bill had become comfortable sitting on a cushion, he thought he had mastered meditation. He was in a comfortable, blissful, dreamy state. When he had his first interview with the monk and described his experience, Bill was surprised by the monk's response. He looked at Bill solemnly and said, "You are guilty of sloth." He went on to say: "Meditation is not naptime, even if you can do it sitting up." He told Bill the purpose of meditation was to observe the mind and be aware, and to have a clear and quiet mind. Bill was stunned, confused, angry, embarrassed, and felt like a failure.

During subsequent meditation sessions, Bill did everything in his power to drive out thoughts so that he could attain an undisturbed mind. During the next interview the monk asked once again how the meditation was proceeding. Bill smiled and, with the pride of a first grader who had just learned his alphabet, told the monk he had driven out all thoughts and had a clear, calm, mind. The monk surprised him with his response. He looked meaningfully at Bill, slowly picked up a small rock, and said, "You are no better than a rock. This rock has no thoughts, and it can do so much longer than you." Bill was truly confused. The monk handed Bill the rock and said, "Meditate on this." Bill left the interview more dazed and confused than ever.

Each meditation session seemed worse than the previous one. His mind was trying to figure out what the monk meant and why he had not been praised for what he had achieved. The next few interviews were similar: no sooner had Bill walked into the room, bowed and kneeled in front of the monk, than the monk would say with a sly grin, "You are fighting with the rock, and the rock is winning." During those interviews, Bill never said a word and was dismissed after the monk's comments. Bill was even more confused than before and wondered why he was on the retreat.

In a subsequent meditation session while staring at the rock, Bill had an epiphany: Meditating was not daydreaming or napping, and while it was a disciplined process, it was not a contest to see if he could drive out all thoughts and thereby earn his teacher's praise. Meditation did not have anything to do with what the Zen master thought of Bill personally. The whole purpose was to be aware of his thoughts: When they arose, let them go, and bring his attention back to the breath. It was as simple and as difficult as that. A calm and undisturbed mind does not clutch at, or overly identify with, its thoughts. Neither is it just peacefully drifting through daydreams. At that moment, it was as if a heavy load had been lifted from Bill's shoulders. Although technique and discipline are important, achieving a clear mind had far more to do with observing one's thoughts and not identifying or fighting with them.

In the next interview, after Bill bowed and kneeled, the Zen master simply asked, "How is your meditation?" Bill described to him how he sat, observed thoughts, and gently brought the mind back to the breath, countless times. He said, "Is there anything else?" Bill replied, "Not right now." The monk looked at him and asked how the rock was doing. Bill picked up the rock, extended his arm to offer it to the monk, and said, "I don't know. You will have to ask the rock." The monk smiled, put his hands together and bowed. Bill did the same in response. The monk then said, "Keep the rock as a reminder," and Bill exited the room.

Bill had learned to take a step back from himself and simply observe his thoughts and emotions. What he observed were his confusion, anger, competitiveness, desire to please, and his need for praise. He learned that a clear and undisturbed mind was not a mind that never experienced such thoughts or feelings. The very act of simply being mindful of them—neither hanging on to them nor fighting them—allowed their quick dissipation. Bill was not his thoughts, however useful they might be. Schwartz and Begley (2002) reported that Buddhist mindfulness practice emphasizes that humans can operate out of 10 different states that range from suffering to anger to enlightenment. As miserable or blissful as they might be, Bill was not any of those states.

The benefits of training the mind are described in both Eastern and Western scriptures. The Dhammapada, a Buddhist scripture tradition-ally ascribed to the Buddha himself, (Thondup, 1996, p. 25) observes:

> Mind leads phenomena.
> Mind is the main factor and forerunner of all actions.
> If one speaks or acts with a cruel mind,
> Misery follows, as the cart follows the horse.
>
> Phenomena are led by the mind.
> Mind is the main factor and forerunner of all actions.
> If one speaks or acts with a pure mind,
> Happiness follows, as a shadow follows its source.

In a similar vein, the Book of Ecclesiastes (Eccl. 30:5), as translated in the New Jerusalem Bible (1985), states:

> Do not abandon yourself to sorrow.
>   Do not torment yourself with brooding.
> Gladness of heart is life to anyone,

> Joy is what gives length of days.
> Give your cares the slip, console your heart,
>> Chase sorrow far away;
> For sorrow has been the ruin of many
>> And is no use to anybody.
> Jealousy and anger shorten your days,
>> And worry brings premature old age.
> A genial heart makes a good trencherman,
>> Someone who enjoys a good meal.

Therapists who work on developing mastery themselves are better able to assist their clients. Not only are clients' states influenced positively, but clients experience an unconscious desire to live in the empowered states that the clinician experiences. Within the therapeutic context, the clinician also models taking one's life to the next level and living more often in peak states.

Case Example: Getting a Jumpstart

After having tried many medications, Jean came to treatment for anxiety and panic attacks. Working with Carol, she started alpha–theta training and immediately began to lower her arousal rate. After 10 sessions she reported experiencing her workplace as much less disturbing, even though she was still responsible for meeting just as many deadlines. After 20 sessions, she noted that she slept better, felt calmer, and felt more in control. All her panic attacks had ceased, and she could remain calm even if her boss became upset with her. By the time Jean had finished roughly 40 sessions and terminated therapy, she had moved from being completely focused on her negative symptoms to having an interest in becoming the best that she could be. As she put it, the therapy had given her "a jumpstart" and, at that point, she was ready to continue her mind–body development on her own. One year later, Jean reported that she still felt great.

Too often clinicians come to see their role as "patching people up enough that they can go back out onto the battlefield of life." To whatever extent possible, we encourage each client to go beyond simply healing dysfunction. Thriving—or "flourishing," as Keyes described it— encourages living more authentically, breaking old patterns of behavioral automaticity, and largely avoiding states of anger and worry. Accessing unconscious resources such as confidence, flexibly changing states of consciousness, calming the mind and feeling at peace regardless of outside event—these are all attainable goals. Such development also gives a person the ability to perceive his or her life situation in a relatively objective manner and to stop fabricating stories about how he or she wishes it were. In our view, a state of joyous thriving is the least that we might wish for our clients—because much more is possible.

Beyond Thriving: Supramental States

Yogi Sri Aurobindo (1872–1950) labeled what we might term higher or exceptional states of mind as the *supramental* states and suggested that they may be a key to evolutionary growth and higher awareness (Aurobindo, 1992). Cade and Coxhead (1991) and Wise (1997) defined the awakened mind as one having the ability to create both the desired mental state and content at will. As a precursor to developing an awakened or exceptional mind, a person needs to learn how to calm the mind and stay more frequently in positive states. Developing one-pointed concentration, flexible and creative thinking, expanded intuition, and a "mind like water" (so fluid that it can simply move around any obstacle) improves a client's ability to deal with life's challenges and builds compassion. These are states of "mental fitness." To achieve the awakened mind—that is, psychological maturation characterized by a nonreactive mind—and maintain it for any appreciable length of time, a client needs to resolve past hurts and yearnings, areas of inadequacy, and participate in ongoing mind training. Meditative practices that promote detaching from thoughts (e.g., Vipassana meditation, Transcendental Meditation, centering prayer) or alpha brain entrainment for 10–20 minutes a day can lead to this level of mind discipline.

During meditation, the electrical activity of the brain shifts to the parietal region where one's sense of self strengthens (Newberg et al., 2001). When the mind is quiet, self-understanding, wisdom, and creativity emerge. Through meditation, a person can move into the state of self-transcendence and into empathy for self and others. From there, the undisturbed mind may open to deeper aspects of the self and develop advanced states of mind where higher states are attained and maintained for increasing periods of time. These exceptional states eliminate chaotic thought and provide access to wisdom, clarity, and bliss.

Development of Supramental States

The intentional development of supramental states of consciousness through alpha–theta biofeedback training, hypnosis, and heart rate coherence training (orderly heart rate variability synchronized with the breath) is a program we suggest to people who want to go further in training the mind and enhancing the quality of their daily lives. In these deep states, people discover the capacity to forgive those who have harmed them in the past and let go of any remnants of feeling victimized. More than that, the training facilitates the exploration of deeper parts of the self and a growing understanding of the interconnectedness and multidimensionality of life. The deep mind learns that solutions to some problems are not solutions per se, but rather new perspectives learned from new levels of awareness. Don Juan, the shaman who trained Carlos Castaneda in *A Separate Reality*, said: "Things don't change. You change your way of looking, that's all. . . . Whenever you look at things you don't see them. You just look at them . . . to make sure that something is there. . . . [But when] you learn to see . . . a thing is never the same every time you see it, and yet it is the same" (Castaneda, 1971, p. 37).

It has been our experience over the last 30 years of therapeutic practice that a qualitatively different experience of life emerges out of a quiet, calm state. To date, we do not know the limitations of the human mind, but neuroscience suggests that the ability of humans to change and flourish is nothing short of remarkable (Cozolino, 2008). People may have an almost unlimited capacity to achieve balance and flexibility and to experience joy. According to Davidson (as cited in Goleman, 2003), by calming the amygdala and activating the left prefrontal cortex and the left middle frontal gyrus (the areas of the brain involved in the experience of happiness), a person can explore and experience what may be an unbounded process of mind- and self-transformation.

State-training in alpha–theta brain rhythms (4–12 Hz), using hypnosis or any of the brain-based technologies, has been shown to accelerate learning, cognitive and musical performance, interpersonal empathy and emotional stability (Hardt, 2007; Kirsch, Montgomery, & Sapirstein, 1995; Stanton, 1993; Rundle, 2009). Shifting into the alpha state also fosters a more relaxed and focused mind. When a person can produce consistent alpha waves, even under potentially stressful situations, profound insights and breakthroughs to greater self-understanding are more likely to occur.

A Glimpse of the Possible

A consistently maintained state of thriving is only the beginning of what is possible. Although different traditions concerned with the development of consciousness employ a variety of systems to categorize the states beyond thriving, they can be broadly summarized hierarchically as follows:

- A witness state—the ability to maintain disengaged equanimity in the face of a situation.
- A state of enduring compassion—the ability to respond to a given situation with positive regard.
- A state that includes an embodied sensation of expansiveness and that frequently reduces the sense of separation between ego and object.
- A state of unity consciousness in which there is no perceived separation between ego and object.

When clients are thriving, they begin to realize that putting up with chronic stressors is not "good enough." Almost certainly, they begin to transform their interactions in the world, become aware of where their emotional energy is blocked, and seek to deal with deeper emotional issues to free up life energy. The ability to relate to deeper aspects of the self is a natural outgrowth from spending increasing amounts of time in a state of thriving and allows the development of deeper personal relationships. Thriving individuals tend to reframe chronic stressors by looking at the world through a different lens, one that appreciates other perspectives rather than feeling threatened by them. Realizing that even a long life is relatively short, the consideration becomes: "How do I want to spend my time? In chronic struggle or focusing on what is really important to me?" And at that point, individuals who value thriving can freely decide either to challenge a problematic situation in order to change it or accept it and move their attention to other things.

The next higher state of mind is the witness state or a state of unwavering calm. This state of mind allows a person to observe the contents of mind without reacting to it even in the midst of what might otherwise have been upsetting events. Emotions, thoughts, and inner conversations can be stimulated by events and yet a person who has trained the mind can notice these and allow them to pass by as if they were butterflies.

A further, more mature mind state developed with training is an enduring sense of compassion. Being able to understand another's struggle promotes loving-kindness, connection, and openness. It can also offer insights into another person's innermost reality. Ultimately, compassion will lead one to live in service to others—be they other people, endangered species, the eco-system of the planet, or perhaps to consciousness itself. In describing his hierarchy of needs and human growth, Abraham Maslow (1975) placed self-actualization at the top of the pyramid. This stage comes *after* a period of generativity, wherein one creatively uses talents and capabilities to serve other people. Along that line, Alfred Adler broke with Freud not just over the drive theory and Adler's theory of the inferiority complex, but also around what he thought was the purpose of life. Adler (1969) believed that the highest form of mental health was not just the alleviation of neurotic suffering, but of social service.

From the inner space of a quiet mind–heart, one can emerge into a state marked by an embodied sensation of expansiveness that is free of all fear. It is loving, nonseeking, joyful, and peaceful. The same inner state, however, can be experienced in either of two different modes. One is a deep, centered inward-drawing stillness; the other is an outward-going momentum of which ecstatic dance is perhaps the best known expression. Although almost everyone has experienced this state at some time, the English language has no single, well understood name for it. People call it "a state of emergence," "presence," "a quality of consciousness," "the Tao," "an experience of the Word," "being filled," "a true state of grace," and literally countless other terms. To reach it, a shift in consciousness—for which there is no single set of directions—needs to occur. For many people, there is a specific piece of music that facilitates its arising; for others it is being out in nature, seeing an extraordinary sunrise, the practice of an "extreme" sport such as rock climbing, or simply falling into one of those few conversations that has such a quality that a person remembers it for the rest of his or her life.

Finally, one of the highest states of development is unity consciousness. This is experienced as a connectivity to all of creation, such that
one perceives the true absence of all boundaries, that there is only One,
while simultaneously being able to distinguish perfectly well the physical
boundaries of both animate and inanimate entities. Unity consciousness
normally takes years of meditation practice to achieve. When subjects
have reported experiences of a dissolution of self into a boundless emp-
tiness, 40 Hz amplitude increases in the right front temporal area commonly have been detected (Lehmann et al., 2001). Forty Hz, although
not in the theta range, may be the "signature" of a transpersonal state
(p. 2). Using alpha–theta training, one client reached an experience of
unity consciousness in 40 sessions. Occasionally when working with people who are highly motivated to develop the mind, we have trained them
to achieve 40 Hz directly; however, they need to follow this transitory
experience with some type of further training at home and/or within
some spiritual tradition if they wish to deepen and maintain the enhanced state of mind.

As Irving Kirsch (2010) suggested, meaning and belief are the foundations of psychotherapeutic change. There is a cognitive aspect to BCT
that is also found in other types of psychotherapy and in meditation retreats: With inner work, a person's beliefs about him- or herself, about
the world around him or her, and about the ultimate nature of reality
may undergo a deepening transformation. Not only do a person's beliefs
and perception of reality influence his or her neural patterning; a person's neural patterning also influences his or her beliefs and perception
of reality. It is a stream that endlessly loops back onto itself—but it is not
a closed loop. Like a stream in nature, one can step into it at many different points. Some people will want to wade in and splash in the stream
briefly—just enough to cool off on a hot summer day and reduce the
distress of dysfunctional life and neural patterns. Others will discover
the joy of swimming, of thriving, and make that a consistent part of their
lives. They may even learn to dive into some of the stream's deeper
pools. And a few will choose to become superb swimmers. No longer
content with the stream, they will keep going until they reach the ocean.

EPILOGUE

We are on the brink of a revolution in psychology and psychotherapy—moving from a medical model of symptom treatment based in Cartesian thinking and linear conceptualization to a model underscored by discoveries in neuroscience. This exciting new model suggests that the human brain–mind is an intersection of local and nonlocal elements with a capacity to access innate healing mechanisms far beyond what we have so far presumed in Western medicine. We truly possess the capacity to live optimally by improving mental, emotional, and spiritual well-being.

By addressing the brain, either directly or through the mind, we have the ability to manage feelings, reduce stress, eliminate unwanted behaviors, and achieve health. Increasingly, neuroscience is discovering ways of "tuning" the brain to stimulate learning, creativity, and memory; to improve sleep, concentration, and pain management; to enhance intuition and problem solving; and to permit the acquisition of deep wisdom. BCT promotes a balancing of the entire brain–mind–body. Included in this balance is the ability to activate the parasympathetic system and achieve states of calm and happiness. When the nervous system is balanced, stressful life events can be managed and a person can remain in a state of thriving for longer periods of time. Using BCT, a therapist can assist an individual in developing a nonreactive mind and reconfiguring defensive patterns that have been blocking internal balance and connection with others.

This book is an invitation to use a new approach to encourage change, growth, and flourishing, an invitation to put aside outmoded ideas of human capacity to explore the realms of the possible both for our clients and for ourselves as clinicians. For it is there—in the realms of the possible—that the future lies. As the scholar and political theorist John Schaar (1995) noted: "The future is not a result of choices among alternative paths offered by the present, but a place that is created—created first in the mind and will, created next in activity. The future is not some place we are going, but one we are creating. The paths to it are not found but made, and the activity of making them changes both the maker and the destination."

REFERENCES

Achterberg, J., & Lawlis, F. (1980). *Bridges of the bodymind.* Chicago: Institute for Personality and Ability Testing.

Adams, D. (1995). *Life, the universe and everything .* Los Angeles, CA: Del Rey.

Ader, R., & Cohen, N. (1975). Behaviorally conditioned immunosuppression. *Psychosomatic Medicine, 37*(4), 333–340.

Adler, A. (1969). *Understanding human nature.* New York, NY: Fawcett.

Alexander, C., & Schneider, R. (1996). Trial of stress reduction for hypertension in older African Americans. *Hypertension, 28,* 228–237.

Alexander, W. (1997). *Cool water, alcoholism, mindfulness and ordinary recovery.* Boston: Shambhala.

Ali, M. (1972). Pattern of EEG recovery under photic stimulation by light of different colors. *Electroencephalography and Clinical Neurophysiology, 3,* 332–335.

Allman, J., Atiya, H., Erwin, E., Nimchinsky, P., & Hof, A. (2001). Anterior cingulate cortex: The evolution of an interface between emotion and cognition. *Annals of the New York Academy of Sciences, 935,* 107–117.

Alvarez de Lorenzana, J. (2008). *Therapists who practice mindfulness meditation: Implications for therapy.* Unpublished master's thesis, University of British Columbia, Vancouver.

Amen, D. (1999). *Change your brain, change your life: The breakthrough program for conquering anxiety, depression, obsessiveness, anger, and impulsiveness.* Three Rivers, MA: Three Rivers Press.

Anderson, D. (1989). The treatment of migraine with variable frequency photostimulation. *Headache,* 29, 154–155.

Anderson, R., Barr, G., Owall, A., & Jacobbson, J. (2004). Entropy during propofol hypnosis, including an episode of wakefulness. *Anesthesia, 59*(1), 52–56.

Archer, R. (2005). *A brief biography of Albert Einstein.* Retrieved from http://ssqq.com/archive/alberteinstein.htm

Arenander, A., Travis, F.T. (2005). Brain patterns of self-awareness. In B. Beitman & J. Nair (Eds.), *Self-awareness deficits* (pp. 24–111). New York, NY: Norton.

Arnsten, A. (1998). The biology of being frazzled. *Science, 280*(5370), 1711–1712.

Ashby, F.G., Isen, A.M., & Turken, A.U. (1999). A neuropsychological theory of positive affect and its influence on cognition. *Psychological Review, 106*, 529–550.

Atkinson, B. (2005). *Emotional intelligence in couples therapy: Advances from neurobiology and the science of intimate relationships.* New York, NY: Norton.

Atwater, F. H. (2001). *Captain of my ship, master of my soul: Living with guidance.* Charlottsville, VA: Hampton Roads.

Austin, J. (2006). *Zen and the brain: Toward an understanding of meditation and consciousness.* Cambridge, MA: MIT Press.

Austin, R. (1991). Shedding light on photic driving. *Mega Brain Report, 2*(2), 1–4.

Aurobindo, S. (1992). *Growing within: Psychology of inner development.* Twin Lakes, WI: Lotus Press.

Axelrod, J., & Felder, C. (1998). Cannabinoid receptors and their endogenous agonist, anandamide. *Neurochemical Research, 23*(5), 575–581.

Baars, B. & Gage, N. (2010). *Cognition, brain and consciousness: introduction to cognitive neuroscience, (2nd Ed.).* New York: Academic Press.

Bachelor, S. (2002). *Living with the devil.* Lecture given at Upaya Zen Center, Santa Fe, NM.

Badenoch, B. (2008). *Being a brain-wise therapist: A practical guide to interpersonal neurobiology.* New York, NY: Norton.

Baker, F. A. (2000). Modifying the melodic intonation therapy program for adults with severe non-fluent aphasia. *Music Therapy Perspectives, 18*(2), 110–114.

Barabasz, A., & Barabasz, M. (Eds.). (1993). *Clinical and experimental restricted environmental stimulation: New developments and perspectives.* New York, NY: Springer-Verlag.

Barber, J., &. Adrian, C. (1982). *Psychological approaches to the management of pain.* New York, NY: Norton.

Baumeister, R., Bratslavsky, E., Finkenauer, C., & Vohs, K. (2001). Bad is stronger than good. *Review of General Psychology, 5*(4), 323–370.

Baumeister, R., DeWall, N., Vohs, K., & Ahlquist, J. (2009). In C.R. Agnew, D. E. Carlston, W. G., Graziano, & J.R. Kelly (Eds.). (2010). *Then a miracle occurs: Focusing on behavior in social psychological theory and research* (pp. 1–11). New York, NY: Oxford University Press.

Benson, H. (1997). *Timeless healing.* New York, NY: Scribner.

Benson, H., & Klipper, M. (2000). *The relaxation response.* New York: HarperCollins.

Berns, G. (2006). *Satisfaction: The science of finding true fulfillment.* New York, NY: Holt.

Berstein, J. (1995). *Handbook of drug therapy in psychiatry.* St. Louis, MO: Mosby.

Biederman, J., Faraone, S., Hirshfeld-Becker, D., Friedman, D., Robin, J., & Rosenbaum, J. (2001). Patterns of psychopathology and dysfunction in high-risk children of parents with panic disorder and major depression. *American Journal of Psychiatry, 158*(1), 49–57.

Blass, E. M. (1986). Interactions between sucrose, pain and isolation distress. *Pharmacology, Biochemistry, and Behavior, 26*, 483–489.

Blass, E. M., & Watt, L. (1999). Suckling- and sucrose-induced analgesia in human newborns. *Pain, 83*(3), 611–623.

Blood, A. J. & Zatorre, R. J. (2001). Intensely pleasurable responses to music correlate with activity in brain regions implicated in reward and emotion. *PNAS, 98*(20), 11818-11823

Bloom, P. (2004, October). *Advances in neuroscience relevant to the clinical practice of hypnosis: A clinician's perspective.* Keynote address to the 16th International Congress of Hypnosis and Hypnotherapy, Singapore.

Blum, K. M., & Tractenberg, M. (1990). Neuronutrient effects on weight loss in carbohydrate bingers: An open clinical trial. *Current Therapeutic Research, 48*, 217–233.

Bowlby, J. (1988). *A Secure Base: Clinical Applications of Attachment Theory.* London: Routledge.

Braverman, E. (2009). *Younger thinner you diet: How understanding your brain chemistry can help you lose weight, reverse aging, and fight disease.* New York, NY: Rodale Books.

Breiling, B. (1996). *Light years ahead: The illustrated guide to full spectrum and colored light in mindbody healing.* Berkley, CA: Celestial Arts.

Bremner, J. (2005). Effects of traumatic stress on brain structure and function: Relevance to early responses to trauma. *Journal of Trauma Dissociation, 6*(2), 51-68.

Brown, F., Graeber, M., & Curtis, R. (Eds.). (1982). *The rhythmic aspects of behavior.* Hillside, NJ: Erlbaum.

Bryant, F. (2009). *Savoring: A new model of positive experience.* New York, NY: Erlbaum.

Bryant, R.A., & Mallard, D. (2002). Hypnotically-induced emotional numbing: A real-simulating analysis. *Journal of Abnormal Psychology, 111*, 203-207.

Buckman, S.E. (1994). *Handbook of humor: Clinical applications in psychotherapy.* Melbourne, FL: Krieger.

Budzynski, T. (1986). Clinical applications of non-drug-induced states. In B. Wolman & M. Ullman (Eds.), *Handbook of states of consciousness* (pp. 428–460). New York, NY: Van Rostrand Reinhold.

Budzynski, T. (1997, February). *The case for alpha–theta: A dynamic hemispheric asymmetry model.* Paper presented at the annual conference of the Society for the Study of Neuronal Regulation. Aspen, CO: Society for the Study of Neuronal Regulation.

Budzynski, T. J. (1999). Academic performance enhancement with photic stimulation and EDR feedback. *Journal of Neurotherapy, 3*, 11–21.

Budzynski, T., & Sherlin, L. (2002). Audio-visual stimulation effects in an Alzheimer's patient as documented by QEEG and LORETA. *Journal of Neurotherapy, 6*, 54–56.

Budzynski, T., Budzynski, H., & Tang, H.-Y. (2006). Brain brightening: Restoring the aging mind. In J. Evans (Ed.), *Handbook of neurofeedback: Dynamics and clinical applications* (pp. 231–266). New York, NY: Haworth Press.

Cade, M., & Coxhead, N. (1991). *The awakened mind: Biofeedback and the development of higher states of awareness.* London: Element Books.

Calaprice, A. & Lipscombe, T. (2005). *Albert Einstein: A Biography.* Westport, CT: Greenwood Press.

Cantor, D. (2007, September). *Pilot study shows audiovisual entrainment therapy stimulates mood centers in brain.* Paper presented at the EEG and Clinical Neuroscience Society Conference, Montreal, Canada.

Carmen, J. (2005). Passive infrared hemoencephalography: Four years and 100 migraines. *Journal of Neurotherapy: Investigations in Neuromodulation, Neurofeedback, and Applied Neuroscience, 8*(3), 23–51.

Capra, F. (1997). *The web of life.* New York, NY: Anchor.

Carroll, D., Smith, G., Sheffield, D., Sweetnam, P., Gallacher, J., & Elwood, P. (1998). Blood pressure reactions to the cold pressor test and the prediction of ischaemic heart disease: Data from the Caerphilly Study. *Journal of Epidemiology and Community Health, 52*, 528–529.

Carroll, L. (1872). *Through the looking glass and what Alice found there.* London: MacMillan.

Castaneda, C. (1971). *A separate reality.* New York, NY: Washington Square Press.

Celsis, P. A. (1997). Age related cognitive decline: A clinical entity? A longitudinal study of cerebral blood flow and memory performance. *Journal of Neurology, Neurosurgery, and Psychiatry, 62,* 601–608.

Centers for Disease Control and Prevention. (2009). *Overweight prevalence: Faststats.* Retrieved from http://www.cdc.gov/nchs/fastats/overwt.htm

Ceriello, A. (2000). Oxidative stress and glycemic regulation. *Metabolism, 49,* 27–29.

Cermak, T. (2003). *Marijuana: What's a parent to Do?* Center City, MN: Hazelden.

Chabot, R. J. (1998). Quantitative EEG profiles of children with attention and learning disorders and the role of QEEG in predicting medication response and outcome. *Journal of Neurotherapy, 2*(3), 61–62.

Chartier, D., Collins, L., & Koons, D. (1997, February). *Peak performance EEG training and the game of golf.* Paper presented at the 5th Annual Conference on Brain Function/EEG, Palm Springs, CA.

Chen, J. (2002). *A quantum theoretical account of linguistics.* Retrieved from http://nats–www.informatik.uni–hamburg.de/joseph/di/dis/node26.html

Childre, D., & Rozman, D. (2007). *Transforming depression: The HeartMath solution to feeling overwhelmed, sad, and stressed.* New York, NY: New Harbinger.

Christensen, L. (1991). The role of caffeine and sugar in depression. *Nutrition Report, 9(3),* 17–24.

Cleary, J. (1996). Naloxone effects on sucrose-motivated behavior. *Psychopharmacology, 176,* 110–114.

Cohen, S., Tyrell, D., & Smith, A. (1991). Psychological stress and susceptibility to the common cold. *New England Journal of Medicine, 325,* 606–612.

Colantuoni, C. (1992, Jul.). Sugar, white flour withdrawal produces chemical response. *The Addiction Letter,* 4.

Colantuoni, C., Rada, P., McCarthy, J., Patten, C., Avena, N., Chadeayne, A., et al. (2002). Evidence that intermittent, excessive sugar intake causes endogenous opioid dependence. *Obesity Research, 10,* 478–488.

Collins, A. (2009). Neurofeedback for addictions: The state of the science. *International Society for Neurofeedback Research on Addiction* [Online]. Retrieved from http://isnr.org/information/addiction.cfm

Cormier, S., Nurius, P., & Osborn (2009). *Interviewing and Change Strategies for Helpers: Fundamental Skills and Cognitive Behavioral Interventions,* (Sixth Edition). Belmont, CA: Brooks/Cole.

Cowan, J. (2006). *A brief history of the 40 Hertz rhythm.* Retrieved from http://PeakAchievement.com

Cowan, N. (2001). The magical number 4 in short-term memory: A reconsideration of mental storage capacity. *Behavioral and Brain Sciences,* 24, 87-185.

Cozolino, L. (2002). *The neuroscience of psychotherapy: Building and rebuilding the human brain.* New York, NY: Norton.

Cozolino, L. (2008). *The healthy aging brain: Sustaining attachment, attaining wisdom.* New York, NY: Norton.

Crawford, H. J. (1998). Hypnotic analgesia: 1. Somatosensory event-related potential changes to noxious stimuli, and 2. Transfer learning to reduce chronic low back pain. *International Journal of Clinical and Experimental Hypnosis, 46,* 92–132.

Crawford, H. & Gruzelier, J. (1992). A midstream view of the neuropsychophysiology of hypnosis: recent research and future directions. In W. Fromm, M. Nash (Eds.) *Hypnosis, Research Developments and Perspectives,* 3rd Ed., New York: Guildford Press, 227–66.

Csikszentmihalyi, M. (1990). *Flow: The psychology of optimal experience.* San Francisco, CA: Harper Perennial.

Cygnet. (2008). *Manual for neurofeedback software.* Los Angeles, CA: Author.

Dalai Lama, & Cutler, H. (1998). *The art of happiness.* New York: Riverhead Books.

Damasio, A. (1999). *The feeling of what happens.* London: Random House.

Damasio, A., Grabowski, T.J., Bechara, A., Damasio, H., Ponto, L., Parvizi, J., et al.

(2000). Subcortical and cortical brain activity during the feeling of self-generated emotions. *Nature Neuroscience, 3*, 1049–1056.

Dandeneau, S. D., & Baldwin, M. W. (2004). The inhibition of socially rejecting information among people with high versus low self-esteem: The role of attentional bias and the effects of bias reduction training. *Journal of Social and Clinical Psychology, 23*, 584–602.

Dandeneau, S. D., Baldwin, M. W., Baccus, J. R., Sakellaropoulo, M., & Pruessner, J. C. (2007). Cutting stress off at the pass: Reducing vigilance and responsiveness to social threat by manipulating attention. *Journal of Personality and Social Psychology, 93*, 651–666.

Dardik, I. (1996). The origin of disease and health, and heart waves: The single solution to heart rate variability and ischemic preconditioning. *Cycles, 46*(3), 67–77.

Dardik, I., & Lewin, R. (2005). *Making waves: Irving Dardik and his superwave principle.* New York, NY: Rodale Books.

Davidson, R. (2000). *Understanding positive and negative emotions.* Retrieved from Library of Congress, http://www.loc.gov/loc/brain/emotion/Davidson.html

Davidson, R.(2001). Prefrontal and amygdala contributions to emotion and affective style. In F. Boller (Ed.), *Handbook of neuropsychology* (2nd ed.). New York: Elsevier.

Davidson, R. (2003). Alterations in brain and immune function produced by mindfulness meditation. *Psychosomatic Medicine, 65*, 564–570.

Davidson, R. (2007, December). *The heart–brain connection: The neuroscience of social, emotional, and academic learning.* Paper presented at the Casel Forum, New York, NY.

Davidson, R., & Lutz, A. (2008). *Buddha's brain: Neuroplasticity and meditation. IEEE Signal Processing, 25*(1), 171–174.

Davidson, R., Scherer, K., & Goldsmith, H. (2002). *Handbook on affective science.* New York, NY: Oxford University Press.

Dawson, G.(1994). *Human behavior and the developing brain.* New York, NY: Guilford Press.

Dawson, G., & Fischer, K. (1994). *Human behavior and the developing brain: How to help your child thrive.* New York: NY, Guilford Press.

Demos, J. (2005). *Getting started with neurofeedback.* New York, NY: Norton.

Derbyshire, S., Whalley, M., Stenger, V., Oakley, D. A. (2009). Fibromyalgia pain and its modulation by hypnotic and non-hypnotic suggestion: An fMRI analysis. *European Journal of Pain, 13: 542-550.*

Desmond, J., & Fiez, J. (1998). Neuroimaging studies of the cerebellum: Language, learning, and memory. *Trends in Cognitive Sciences, 2*(9), 355–362.

Devane, W. A., & Axelrod, J. (1994). Enzymatic synthesis of anandamide, an endogenous ligand for the cannabinoid receptor, by brain membranes. *Proceedings of the National Academy of Sciences, USA, 91*(14), 6698–6701.

Dias-Ferreira, E., Sousa, J., Melo, I., Morgado, P., Mesquita, A., Cerqueira, A., et al. (2009). Chronic stress causes frontostriatal reorganization and affects decision-making. *Science, 325*(5940), 621–625. doi: 10.1126/science.1171203

Dickinson, E. (1955). *The complete poems of Emily Dickinson.* Boston, MA: Little, Brown.

Didion, J. (1979). *The white album.* New York, NY: Simon & Schuster.

Dikjsterhuis, A. (2004). Think different: The merits of unconscious thought in preference development and decision making. *Journal of Personality and Social Psychology, 87*(5), 586–598.

Dillon, K. M., Minchoff, F., & Baker, K. (1985). Positive emotional states and enhancement of the immune system. *International Journal of Psychiatry in Medicine, 15*, 13–17.

Dingfelder, S.F. (2008). Mind games: Elite athletes are using EEG feedback to hone their mental states—but does it work? *Monitor on Psychology, 39*(7), 58–59.

Driesen, N., & Raz, N.(1995). The influence of sex, age, and handedness on corpus callosum morphology: A meta-analysis. *Psychobiology, 23*(3), 240–224.

Driscoll, R. (1987). Humor in pragmatic psychotherapy. In *Handbook of Humor and Psychotherapy.* William Fry and Waleed Salameh (Eds.). Sarasota, FL: Professional Resource Exchange, 127-48.

Easton, J. (1999). Lack of sleep alters hormones, metabolism. *University of Chicago Chronicle, 19*, 6. Retrieved from http://chronicle.uchicago.edu/991202/sleep.shtml

Eisenberger, N., Lieberman, M., & Williams, K. (Oct., 2003). Does rejection hurt? An fMRI study of social exclusion. *Science, 302*(5643), 290–292. Retrieved from DOI: 10.1126/science.1089134

Egner, T., & Hirsch, J. (2005). Cognitive control mechanisms resolve conflict through cortical amplification of task-relevant information. *Nature Neuroscience, 8*, 1784–1790.

Emory, W., Schiller M., & Suffin S. (2004, June). *Referenced-EEG in the treatment of eating disorders.* Paper presented at the 44th annual meeting of the National Institute of Mental Health, National Clinical Drug Evaluation Unit, Phoenix, AZ. Available online at http://www.nimh.nih.gov/ncdeu/ncdeu2004 abstracts.pdf, Poster No. 221

Erickson, M. (1972). Deep hypnosis and its induction. In L. LeCron (Ed.), *Experimental hypnosis* (pp. 70–112). Secaucus, NJ: Citadel Press.

Erickson, M. (1980). *The collected papers of Milton Erickson on hypnosis* (4 Vols., E. Rossi, Ed.). *1. The nature of hypnosis and suggestion. 2. Hypnotic alteration of sensory perceptual and psychophysiological processes. 3. Hypnotic investigation of psychodynamic processes. 4. Innovative hypnotherapy.* New York, NY: Irvington.

Erickson, M. (2008). The burden of effective psychotherapy. In E. Rossi, R. Erickson-Klein, & K. Rossi (Eds.), *The complete works of Milton H. Erickson, M.D., on therapeutic hypnosis, psychotherapy, and rehabilitation: The neuroscience edition: Vol. 3. Open minds: Innovative psychotherapy.* Phoenix: The MHE Press. (Original work published 1964)

Erickson, M. (2008). Further clinical techniques of hypnosis: Utilization techniques. In E. Rossi, R. Erickson-Klein, & K. Rossi (Eds.), *The complete works of Milton H. Erickson, M.D., on therapeutic hypnosis, psychotherapy, and rehabilitation: The neuroscience edition: Vol. 1. The nature of hypnosis.* Phoenix: MHE Press. (Original work published 1958)

Erickson, M. (2008). Hypnosis: Its renascence as a treatment modality. *American Journal of Clinical Hypnosis, 13*, 71–89. In E. Rossi, R. Erickson-Klein, & K. Rossi (Eds.), *The complete works of Milton H. Erickson, M.D., on therapeutic hypnosis, psychotherapy, and rehabilitation: The neuroscience edition: Vol. 2. Basic hypnotic induction and suggestion.* Phoenix: MHE Press. (Original work published 1970)

Erickson, M. (2008). Hypnotic psychotherapy. In E. Rossi, R. Erickson-Klein, & K. Rossi (Eds.), *The complete works of Milton H. Erickson, M.D., on therapeutic hypnosis, psychotherapy, and rehabilitation: The neuroscience edition: Vol. 2. Basic hypnotic induction and suggestion.* Phoenix: MHE Press. (Original work published 1970)

Erickson, M. (2008). Naturalistic techniques of hypnosis. In E. Rossi, R. Erickson-Klein, & K. Rossi (Eds.), *The complete works of Milton H. Erickson, M.D., on therapeutic hypnosis, psychotherapy, and rehabilitation: The neuroscience edition: Vol. 1. The nature of hypnosis.* Phoenix: MHE Press. (Original work published 1958)

Erickson, M., & Rossi, E. (1979). *Hypnotherapy: An exploratory casebook.* New York, NY: Irvington.

Erickson, M., & Rossi, E. (1981). *Experiencing hypnosis: Therapeutic approaches to altered states.* New York, NY: Irvington.

Erickson, M. & Rossi, E. (1989). *The February Man: Evolving Consciousness and Identity in Hypnotherapy.* New York: Brunner/Mazel.

Erickson, M., Rossi, E., & Rossi, S. (1976). *Hypnotic realities: The induction of clinical hypnosis and forms of indirect suggestion.* New York, NY: Irvington.

Erickson, M., & Rossi, E., Ryan, M., & Sharp, V. (1983). *The seminars, workshops, and lectures of Milton H. Erickson.* New York, NY: Irvington.

Eriksson, E. P. (1998). Neurogenesis in the adult human hippocampus. *Nature Medicine, 4*(11), 1313–1217.

Evans, J. (1999). *Introduction to quantitative EEG and neurofeedback.* New York, NY: Academic Press.

Ewin, D. (1994, January). *Using hypnosis with burn patients.* Session presented at the American Society of Clinical Hypnosis, Atlanta, GA.

Fahrion, S. L. (1995). Human potential and personal transformation. *Subtle Energies, 6*, 55–88.

Farmer, S. (2002) Neural rhythms in Parkinson's disease. *Brain Journal of Neurology, 125*(6), 1176–1176.

Fehmi, L., & Robbins, J. (2007). *Open-focus brain: Harness the power of attention to heal mind and body.* Boston: Trumpeter.

Felder, C.C., & Glass, M. (1998). Cannabinoid receptors and their endogenous agonists. *Annual Review of Pharmacology and Toxicology, 38*, 179–200.

Field, T., Diego, M., & Maria Hernandez-Reif, M.(2006). Prenatal depression effects on the fetus and newborn: A review. *Infant Behavior and Development 29*(3), 445–455.

Fields, M.(1983). Effect of copper deficiency on metabolism and mortality in rats fed sucrose or starch diets. *Journal of Clinical Nutrition, 113*, 1335–1345.

Fisch, B. J. (1999). *Fisch and Spelhmann's EEG primer: Basic principles of digital and analog EEG.* Philadelphia, PA: Elsevier.

Fisher, H. (2009). *Why him, why her?* New York, NY: Holt.

Fletcher, B. P. (2007). *The no diet diet.* London: Orion.

Fonagy, P., Gergey, G., Jurist, E., & Target, M. (2005). *Affect regulation, mentalization, and the development of self.* New York, NY: Other Press.

Frampton, M. (2008). *Embodiments of will: Anatomical and physiological theories of voluntary animal motion from Greek antiquity to the Late Middle Ages, 400 B.C.–A.D. 1300.* Saarbrücken, Germany: VDM Verlag.

Friedman, B., & Thayer, J. (1998). Anxiety and autonomic flexibility: A cardiovascular approach. *Biological Psychology, 47*, 243–263.

Friedman, J. E. (2001). *Mapping the brain's food intake circuitry.* Retrieved from http//:www.hhmi.org/new/hormone.html

Fredrickson, B. L. (2001). The role of positive emotions in positive psychology: The broaden-and-build theory of positive emotions. *American Psychologist, 56*, 218–226.

Gallmann, D., & Grawe, H. (2006). General change mechanisms: The relation between problem activation and resource activation in successful and unsuccessful therapeutic interaction. *Clinical Psychology and Psychotherapy, 13*(1), 1–11.

Gallwey, W. (2009). *The inner game of stress: Outsmart life's challenges, fulfill your potential, enjoy yourself.* New York, NY: Random House.

Ganisa, G. (2004). Brain areas underlying visual mental imagery and visual perception. *Cognitive Brain Research, 20*, 226–241.

Gerrig, R. (1993). *Experiencing narrative worlds: On the psychological activities of reading.* New Haven, CT: Yale University Press.

Gerson, M. (1999). *The second brain: A groundbreaking new understanding of nervous disorders of the stomach and intestine.* New York, NY: Harper Paperbacks.

Goleman, D. (1988). *The meditative mind.* New York, NY: Putnam.

Goleman, D. (2003). *Destructive emotions: How we can overcome them.* New York, NY: Bantam Dell.

Gómez-Pinilla F. (2008). Brain foods: The effect of nutrients on brain function. *Nature Reviews Neuroscience, 9*(7), 568–578.

Gordon, E., Barnet, K., & Cooper, N., Tran, N., & Williams, L. (2008). An integrative neuroscience platform: Applications to profiles of negativity and positivity bias. *Journal of Integrative Neuroscience, 7*(3), 345–366.

Gottman, J. (1995). *Why marriages succeed or fail, and how you can make yours last.* Simon & Schuster: New York, NY.

Gottman, J.M. (1999). *The marriage clinic.* New York, NY: Norton.

Grawe, K. (2004). *Psychological therapy.* Cambridge, MA: Hogrefe & Huber.

Grawe, K. (2007). *Neuropsychotherapy: How the neurosciences effectively inform psychotherapy.* New York, NY: Routledge.

Green, E., & Green, A.M. (1971). On the meaning of the transpersonal: Some metaphysical perspectives. *Journal of Transpersonal Psychology, 3*, 27–46.

Green, E., & Green, A.M. (1977). *Beyond biofeedback and self-control.* San Francisco: Delacorte Press.

Greene, D. (1998). *Audition success.* New York, NY: ProMind Music.

Grigsby, J., & Stevens, D. (2000). *Neurodynamics of personality.* New York, NY: Guilford Press.

Gross, C. (1995). Aristotle on the brain. *The Neuroscientist, 1*(4), 245–250. Retrieved from http://www.princeton.edu/cggross/Neuroscientist_95–1.pdf

Grunwald, F., Schrock, H., Kuschinsky, W. (1991). The influence of nicotine on local cerebral blood flow in rats. *Neuroscience Letters, 124*(1), 108–110.

Gruzelier, J. (2006). Altered states of consciousness and hypnosis in the twenty-first century. *Contemporary Hypnosis, 22*(1), 1–7.

Gurnee, R. (2003, September). *Central 12–15 Hz activity in ADHD.* Paper presented at the conference of the International Society for Neuronal Regulation, Houston, TX.

Guyton, A., & Hall, A. (2005). *Textbook of medical physiology.* Carlsbad, CA: Saunders.

Haidt, J. (in press). *The righteous mind: Why good people are divided by politics and religion.* New York: Pantheon Books.

Hammond, C. (2007). *LENS: The low energy neurofeedback system.* New York, NY: Routledge.

Hardt, J. (2007). *The art of smart thinking.* Victoria, BC: Biocybernaut Press.

Hayashi, T., Urayama, O., Kawai, K., Hayashi, K., Iwanaga, S., Ohta, M., et al. (2006). Laughter regulates gene expression in patients with type 2 diabetes. *Psychotherapy and Psychosomatics, 75*, 62–65.

Heath, T., Melichar, J., Nutt, D., & Donaldson, L. (2006). Human taste thresholds are modulated by serotonin and noradrenaline. *Journal of Neuroscience, 26*(49), 12664–12671.

Heller, W., & Nitsche, J. (1998). The puzzle of regional brain activity in depression and anxiety: The importance of subtypes and comorbidity. *Cognition and Emotion, 12*, 421–447.

Hiew, C. C. (1995). Hemi-sync into creativity. *Hemi-Sync Journal, 13*(1), 3–5.

Hitt, E. (2003). *Dean Ornish: Lifestyle stops/reverses progression.* Delray Beach, FL: Medscape Medical News.

Horney, K. (1991). *Neurosis and human growth.* New York, NY: Norton. (Original work published 1950)

Huang, T., & Charyton, C. (2008). A comprehensive review of the psychological effects of brainwave entrainment. *Alternative Therapies and Health Medicine, 14*(5), 38–49.

Hughes, J.R., & John, E.R. (1999). Conventional and quantitative electroencephalography in psychiatry. *Journal of Neuropsychiatry and Clinical Neurosciences, 11*, 190–208.

Hutterer, J., & Liss, M. (2006). Cognitive development, memory, trauma, treatment: An integration of psychoanalytic and behavioral concepts in light of current of the American Academy of Psychoanalysis and Dynamic Psychiatry neuroscience research. *Journal of the Academy of Psychoanalysis and Dynamic Psychiatry, 34*, 287–302.

Iacoboni, M. (2008). *Mirroring people: The new science of how we connect with others.* New York, NY: Farrar, Straus & Giroux.

Imai, M. (1986). *Kaizen: The key to Japan's competitive success.* New York, NY: McGraw-Hill.

Ito, Y., Teicher, M. H., Glod, C. A., Harper, D., Magnus, E., & Gelbard, H. A. (1993). Increased prevalence of electrophysiological abnormalities in children with psychological, physical, and sexual abuse. *Journal of Neuropsychiatry and Clinical Neurosciences, 5*, 401–408.

Jackson, S. A. (1996). Toward a conceptual understanding to the flow experience in elite athletes. *Research Quarterly for Exercise and Sport, 67*(1), 76–90.

James, W. (1950). *The principles of psychology: Vol. 1.* New York, NY: Dover Publications. (Original work published 1890)

Jamieson, G. A. (Ed.). (2007). *Hypnosis and conscious states: The cognitive neuroscience perspective.* New York, NY: Oxford University Press.

Johnson, D. (1996). Ultraweak photon emission and transcendental meditation. *Hypertension, 28*, 227–238.

Joseph, J. (2008). *Finding the garden of youth: New study shows spinach, strawberries protect against age-related brain decline.* Retrieved from: http://www.sciencedaily.com¬ /releases/1998/09/980929072709.htm

Jung, C. (2006). *The undiscovered self* [Reprint]. New York, NY: Signet.

Justice, B., & Justice, R. (2008). The liminal space. *University of Texas Health Science Center Insight Newsletter.* Retrieved May 18, 2008, from http://www.healthleader.uthouston.edu/archive/mind_body_soul/2004/liminalspace-0126.html

Kaiser, D. O. (1999). The QEEG. *EEG Spectrum Newsletter, 1*, 1.

Kamiya, J. (1968). Conscious control of brain waves. *Psychology Today, 1*(April), 57–60.

Kennerly, R. C. (1994). *An empirical investigation into the effect of beta fre-*

quency binaural beat audio signals on four measures of human memory [Research paper]. Carrolton, GA: Department of Psychology, West Georgia College.

Kershaw, C. (1979). *Imagery and visualization in adult diabetics.* Doctoral dissertation, Texas A&M University, Commerce, TX.

Kershaw, C. (1980). Learning to think for an organ. In J. Achterberg, & F. Lawlis (Eds.), *Bridges of the bodymind* (pp. 51–64), Chicago, IL: IPAT.

Kershaw, C. (1982). Therapeutic metaphor in the treatment of childhood asthma: A systemic approach. In S. Lankton (Ed.), *Central themes and principles of Ericksonian therapy* (pp. 83–95). New York, NY: Brunner/Mazel.

Kershaw, C. (1987). Therapeutic metaphor in the treatment of childhood asthma: A systemic approach. In S. Lankton, *Central themes and principles of Ericksonian therapy* (pp. 83-95). New York: Brunner/Mazel.

Kershaw, C. (1992). *The couple's hypnotic dance: Creating Ericksonian strategies in marital therapy.* New York, NY: Brunner/Mazel.

Keyes, C. & Haidt, J. (Eds). (2002). *Flourishing: Positive psychology and the life well-lived.* Washington, DC: American Psychological Association.

Khalsa, D. (1997). *Brain longevity.* New York, NY: Time Warner.

Kiecolt-Glaser, J. G., Marucha, P., Atkinson, C., & Glaser, R. (2001). Hypnosis as a modulator of cellular immune dysregulation during acute stress. *Journal of Consulting and Clinical Psychology, 69*(4), 674–682.

Kikuchi, M. (2002). EEG harmonic responses to photic stimulation in normal aging and Alzheimer's disease: Differences in interhemispheric coherence. *Clinical Neurophysiology, 113*(7), 1045.

Kirsch, I. (2010). *The emperor's new drugs: Exploding the antidepressant myth.* New York, NY: Basic Books.

Kirsch, I., Montgomery, G., & Sapirstein, G. (1995). Hypnosis as an adjunct to cognitive–behavioral psychotherapy: A meta-analysis. *Journal of Consulting and Clinical Psychology, 63*, 214–220.

Kjaer, T., Nowak, M., & Lou, H. (2002). Reflective self-awareness and conscious states: PET evidence for a common midline parietofrontal core. *NeuroImage, 2*(2), 1080–1086.

Klein, S. (2006). *The science of happiness: How our brains make us happy and what we can do to get happier.* New York, NY: Avalon.

Komatsu, H. (1987). Studies on the temporal frequency characteristics of vision by photic driving method: III. Temporal frequency characteristics of color vision. *Tohoku Psychologica Folia, 46*(1–4) , 1–12.

Koob, G. (2008). The neurobiology of addiction. In M. Galanter & H. Kleber (Eds.), *The American Psychiatric Publishing textbook of substance abuse treatment* (pp. 3–16). Arlington, VA: American Psychiatric Publishing.

Kosslyn, S., Thompson, W., Costantini-Ferrando, M., Alpert, N., & Spiegel, D. (1999). The role of area 17 in visual imagery: Convergent evidence from PET and rTMS. *Science, 284*, 167–170.

Kosslyn, S., Thompson, W., Costantini-Ferrando, M., Alpert, N., & Spiegel, D. (2000). Hypnotic visual illusion alters color processing in the brain. *American Journal of Psychiatry, 157*, 1279–1284.

Kristal-Boneh, E., Raifel, M., Froom, P., & Ribak, J. (1995.) Heart rate variability in health and disease. *Scandinavian Journal of Work, Environment and Health, 2*, 85–95.

Kubie, L. (1943). Dream with distortion. *Bulletin of the Menninger Clinic, 7*, 172–182.

Kumano, H. (1996). Treatment of a depressive disorder patient with EEG-driven photic stimulation. *Biofeedback and Self-Regulation, 21*(4), 323–334.

Kumano, H., Horie, H., Kuboki, T., Hiroyuki, S., Hiroshi, S. & Yasushi, M. et al. (1997). EEG-driven photic stimulation effect on plasma cortisol and beta-endorphin. *Applied Psychophysiological Biofeedback, 3*, 193–208.

Lai, C., Daini, S., Calgagni, M., Bruno, I., & Risio, S. (2007). Neural correlates of psychodynamic psychotherapy in borderline disorders: A pilot study. *Psychotherapy and Psychosomatics, 76*, 403–405.

Landers, D. (1991). Optimizing individual performance. In D. Druckman & R. Bjork (Eds.), *In the Mind's Eye: Enhancing Human Performance* (pp. 193–246). Washington, D.C.: National Academies Press.

Lane, R., & Nadel, J. (Eds.). (2002). *Cognitive neuroscience of emotion.* New York, NY: Oxford University Press.

Lankton, S. (2003). *Assembling Ericksonian therapy.* Redding, CT: Zeig, Tucker, & Thiesen.

Lankton, S., & Lankton, C. (1983). *The answer within.* New York, NY: Brunner/Mazel.

Lankton, S., & Lankton, C. (1989). *Tales of enchantment: An anthology of goal-directed metaphors for adults and children in therapy.* New York, NY: Brunner/Mazel.

Lao Tzu. (2008). *Brainyquote.* Retrieved from http://www.brainyquote.com/quotes/authors/l/lao_tzu.html

LeDoux, J. (1996). *The emotional brain: The mysterious underpinnings of emotional life.* New York, NY: Simon & Schuster.

LeDoux, J. (2002). *The synaptic self: How our brains become who we are.* New York, NY: Viking.

Lehmann, D., Faber, P.L., Achermann, P., Jeanmonod, D., Lorena R., Gianotti, L., et al. (2001). Brain sources of EEG gamma frequency during volitionally meditation-induced, altered states of consciousness, and experience of the self. *Psychiatry Research, 108*(2), 111–121.

Lenoir, M. S. (2007). Intense sweetness surpasses cocaine reward. *PLoS ONE 2*(8), e698. doi:10.1371/journal.pone.0000698

Leonard, G., & Murphy, M. (2005). *The life we are given (inner workbook).* New York, NY: Tarcher/Putnam.

Levine, P. (1997). *Waking the tiger.* Berkeley, CA: North Atlantic Books.

Lilly, J. (1977). *The deep self*. New York, NY: Simon & Schuster.

Lipton, B. (2005). *The biology of belief*. Fulton, CA: Elite Books.

Lubar, J. (1997). Neocortical dynamics: Implications for understanding the role of neurofeedback and related techniques for the enhancement of attention. *Applied Psychophysiological Biofeedback, 2*, 111–126.

Lubar, J., Swartwood, M., Swartwood, J., & O'Donnell, P. (1995). Evaluation of the effectiveness of EEG neurofeedback training for ADHD in a clinical setting as measured by changes in TOVA scores, behavioral ratings, and WISC-R performance. *Applied Psychophysiology and Biofeedback, 20*(1), 83–99.

Lutz, A., Greischar, L., Rawlings, N., Ricard, M., & Davidson, R. (2004). Long-term meditators self-induce high amplitude gamma synchrony during mental practice. *Proceedings of the National Academy of Sciences, 101*, 16369–16373.

Lyonfields, J., Borkovec, T., & Thayer, J. (1995). Vagal tone in generalized anxiety disorder and the effects of aversive imagery and worrisome thinking. *Behaviour Therapy, 26*, 457–466.

Lyubomirsky, S. (2008). *The how of happiness: A scientific approach to getting the life you want*. New York: Penguin Press.

MacArthur, J., & MacArthur, C. (2000). *Heart rate variability*. Research Network on Socioeconomic Status and Health. Retrieved from http://www.macses.ucsf .edu/Research/Allostatic/notebook/heart.rate.html

MacIver, K., Lloyd, D., Kelly, S., Roberts, N., & Nurmikko, T. (2008). Phantom limb pain, cortical reorganization, and the therapeutic effect of mental imagery. *Brain, 131*(8), 2181–2191.

MacKinnon, D. (1971). Creativity and transliminal experiences. *Journal of Creative Behavior*, 5, 227–241

Mahr, K. (2007, November). How stress harms your heart. *Time Magazine* [Online]. Retrieved from http://www.time.com/time/magazine/article/0,9171,1678678, 00.html

Manstead, A. F. (2001). *Feelings and emotions*. Amsterdam: University of Amsterdam.

Maquet, P., Faymonville, M., Degueldre, C., Delfiore, G., Franck, G., Luxen, A., et al. (1999). Functional neuroanatomy of hypnotic state. *Biological Psychiatry, 45*, 327–333.

Markova, D. (1994). *No enemies within*. Berkeley, CA: Conari Press.

Mars, D. (1998). Biofeedback assisted psychotherapy using multimodal biofeedback including capnography. *Biofeedback, 26*, 4–7.

Maslow, A. (1975). *Toward a psychology of being*. New York, NY: Van Nostrand Reinhold.

Matsuoka, Y., Yosikawa, Y., Yamasue, H., Inagaki, M., Nakano, T., Akechi, T., et al. (2003). Prefrontal cortex and amygdala volume in first minor or major depressive episode after cancer diagnosis. *Biological Psychiatry, 59*(8), 707–712.

Mavromatis, A. (1987). *Hypnagogia: The unique state of consciousness between wakefulness and sleep*. London: Routledge & Kegan Paul.

McCraty, R. (2002). Heart rhythm coherence: An emerging area of biofeedback. *Biofeedback, 23*, 23–25.

McCraty, R. (2008). From depletion to renewal: Positive emotions and heart rhythm coherence feedback. *Biofeedback, 36*(1), 30–34.

McCraty, R., Atkinson, M., & Tiller, W. (1995). The effects of emotions on short-term power spectrum analysis of heart rate variability. *American Journal of Cardiology, 76*, 1089–1093.

McCraty, R., Atkinson, M., Tomasino, D., & Bradley, R. (2006). *The coherent heart: Heart–brain interactions, psychophysiological coherence, and the emergence of system-wide order.* HeartMath Research Center, Institute of HeartMath (Publication No. 06–022), Boulder Creek, CO.

McCraty, R., Atkinson, M., Tomasino, D., & Tiller, W. (1998). The electricity of touch: Detection and measurement of cardiac energy between people. In K. Pribram (Ed.) *Brain and values: Is a biological value of science possible?* (pp. 359–379) Mahwah, NJ: Erlbaum.

McCraty, R., & Tomasino, D. (2006).Emotional stress, positive emotions, and psychophysiological coherence. In B. B. Arnetz & R. Ekman (Eds.), *Stress in health and disease* (pp. 342–365). Weinheim, Germany: Wiley-VCH.

McEwen, B. (2002). *The end of stress as we know it.* New York, NY: National Academies Press.

McFadden, J. (2002). The conscious electromagnetic (CEMI) field theory: The hard problem made easy? *Journal of Consciousness Studies, 9*, 45–60.

McTaggart, L. (2002*). The field: The quest for the secret force of the universe.* New York, NY: HarperCollins.

Meares, R. (2005). *The metaphor of play* (3rd ed.). London and New York, NY: Routledge.

Mehl-Madrona, L. (2003, September). *QEEG changes in the recipients of ceremony and prayer.* Paper presented at the International Society for Neurofeedback and Research, Houston, TX.

Mendelsohn, A., Chalamish,Y., Solomonovich, A., & Dudai, Y. (2008). Mesmerizing memories: Brain substrates of episodic memory suppression in posthypnotic amnesia. *Neuron, 57*(1), 159–170.

Merton, T., & Montaldo, J. (2004). *A year with Thomas Merton: Daily meditations from his journals.* New York, NY: HarperOne.

Mignot, E. (2004). *Stanford study links obesity to hormonal changes from lack of sleep.* Retrieved from http://www.sciencedaily.com/releases/2004/12/041206194344.htm

Miller, S., & Miller, P. (1997). *Core communication: Skill and processes.* Minneapolis, MN:ICP.

Miller, W., & Rollnick, S. (2002). *Motivational interviewing: Preparing people for change* (2nd ed.), New York, NY: Guilford Press.

Milne, A. A. (1926). *Winnie-the-Pooh.* London: Methuen.

Mingyur, Y. (2008). *The joy of living: Unlocking the secret and science of happiness.* New York, NY: Three Rivers Press.

Mipham, S. (2005). *Ruling your world*. New York, NY: Broadway Books.

Molteni, R. (2002). A high-fat, refined sugar diet reduces hippocampal brain-derived neurotrophic factor, neuronal plasticity, and learning. *Neuroscience, 112*(4), 803–814.

Moroz, N., Tong, M., Longato, L., Xu, H., & de la Monte, S. (2008). Limited Alzheimer-type neurodegeneration in experimental obesity and Type 2 diabetes mellitus. *Journal of Alzheimer's Disease, 15*(1), 29–44.

Moss, D. (2003). Anxiety disorders. In D. M. Moss (Ed.), *Handbook of mind–body medicine in primary care* (pp. 359–376). Thousand Oaks, CA: Sage.

Moushegian, G. R. (1978). Evaluation of frequency-following potentials in man: Masking and clinical studies. *Electroencephalography and Clinical Neurophysiology, 45*, 711–718.

Murakami, K. (2006). *The divine code of life: Awaken your genes and discover hidden talents*. Hillsboro, OR: Beyond Words.

Nagel, J. (1998). Pain and injury in performing musicians: A psychodynamic approach. In R. Sataloff, A. Brandfonbrener, & R. Lederman (Eds.), *Performing arts medicine* (2nd ed., pp. 291–299). San Diego, CA: Singular.

National Center for Chronic Disease Prevention and Health Promotion (2010). *Obesity: Halting the epidemic by making health easier: At a glance 2010*. Retrieved from: http://www.cdc.gov/chronicdisease/resources/publications/aag/obesity.htm

National Institute on Drug Abuse. (2008). *Drugs, brains, and behavior: The science of addiction*. NIH Publication No. 10–5605. Washington, DC: Author.

Needleman, J. (1983). *Consciousness and tradition*. Bellville, MI. Crossroad.

Newberg, A. (2006). *Why we believe what we believe*. New York, NY: Free Press.

Newberg, A., Alavi, A., Baime, M., Pourdehnad, M., Santanna, J., & Aquili, E. (2001). The measurement of cerebral blood flow during the complex cognitive task of meditation: A preliminary SPECT study. *Psychiatric Research: Neuroimaging Section, 106*, 113–122.

Nhat Hanh, T. (1999). *Miracle of mindfulness*. Boston, MA: Beacon Press.

Nideffer, R. S. (1993). Concentration and attention control training. In J. W. (Ed.), *Applied sport psychology* (pp. 243–262). Palo Alto, CA: Mayfield.

Nideffer, R. S. (2001). *Assessment in sport psychology*. Morgantown, WV: Fitness Information Technology.

Oakley, D. A., & Halligan, P. W. (2008). Hypnotic suggestion and cognitive neuroscience. *Trends in Cognitive Sciences, 13*, 264–270. doi:10.1016/j.tics.2009.03.004

Oberman, L., Hubbard, E., McCleery, J., Altschuler, E., Ramaschandran, V., & Pineda, J. (2005). EEG evidence for mirror neuron dysfunction in autism spectrum disorders. *Cognitive Brain Research, 24*, 190–198.

Oh, S., & Faulkner, D. (1985). *Sadaharu Oh: A Zen way of baseball*. New York, NY: New York Time Books.

Olesen, E. (2004). What is the Roshi? *The Roshi, 1*(10), 1–5.

O'Mahoney, M. (2007). Taste perception, food quality, and consumer acceptance. *Journal of Food Quality, 14(1)*, 9–31.

Orlock, C. (1995). *Know your body clock: Discover your body's inner cycles and rhythms and learn the best times for creativity, exercise, sex, sleep, and more.* New York, NY: Carol Publishing.

Orloff, J. (1997). *Second sight.* New York, NY: Grand Central Publishing.

Ornish, D., Weiner, G., & Fair, W. (2005). Intensive lifestyle changes may affect the progression of prostate cancer. *Journal of Urology, 174*, 1065–1070.

Ortega y Gasset, J. G. (1962). *Man and crisis.* New York, NY: Norton.

Oschman, J. (2000). *Energy medicine: The scientific basis.* New York, NY: Harcourt.

Oster, G. (1973). Auditory beats in the brain. *Scientific American,* 229(4), 94–102.

Othmer, S. (2008). *Protocol guide: Optimizing electrode placements and reward frequencies through assessment and training.* Woodland Hills, CA: EEG Institute.

Othmer, S. (2009). Implications of network models for neurofeedback. In J. Evans (Ed.), *Handbook of neurofeedback: Dynamics and clinical applications* (25–60). New York, NY: Informa.

Overton, D. (1968). Dissociated learning in drug states (statedependent learning). In D. Efron, J. Cole, J. Levine, & J. Wittenborn (Eds.), *Psychopharmacology: A review of progress, 1957–1967* (pp. 918–930). Washington, DC: U. S. Government Printing Office.

Overton, D. (1982). Memory retrieval failures produced by changes in drug state. In R. Isaacson (Ed.), *The expression of knowledge* (pp. 113–139). New York, NY: Plenum Press.

Panksepp, J. (1982). Toward a general psychobiological theory of emotions. *Behavioral and Brain sciences, 5*, 407–468.

Panksepp, J. (1998). *Affective neuroscience: The foundations of human and animal emotions.* London: Oxford University Press.

Panksepp, J. (2003). At the interface between the affective, behavioral and cognitive neurosciences: Decoding the emotional feelings of the brain. *Brain and Cognition, 52*, 4–14.

Panksepp, J. (Ed.). (2004). *A textbook of biological psychiatry.* New York: Wiley.

Panksepp, J. (2006). Emotional endophenotypes in evolutionary psychiatry. *Progress in Neuro-Psychopharmacolgy & Biological Psychiatry, 30*, 774-784.

Panksepp, J., & Burgdorf, J. (1999). Laughing rats? Playful tickling arouses high frequency ultrasonic chirping in young rodents. In S. Hameroff, D. Chalmers, & A. Kazniak (Eds.), *Toward a science of consciousness* (Vol. III, pp. 231–244). Cambridge MA: MIT Press.

Panksepp, J., & Panksepp, J.B. (2001). A continuing critique of evolutionary psychology: Seven sins for seven sinners, plus or minus two. *Evolution and Cognition, 7*, 56–80.

Parvin, P. (2008). Why is this man smiling? *Emory Magazine*, Winter, 1. Emory University, Atlanta, GA.

Pasternak, B. (1957). *Doctor Zhivago*. New York, NY: Pantheon.

Patrick, G. J. (1996). Improved neuronal regulation in ADHD: An application of 15 sessions of photic-driven EEG neurotherapy. *Journal of Neurotherapy, 1*(4), 27–36.

Pelphrey, K., Singerman, J., Allison, T., & McCarthy, G. (2003). Brain activation evoked by perception of gaze shifts: The influence of context. *Neuropsychologia, 41*(2), 156–170.

Pembrey, M., Bygren, L., Kaati, G., Edvinsson, S., Northstone, K., Sjöström, M., et al., and the ALSPAC Study Team (2006). Sex-specific, male-line transgenerational responses in humans. *European Journal of Human Genetics, 14*, 159–166. doi: 10.1038/sj.ejhg.5201538

Peniston, E., & Kulkosky, P. (1989). Alpha–theta brainwave training and beta endorphin levels in alcoholics. *Alcoholism: Clinical and Experimental Results, 13*, 271–279.

Peniston, E.G., & Kulkosky, P.J. (1991). Alpha–theta brainwave neurofeedback therapy for Vietnam veterans with combat-related posttraumatic stress disorder. *Medical Psychotherapy: An International Journal, 4*, 47–60.

Pert, C. (1999). *Molecules of emotion: The science behind mind–body medicine*. New York, NY: Simon & Schuster.

Pettigrew, J., & Miller, S. (1998). A "sticky" interhemispheric switch in bipolar disorder? *Proceedings of the Royal Society of London (B), 265*, 2141–2148.

Peykar, M. (2008). *How lack of sleep can affect your diabetes*. Retrieved from http://www.online–diabetes–information.com/diabetes–risk–factors/how–lack–of–sleep–can–effect–your–diabetes

Pieron, H. (1982). Melanges dedicated to Monsieur Pierre Janet. *Acta Psychiatrica Belgica, 1*, 7–112.

Piomelli, D., Giuffrida, A., Calignano, A., & Rodriguez de Fonseca, F. (2000). The endocannabinoid system as a target for therapeutic drugs. *Trends in Pharmacological Science, 2*(6), 218–224.

Porges, S. (2007). The polyvagal perspective. *Biological Psychology, 74*(2), 116–143

Prabhavananda, Swami, & Isherwood, C. (1953). *How to know God: The Yoga aphorisms of Patanjali*. New York, NY: Harper & Row.

Pribram, K. (1982). Localization and distribution of function in the brain. In J. Orbach (Ed.), *Neuropsychology after Lashley* (pp. 273–296). Hillsdale, NJ: Erlbaum.

Pribram, K. (1994). *Origins: Brain and self-organization*. New York, NY: Erlbaum.

Pribram, K. (1997, March). *Holonomic brain theory and motor gestalts: Recent experimental results*. Keynote lecture given at the 10th Scientific Convention of the Society for Gestalt Theory and its Applications (GTA), Vienna, Austria. Retrieved from http://gestalttheory.net/conv/prib.html

Prichep, L., & John, E. (1992). QEEG profiles of psychiatric disorders. *Brain Topography, 4*(4), 249–257.

Prigogine, I. (1983). *Order out of chaos.* New York, NY: Bantam.

Prochaska, J.O., & DiClemente, C. (1982). Transtheoretical therapy toward a more integrative model of change. *Psychotherapy: Theory, Research and Practice,* 19(3), 276–287.

Prunet-Marcassas, B., Desbazeille, M., Bros, A., Louche, K., Delegrange, P., Renard, P., et al. (2003). Melatonin reduces body weight gain in Sprague Dawley rats with diet-induced obesity. *Endrocrinology, 144*(12), 5347–5322. doi: 10.1210/en.2003–0693

Pulos, L. (2003). *The biology of empowerment.* New York, NY: Nightengale-Conant.

Rainville, P. (2002). Brain mechanisms of pain affect and pain modulation. *Current Opinion in Neurobiology, 12,* 195–204.

Rainville, P., Hofbauer, R., Paus, T., Duncan, G., Bushnell, M., & Price, D. (1999). Cerebral mechanisms of hypnotic induction and suggestion. *Journal of Cognitive Neuroscience, 11*(1), 110–125.

Ratey, J. (2002). *A user's guide to the brain.* New York, NY: Vintage.

Raz, A. (2004). Anatomy of attentional networks. *Anatomical Record, Part B, New Anatomist, 281*(1), 21–36.

Raz, A., Fan, J., & Posner, M. (2005). Hypnotic suggestion reduces conflict in the human brain. *PNAS.* doi: 10.1073/pnas.0503064102

Raz, A., & Shapiro, T. (2002). Hypnosis and neuroscience: A cross talk between clinical and cognitive research. *Archives of General Psychiatry, 59,* 85–90.

Restak, R. (2001). *The secret life of the brain.* New York, NY: Joseph Henry Press.

Ricard, M. (2008, July 28). *Happiness.* Presentation given at Rothko Chapel, Houston, TX.

Rilke, M. (1993). *Letters to a young poet.* New York, NY: Norton.

Robertson, J. (1996). *Peak performance living.* San Francisco: Harper.

Rock, D., & Schwartz, J. (2007a). Attention density: New big thing? *Consulting Today.* Retrieved from http://www.resultsworkplacecoaching.co.za/pdf/Attention%20density.%20DR%20and%20JS.pdf

Rock, D., & Schwartz, J. (2007b). *The neuroscience of leadership.* Retrieved from http://www.scribd.com/doc/33244597/The-Neuroscience-of-Leadership-Rock-Schwartz

Rossi, E. (1986). Altered states of consciousness in everyday life: The ultradian rhythms. In B. Wolman (Ed.), *Handbook of states of consciousness* (pp. 97–132). New York, NY: Van Nostrand Reinhold.

Rossi, E. (1993). *Psychobiology of mind–body healing: New concepts of therapeutic hypnosis* (Rev. ed.). New York, NY: Norton.

Rossi, E. (1996). *The symptom path to enlightenment.* Redding, CT: Zeig, Tucker, & Thiesen.

Rossi, E. L. (2002). *The psychobiology of gene expression: Neuroscience and neurogenesis in therapeutic hypnosis and the healing arts.* New York, NY: Norton.

Rossi, E. (2003). Gene expression, neurogenesis, and healing: Psychosocial genomics of therapeutic hypnosis. *American Journal of Clinical Hypnosis, 45* (3), 197–216.

Rossi, E. (2006). The neuroscience of observing consciousness and mirror neurons in therapeutic hypnosis. *American Journal of Clinical Hypnosis, 48*(4), 263–278.

Rossi, E., & Cheek, D. (1994). *Mind–body therapy: Methods of ideodynamic healing in hypnosis.* New York, NY: Norton.

Rousch, W. (1995). Can resetting hormonal rhythms treat illness? *Science, 269,* 1220–1221.

Rowe, C.E., & Mac Isaac, D.S. (1991). *Empathic attunement: The technique of psychoanalytic self-Psychology.* Northvale, NJ: Jason Aronson

Rugg, H. (1963). *Imagination.* New York, NY: Harper & Row.

Rundle, M. (2009). *Empathy and hypnotic susceptibility in volunteers and nonvolunteers.* Doctoral dissertation, Adler School of Psychology. Retrieved from www.docstoc.com/docs/47049219.

Russell, H. (1997a). *EEG driven audio-visual stimulation unit for enhancing cognitive abilities of learning disordered boys: Final report.* Washington, DC: U.S. Department of Education SBIR Phase II Contract Number: RA94130002.

Russell, H. (1997b). Intellectual functioning, auditory and photic stimulation, and changes in functioning in children and adults. *Biofeedback, 25,* 16–27.

Salmon, D., & Maslow, J. (2007). *Yoga psychology and the transformation of consciousness: Seeing through the eyes of infinity.* St. Paul, MN: Paragon.

Sams, M. (2006). *The winner's circle.* Retrieved from http// www.GreatBrain .com

Sapolsky, R. (2003). Taming stress. *Scientific American, 289*(3), 87–91.

Sapolsky, R. (2004). *Why zebras don't get ulcers.* New York, NY: Holt.

Schaar, J. (1995). *World of quotes.* Retrieved from http://www.worldofquotes .com/author/John-Schaar/1/index.html

Scharmer, O. (2007). *Theory U: Leading from the future as it emerges.* Cambridge, MA: Society for Organizational Learning.

Schmid, A., & Peper, E. (1998). Strategies for training concentration. In J. M. Williams (Ed.), *Applied sport psychology* (pp. 316–328). Mountain View, CA: Mayfield.

Schmidt, P. H. (1989). Seizure disorder misdiagnosed as borderline syndrome. *Amercian Journal of Psychiatry, 146,* 400–401.

Schore, A. (1994). *Affect regulation and the origin of the self: The neurobiology of emotional development.* Mahwah, NJ: Erlbaum.

Schore, A. (1997). Early organization of the nonlinear right brain development of a predisposition to psychiatric disorders. *Development and Psychopathology, 9,* 595–631.

Schore, A. (2003a). *Affect regulation and the repair of the self.* New York, NY: Norton.

Schwartz, G. (2003). *The afterlife experiments: Breakthrough scientific evidence of life after death.* New York, NY: Atria Publishing.

Schwartz, J., & Begley, S. (2002). *The mind and the brain: Neuroplasticity and the power of mental force.* New York, NY: Harper.

Schwartz, J., Stapp, H., & Beauregard, M. (2004). Quantum physics in neuroscience and psychology: A neurophysical model of mind–brain interaction. *Philosophical Transactions of the Royal Society (B).* doi: 10.1098/rstb.1598

Schwartz, T. (1995). *What really matters: Searching for wisdom in America.* New York, NY: Bantam.

Selye, H. (1978). *The stress of life.* New York, NY: McGraw Hill.

Shapiro, S., Walsh, R., & Britton, W. (2003). An analysis of recent meditation research and suggestions for future directions. *Journal for Meditation and Meditation Research, 3,* 69–90.

Shealy, C. A. (1990). Multidisciplinary pain clinics. In E. R. Weiner (Ed.), *Innovations in pain management* (Vol. 1, pp. 4–20). Orlando, FL: Deutsch Press.

Shibata, D. (2001, November). Decision-making requires both analysis and emotion. Paper presented at the annual meeting of the Radiological Society of North America, University of Washington, Seattle.

Siegel, D. (1999). *The developing mind: Toward a neurobiology of interpersonal experience.* New York, NY: Guilford Press.

Siegel, D. (2006, January 10). Cells that read minds. *New York Times,* pp. 1–3.

Siegel, D. (2007). *The mindful brain.* New York, NY: Norton.

Siegman, A., Townsend, S., Blumenthal, R., Sorkin, J., & Civelak, C. (1998). Dimensions of anger and CHD in men and women: Self-ratings versus spouse ratings. *Journal of Behavioral Medicine, 21*(4), 315–336.

Siever, D., (2000). *The rediscovery of audio-visual entrainment technology.* Unpublished manuscript. Available from Mind Alive Inc.

Siever, D. (2004). The neurobiology of childhood trauma. *Journal of Neurotherapy, 8,* 113–114.

Siever, D. (2009). *Audio–visual entrainment: The application of audio–visual entrainment for the treatment of seniors' issues.* Retrieved from http://www.mindalive.com/articlesix.htm

Silvers, J., & Haidt, J. (2008). Moral elevation can induce lactation. *Emotion, 8,* 291–295.

Spiegel, D. (1991). A psychosocial intervention and survival time of patients with metastatic breast cancer. *Advances, 7*(3), 10–19.

Spiegel, K., Leproult, R., & Van Cauter, E. (1999). Impact of sleep debt on metabolic and endocrine function. *Lancet, 354*(9188), 1435–1439.

Stanton, H. (1993). Research note: Alleviation of performance anxiety through hypnotherapy. *Psychology of Music, 21*(1), 78–82

Sterman, M. B. (1995). Physiological origins and functional correlates of EEG rhythmic activities: Implications for self-regulation. *Applied Psychophysiology and Biofeedback, 21*(1), 3–33.

Strauch, B. (2004). *The primal teen: What the new discoveries about the teenage brain tell us about our kids.* New York, NY: Anchor Books.

Suedfeld, P. (1993). Stimulus and theoretical reductionism: What underlies REST effects? In A. Barabasz & M. Barabasz (Eds.), *Clinical and experimental restricted environmental stimulation* (pp. 3–10). New York: Springer-Verlag.

Suffin, S., & Emory, W. (1996). *Neurometric EEG classifiers and response to medicine: Syllabus and proceedings summary, American Psychiatric Association 1996 annual meeting* (pp. 87–88). Washington, DC: American Psychiatric Association.

Suffin, S., Emory, W., Guiterrez, N., Arora, G., Schiller, M., & Kling, A. (2007). A QEEG database method for predicting psychotherapeutic outcome in refractory major depressive disorders. *Journal of American Physicians and Surgeons, 12*(4), 104–108.

Suffin, S., Emory, W., & Proler, M. (1997). *Neurometric EEG predictors of response to medication in psychiatric patients.* American Clinical Neurophysiology Society Program and Proceedings Booklet, Bloomfield, CT.

Taheri, S., Lin, L., Austin, Young, T. & Mignot, E. (2004). Short sleep duration is associated with reduced leptin, elevated threlin, and increased body mass index. *PLoS Med., 1*(3). Retrieved from doi:10.10371/journal.pmed.0010062.

Tatkin, S. (2003). Marital therapy and the psychobiology of turning toward and turning away: Part 1. *The Therapist, 15*(5), 75–78.

Taveras, E. (2008). Short sleep duration in infancy and risk of childhood overweight. *Archives Pediatric Adolescent Medicine, 162*(4), 305–311.

Thatcher, R. (1997). Neural coherence and the content of consciousness. *Consciousness and Cognition, 6*(1), 42–49.

Thayer, R. (2001). *Calm energy: How people regulate mood with food and exercise.* New York, NY: Oxford University Press.

Thomas, R., Grimshaw, J., Mollison, J., McClinton, S., McIntosh, E., Deans, H., et al. (2003). Cluster randomised trial of a guideline-based open access urological investigation service. *Family Practice, 20,* 646–654.

Thompson, J. (2006). *Acoustic brainwave entrainment with binaural beats.* Retrieved from http://www.neuroacoustic.com/entrainment.html

Thondup, T. (1996). *The healing power of the mind.* Boston: Shambhala.

Townsend, A. (2001). QEEG and MMPI-2 of adults reporting childhood sexual abuse: Determining differences and predictor models. Unpublished doctoral dissertation, University of North Texas, Denton, TX.

Travis, F. (2009). Relationship between meditation practice and transcendent states of consciousness. *Biofeedback, 32*(3), 33–36.

Travis, F.T. & Pearson, C. (2000). Pure consciousness: Distinct phenomenological and physiological correlates of "consciousness itself." *International Journal of Neuroscience,* 100, 77-88.

Trudeau, D. M. (1999). A pilot study of the effect of 18 Hz audiovisual stimulation (AVS) on attention and concentration symptoms and on quantitative EEG (QEEG) in long term chronic fatigue (CFS). *Journal of Neurotherapy, 3,* 76.

Tulving, E. (1993). Varieties of consciousness and levels of awareness in memory. In A. Baddeley & L. Weiskrantz (Eds.), *Attention, selection, awareness, and control: A tribute to Donald Broadbent* (pp. 283–299). London: Oxford University Press.

Turner, J., & Fine, T. (1987). *Second International Conference on REST.* Toledo, OH: Iris Publishing.

van der Kolk, B. (2006). Clinical implications of neuroscience research in post traumatic stress disorder. *Annals of the New York Academy of Sciences, 821,* 1–17.

Wake, L. (2008). *Neurolinguistic psychotherapy: A postmodern perspective.* London: Routledge.

Wallace, B. A. (2006). *Contemplative science: Where Buddhism and neuroscience converge.* New York, NY: Columbia University Press.

Wansbrough, H. (1985). *The new Jerusalem Bible.* New York, NY: Double Day.

Waterland, R., & Jirtle, R. (2003). Transposable elements: Targets for early nutritional effects on epigenetic gene regulation. *Molecular and Cellular Biology, 23*(15), 5293–5300.

Weedman, M. (1997). *Hypothalamus and autonomic nervous system.* Neuroscience tutorial, Washington University School of Medicine. Retrieved May 19, 2007, from http://www.newworldencyclopedia.org/entry/Hypothalamus

Wegner, D. (2002). *The illusion of conscious will.* Cambridge, MA: MIT Press.

Wells, S., Polglase, K., Andrews, H.B., Carrington, P., & Baker, H.A. (September, 2003). Evaluation of a meridian-based intervention, emotional freedom techniques (EFT), for reducing specific phobias of small animals. *Journal of Clinical Psychology, 59*(9), 943–966.

White, N. (1995). Alpha–theta training for chronic trauma disorder: A new perspective. *Journal of Mind Technology and Optimal Performance, Mega Brain Report, 2*(4), 44–50.

Wiener, B., & Graham, S. (1989). Understanding the motivational role of affect: Life-span research from an attributional perspective. *Cognition and Emotion, 3,* 401–419.

Wilber, K. (1993). *The spectrum of consciousness.* New York, NY: Quest Books.

Wild, B., Rodden, F., Grodd, W., & Ruch, W. (2003). Neural correlates of laughter and humor. *Brain, 126*(10), 2121–2138.

Williams, L.M., Gatt, J.M., Hatch, A., Palmer, D.M., Nagy, M., Rennie, C., et al. (2008). The integrated model of emotion, thinking, and self-regulation: An application to the "paradox of aging." *Journal of Integrative Neuroscience, 7*(3), 367–404.

Wilson, Timothy D. (2002). *Strangers to ourselves: Discovering the adaptive unconscious.* Cambridge, MA: Belknap Press of Harvard University Press.

Winnicott, D. W. (1958). The capacity to be alone. In A. Phillips (Ed.), *Maturational processes and the facilitating environment* (pp. 29–36). New York, NY: International Universities Press.

Wise, A. (1997). *The high performance mind.* New York, NY: Tarcher.

Wisneski, L., & Anderson, L. (2005). *The scientific basis of integrative medicine.* New York, NY: CRC Press.

Wolf, F. (1990). *Parallel universes.* New York, NY: Simon & Schuster.

Yerkes, R., & Dodson, J. (1908). The relation of strength of stimulus to rapidity of habit-formation. *Journal of Comparative Neurology and Psychology, 18,* 459–482.

Young, G. B., Chandarana, P., Blume, W., McLachman, R., Munoz, D., & Girvin, J. (1995). Mesial temporal lobe seizures presenting as anxiety disorders. *Journal of Neuropsychiatry and Clinical Neuroscience, 7,* 352–357.

Young, J., & Kloska, J. (1999). *Reinventing your life.* New York, NY: Plume Books.

Yudkin, J., Kang, S., & Bruckdorfer, K. (1980). Effects of high dietary sugar. *British Journal of Medicine, 281*(1396) 127–132.

Zeig, J. (1992). *Ericksonian methods: The essence of the story.* New York, NY: Routledge.

Zhang, X., Zhang, G., Zhang, H., Karin, M., Bai, H., & Cai, D. (2008). Hypothalamic IKKβ/NF–κB and ER stress link over nutrition to energy imbalance and obesity. *Cell, 135,* 61–73.

Zinn, M., & Zinn, M. (2003). Psychophysiology for performing artists. In M. Schwartz & F. Andrasik (Eds.), *Biofeedback: A practitioner's guide* (3rd ed., pp. 545–559). New York, NY: Guilford Press.

INDEX